Laboratory Diagnosis in Microbial Diseases

Laboratory Diagnosis in Microbial Diseases

Editor

Hsin-Yao Wang

MDPI

Basel • Beijing • Wuhan • Barcelona • Belgrade • Novi Sad • Cluj • Manchester

Editor
Hsin-Yao Wang
Chang Gung Memorial
Hospital, Linkou Branch
Taoyuan
Taiwan

Editorial Office
MDPI
St. Alban-Anlage 66
4052 Basel, Switzerland

This is a reprint of articles from the Special Issue published online in the open access journal *Diagnostics* (ISSN 2075-4418) (available at: https://www.mdpi.com/journal/diagnostics/special_issues/01I7A53F1A).

For citation purposes, cite each article independently as indicated on the article page online and as indicated below:

Lastname, A.A.; Lastname, B.B. Article Title. *Journal Name* **Year**, *Volume Number*, Page Range.

ISBN 978-3-7258-0361-3 (Hbk)
ISBN 978-3-7258-0362-0 (PDF)
doi.org/10.3390/books978-3-7258-0362-0

Contents

diagnostics

MDPI

Article

Identification of Intestinal Microbial Community in Gallstone Patients with Metagenomic Next-Generation Sequencing

Li Ding [1,2,3,†], Su Wang [1,2,3,†], Wenrong Jiang [1,2,3], Yingxin Miao [1,2,3], Wenjian Liu [1,2,3], Feng Yang [1,2,3], Jinghao Zhang [1,2,3], Wenjing Chi [1,2,3], Tao Liu [1], Yue Liu [1,2,3], Shiwen Wang [1,2,3,*], Yanmei Zhang [1,2,3] and Hu Zhao [1,2,3,*]

1 Department of Laboratory Medicine, Huadong Hospital Affiliated to Fudan University, Shanghai 200040, China
2 Department of Laboratory Medicine, Research Center on Aging and Medicine, Fudan University, Shanghai 200040, China
3 Department of Laboratory Medicine, Huadong Hospital, Shanghai 200040, China
* Correspondence: wangshiwen@fudan.edu.cn (S.W.); hdyyzhaohu@fudan.edu.cn (H.Z.)
† These authors contributed equally to this work.

Abstract: Gallstone disease (GD) is one of the most common gastrointestinal diseases worldwide. Nowadays, intestinal microbiota are thought to play important roles in the formation of gallstones. In our study, human fecal samples were extracted for metagenomic next-generation sequencing (mNGS) on the Illumina HiSeq platform, followed by bioinformatics analyses. Our results showed that there was a particular intestinal micro-ecosystem in GD patients. In contrast to healthy people, the sequences of *Bacteroidetes*, *Bacteroides* and *Thetaiotaomicron* were obviously more abundant in GD patients at phylum, genus and species levels, respectively. On the other hand, the glycan metabolism and drug resistance, especially for the β-lactams, were the most profound functions of gut microbes in GD patients compared to those in normal subjects. Furthermore, a correlation analysis drew out that there existed a significant relationship between the serum levels of biochemical indicators and abundances of intestinal microbes in GD patients. Our results illuminate both the composition and functions of intestinal microbiota in GD patients. All in all, our study can broaden the insight into the potential mechanism of how gut microbes affect the progression of gallstones to some extent, which may provide potential targets for the prevention, diagnosis or treatment of GD.

Keywords: intestinal microbial community; gallstone disease (GD); species composition; microbial function

Citation: Ding, L.; Wang, S.; Jiang, W.; Miao, Y.; Liu, W.; Yang, F.; Zhang, J.; Chi, W.; Liu, T.; Liu, Y.; et al. Identification of Intestinal Microbial Community in Gallstone Patients with Metagenomic Next-Generation Sequencing. *Diagnostics* **2023**, *13*, 2712. https://doi.org/10.3390/diagnostics13162712

Academic Editors: Laurent Bélec and Hsin-Yao Wang

Received: 3 July 2023
Revised: 14 August 2023
Accepted: 16 August 2023
Published: 21 August 2023

1. Introduction

Gallstone disease (GD), also known as cholelithiasis, is a common disease which can stimulate the gallbladder mucosa and result in acute/chronic cholecystitis or even gallbladder carcinoma [1]. The cholesterol gallstone is the most familiar type of GD in cholecystectomy [2]. The prevalence of GD is extremely high in Western countries with the rate of about 10~20% [3]. Nowadays, GD has become more and more prevalent in China, ranging from 10 to 15% [4]. The majority of the population with the disease are women and elderly people. Generally, the morbidity of GD can be impacted by a great deal of factors, including heredity, lifestyle, dyslipidemia and especially a high-cholesterol diet [5,6]. The abnormal metabolism or supersaturated secretion of cholesterol and bile acids is commonly believed to induce the formation of gallstones [7,8].

It is universally acknowledged that intestinal microbial communities participate in regulating the endocrine and biological metabolism in human bodies [9–11], which are intimately associated with various diseases, such as adiposity, diabetes, inflammation, depression or even some kinds of tumors [12–15]. In recent years, several researchers have suggested that intestinal microbiota may play a vitally important role in gallstone pathogenesis [16,17]. Wang et al. supposed that a lithogenic diet could lead to dramatic alteration in the abundance and composition of gut microbiota, which might contribute to the metabolic disorders of cholesterol and bile acid [17]. Wu et al. found an overgrowth of the bacterial phylum *Proteobacteria* within the gut of GD patients, while three gut bacterial genera, including *Faecalibacterium*, *Lachnospira* and *Roseburia*, significantly decreased [18]. Interestingly, Keren et al. pointed out that the intestinal genus *Roseburia* and the species *Bacteroides* were reduced, but the family *Ruminococcaceae* and the genus *Oscillospira* increased in GD patients [19]. However, the pathogenesis of GD affected by intestinal microbiota still remained unclear up until now. The most common hypothesis could be concluded that bile acids' metabolism is mediated by intestinal bacteria via the activation of bile salt hydrolases (BSH), existing in genera *Bifidobacterium*, *Lactobacillus*, *Clostridium*, etc. BSH might further dissociate both 7α-dehydroxylase and bile acids, thereby turning primary bile acids into secondary bile acids. The high level of secondary bile acids is considered to cause an increased secretion of biliary cholesterol and formation of gallstones [20–22]. On the whole, the available studies usually focused on the description of species in cholelithic gut microbiota with 16S rRNA sequencing. Very few of them laid emphasis on the detailed function of those differential microbes. In view of the intestinal microbial community being a complex and crucial ecosystem, more and more research should be conducted to reveal the intrinsic effect of gut microbiota on the occurrence and development of GD.

In our study, metagenomic next-generation sequencing (mNGS) was performed on the Illumina HiSeq platform so as to undertake a relatively comprehensive analysis of the relationship between intestinal microbiota and GD. In summary, we attempted to draw a clear illustration of four important and key issues: (1) The characteristics of the intestinal microbial community in GD patients compared with those in healthy individuals. (2) The functions of differential gut microbiota in GD patients. (3) The relationship between intestinal microbiota and traditional biochemical markers in patients with cholelithiasis. (4) The potential mechanism of how the intestinal microbial community affects the formation of gallstones.

2. Materials and Methods

2.1. Patient Cohorts

GD patients and healthy individuals in our study were all recruited from Huadong Hospital affiliated with Fudan University. The criteria used for the selection of patients were as follows: (1) The diagnostic criteria were according to the European Association for the Study of the Liver (EASL) guidelines. (2) None of the patients indicated they had suffered gastrointestinal diseases except GD. (3) All the patients were excluded from chronic diseases, such as cirrhosis, diabetes, cardiovascular disease, etc. (4) None of the patients had taken antibiotics or probiotics within the previous 3 months prior to this study. (5) None of the patients underwent surgery prior to this study.

In all selected cases, the characteristics of healthy individuals were as follows: (1) None of the healthy individuals had suffered any diseases of the gastrointestinal tract or other chronic diseases. (2) None of them had been subjected to surgical procedures for several years prior to this study. (3) None of them had taken antibiotics or probiotics within the previous 3 months prior to this study.

Our study was approved by the committee for ethical review of research involving human subjects (Ethical Project No. 2018k045), Huadong Hospital affiliated with Fudan University, Shanghai, China. All participants signed informed consent forms.

2.2. Fecal Samples' Collection

Fresh fecal samples were obtained from the GD patients or healthy individuals. The collection procedures were followed by our previously published methods [23,24]. All the fecal samples were placed in cryovials without a preservative, then immediately snap-frozen in liquid nitrogen and stored at −80 °C. Afterwards, the samples were kept on dry ice for the subsequent sequencing analysis. All samples were stored in their original tubes at −80 °C until further processing.

2.3. DNA Extraction and Sequencing

A DNeasy PowerSoil Kit (QIAGEN, Inc., Dusseldorf, Germany) was used for extracting the total microbial genomic DNA from fecal samples. The extraction procedure was conducted under the guidance of the manufacturer's instructions. Then, the quality and quantity of extracted DNA were estimated with agarose gel electrophoresis and a NanoDrop spectrophotometer (ND-1000, Thermo Fisher Scientific, Waltham, MA, USA), respectively. After that, an Illumina TruSeq Nano DNA LT Library Preparation Kit (Illumina, San Diego, CA, USA) was used to set up metagenome shotgun sequencing libraries with insert sizes of 400 bp using extracted microbial DNA. Finally, the sequencing processes of constructed libraries were performed on the Illumina HiSeq X-ten platform (Illumina, USA) with a PE150 strategy at Personal Biotechnology Co., Ltd. (Shanghai, China).

2.4. Sequence Analysis

Raw sequencing reads were processed to obtain quality-filtered reads for the further analysis. First of all, Cutadapt (v1.2.1) was used to eliminate sequencing adapters from sequencing reads [25]. Then, low-quality reads were cleaned up with a sliding-window algorithm. Thirdly, qualified reads were aligned to the host genome with a Burrows Wheeler Alignment (BWA) Tool (http://bio-bwa.sourceforge.net/) (accessed on 18 April 2022) to clear host contamination [26]. The reads were further applied to construct the metagenome for each sample when they were de novo assembled with an iterative De Bruijn graph assembler for sequencing data with a highly uneven depth (IDBA-UD) [27]. Finally, the coding regions (CDS) of metagenomic scaffolds (>300 bp) were predicted with MetaGeneMark (http://exon.gatech.edu/GeneMark/metagenome) (accessed on 18 April 2022) [28], followed by CDS sequence clustering so as to obtain a non-redundant gene catalog [29].

The sequence data analyses were mainly performed using R packages (v3.2.0). Operational Taxonomic Units (OTU)-level alpha diversity indices, such as the Chao1 richness estimator, abundance-based coverage estimator metric (ACE), Shannon diversity index and Simpson index, were calculated using the OTU table in Quantitative Insights Into Microbial Ecology (QIIME). Meanwhile, a beta diversity analysis was performed to investigate the compositional and functional variation of microbial communities of all samples using Bray–Curtis distance metrics and visualized via a principal coordinate analysis (PCoA) [30], nonmetric multidimensional scaling (NMDS) and the unweighted pair-group method with arithmetic means (UPGMA) hierarchical clustering [31]. Additionally, the functional profiles of the non-redundant genes were obtained by annotating against the Gene Ontology (GO), Kyoto Encyclopedia of Genes and Genomes (KEGG), Evolutionary genealogy of genes: Non-supervised Orthologous Groups (EggNOG) and Carbohydrate-Active enzymes (CAZy) databases, respectively, by using the double index alignment of next-generation sequencing data (DIAMOND) alignment algorithm [32]. Based on the taxonomic and functional profiles of non-redundant genes, linear discriminant analysis effect size (LEfSe) was used to detect differentially abundant taxa and functions across groups using the default parameters [33]. Moreover, a random forest analysis was applied for discriminating different samples using the R package "random Forest" with 1000 trees and all default settings [34,35]. The generalization error was estimated using 10-fold cross-validation. The expected "baseline" error was also included, which was obtained with a classifier that simply predicted the most common category label.

2.5. Data Access

All raw sequences were deposited in the NCBI Sequence Read Archive (SRA) under the accession number PRJNA999028.

2.6. Statistical Analysis

Statistical analyses were performed with R packages (v3.2.0) and SPSS version 20.0 (SPSS, Chicago, IL, USA). The comparisons of species and related functions between groups were displayed with the LEfSe method. Differences of clinical features between groups were analyzed with a one-way ANOVA or Chi-square test. Correlation analyses were conducted with a Pearson's correlation test. The degree of correlation was evaluated with the Pearson correlation coefficient. In all cases, $p < 0.05$ was considered to be statistically significant.

3. Results

3.1. Analysis of Intestinal Microbial Community in GD Patients

A total of 62 fecal samples from 42 GD patients (16 males/26 females) and 20 healthy individuals (12 males/8 females) were included in our study. The values of serum biochemical markers and parameter distribution of all samples are shown in Table 1. The Scaffolds/Scaftigs of each sample were aligned using BLASTN with the sequences of Bacteria, Archaea, Fungi and Viruses in the NCBI-NT database (Nucleotide collection, ftp://ftp.ncbi.nih.gov/blast/db/) (accessed on 21 February 2023), followed by an analysis of species classification from phylum to species on the MEtaGenome Analyzer platform (http://ab.inf.uni-tuebingen.de/software/megan5) (accessed on 21 February 2023) according to the lowest common ancestor (LCA) algorithm [36,37].

Table 1. Clinical features of the samples.

	GD Patients	Healthy People	p-Value
Age (years)	49.69 ± 7.37	46.10 ± 6.32	0.066
Gender			
Male	16	12	0.105
Female	26	8	
Glutamate Dehydrogenase (μmol/L)	3.39 ± 2.10	-	-
Total Protein/Albumin	1.62 ± 0.46	-	-
Total Protein (μmol/L)	71.89 ± 5.00	-	-
Albumin (μmol/L)	45.08 ± 3.52	-	-
Prealbumin (μmol/L)	233.37 ± 41.85	-	-
Alanine Aminotransferase (μmol/L)	25.16 ± 18.51	-	-
Aspartate Aminotransferase (μmol/L)	22.73 ± 18.64	-	-
Lactate Dehydrogenase (μmol/L)	168.81 ± 25.12	-	-
Total Bile Acid (μmol/L)	4.10 ± 3.10	-	-
γ-Glutamyl Transpeptidase (μmol/L)	45.69 ± 23.96	-	-
Direct Bilirubin (μmol/L)	4.49 ± 2.40	-	-
Total Bilirubin (μmol/L)	11.45 ± 5.01	-	-
Alpha-l-fucosidase (μmol/L)	19.85 ± 5.47	-	-
Cystatin C (μmol/L)	0.73 ± 0.18	-	-

In general, the intestinal microbial composition of GD patients was described with taxonomic profiling. At the phylum level, we noticed *Firmicutes* (36.13%), *Bacteroidetes* (31.85%), *Proteobacteria* (10.71%) and *Actinobacteria* (1.66%) accounted for the majority of the sequences (Figure 1A). When it comes to the genus level, *Bacteroides* (26.17%), *Faecalibacterium* (6.99%), *Escherichia* (5.12%), *Blautia* (2.30%) and *Lachnoclostridium* (2.44%) were found to be the main gut genera for GD patients (Figure 1B). Furthermore, *Faecalibacterium prausnitzii* (6.9%), *Escherichia coli* (5.1%), *Bacteroides vulgatus* (3.5%), *Bacteroides thetaiotaomicron* (2.7%), *Bacteroides dorei* (2.5%), *Bacteroides fragilis* (2.3%), *Roseburia intestinalis* (1.5%) and *Bacteroides cellulosilyticus* (1.4%) were the dominant gut microbes (>1% of all sequences) at the species level (Figure 1C). Additionally, no matter in the GD patients or in the healthy individuals, there are no newly identified microbes.

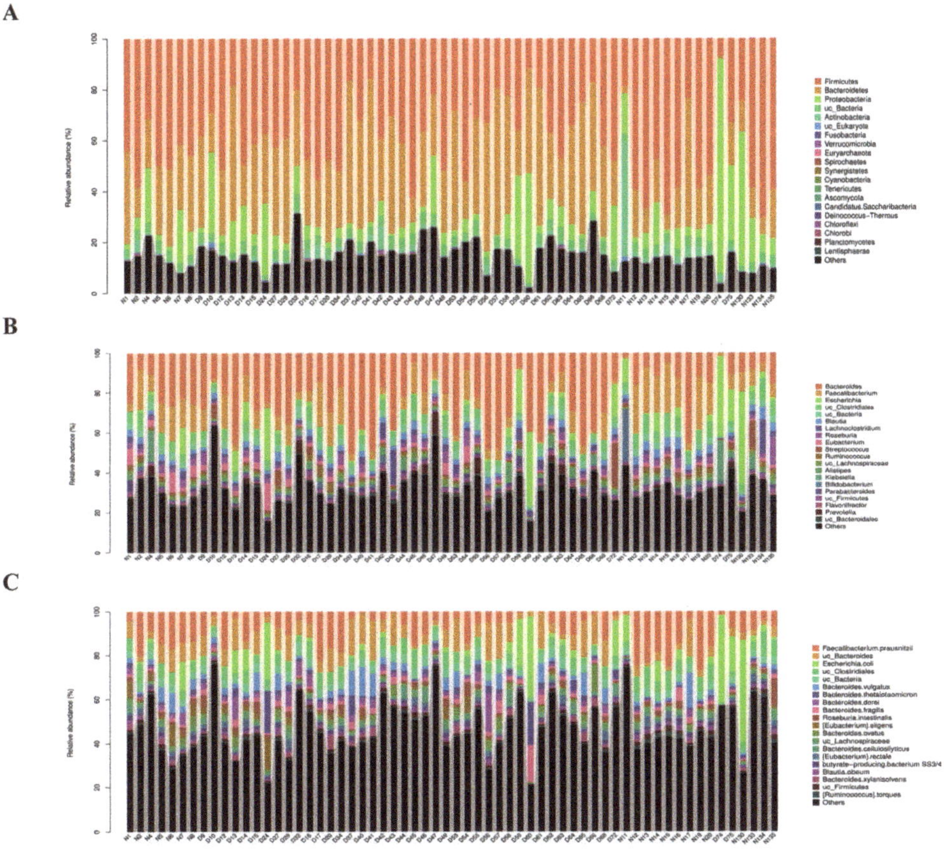

Figure 1. The composition of intestinal microbiota in GD patients and healthy individuals. (**A**) The composition of intestinal microbiota at the phylum level. (**B**) The composition of intestinal microbiota at the genus level. (**C**) The composition of intestinal microbiota at the species level. Note: N: healthy individuals, D: GD patients.

Moreover, the beta diversity of species composition was estimated with Bray–Curtis-distance-based PCoA. The result revealed the fecal samples from GD patients were grouped together showing obviously less similarities to each other than to those samples from healthy individuals (Figure 2).

3.2. The Intestinal Microbiota in GD Patients Were Extraordinarily Different from Those in Healthy Individuals

To elucidate the specific gut microbiota of GD patients, the LEfSe method was conducted on the Galaxy online analysis platform (http://huttenhower.sph.harvard.edu/galaxy/) (accessed on 21 February 2023) according to the species composition spectra. The results showed that there were several kinds of intestinal microbes with a significant difference in the patient group compared to those in healthy individuals at the phylum, genus and species levels, respectively. To be specific, the member of phylum *Bacteroidetes* (logarithm value: 5.515, $p = 0.001$) was the only differential species in GD patients. At the genus level, *Bacteroides* (5.418, $p = 0.004$), *Prevotella* (4.075, $p < 0.001$), *Odoribacter* (3.636, $p = 0.027$), *Barnesiella* (3.091, $p = 0.003$), *Tannerella* (2.557, $p < 0.001$), etc., were more frequently detected in GD patients. In addition, the main bacterial species were represented by *Thetaiotaomicron* (4.430, $p < 0.01$), *Dorei* (4.407, $p < 0.05$), *Fragilis* (4.359, $p < 0.01$), *Cellulosi-*

lyticus (4.167, $p < 0.05$), *Salanitronis* (3.761, $p < 0.01$), etc., in the fecal microecosystem of the patients (Figure 3).

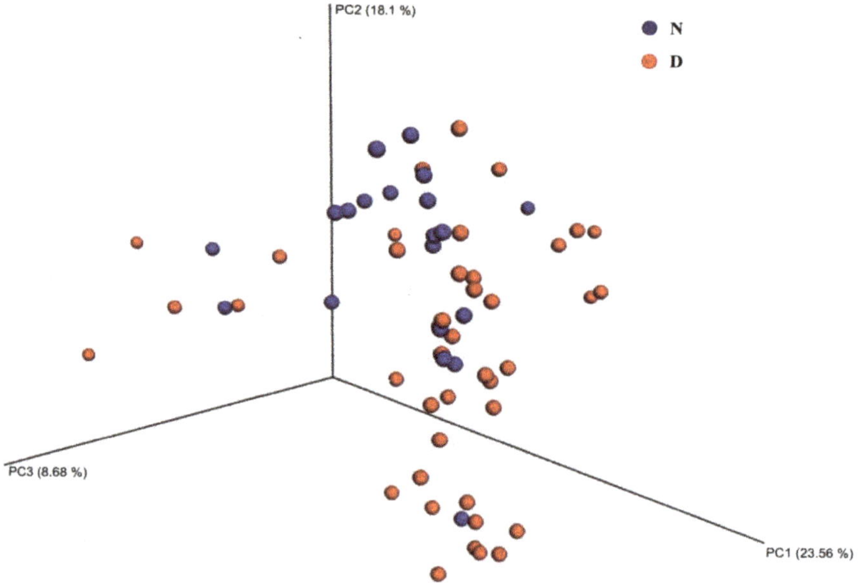

Figure 2. Bray–Curtis-distance-based PCoA of species composition dissimilarity between GD patients and healthy people. The percentages in the axes represent the proportion of differences in the original data, which the corresponding principal coordinates can explain. Each point represents a sample and points of different colors belong to different groups. Note: N: healthy individuals, D: GD patients.

3.3. The Functions of Intestinal Microbiota in GD Patients Varied from Those in Healthy Individuals

The LEfSe method was used to further explore the functions of differential gut microbes in GD patients according to the abundance spectra of basic functional groups of all samples annotated in the KEGG database [38]. The results revealed that the gut microbial function could be divided into several sections, including metabolism, human diseases, cellular processes and organismal systems.

In the GD group, within the metabolism section, glycan biosynthesis (logarithm value: 4.554, $p < 0.001$), amino sugar and nucleotide sugar metabolism (4.348, $p = 0.023$), sphingolipid metabolism (3.777, $p = 0.004$), folate biosynthesis (3.775, $p = 0.008$) and glycosaminoglycan degradation (3.479, $p = 0.004$), etc., showed a remarkably higher proportion compared with those in healthy individuals. When it comes to the human diseases section, only the antimicrobial resistance class exhibited an obviously higher representation in GD patients. Moreover, the β-lactam resistance (3.884, $p < 0.014$) and cationic antimicrobial peptide (CAMP) resistance (3.727, $p = 0.007$) were the two sub-classes with significant differences. When it comes to the cellular processes section, the cholelithic gut microbiota were involved in cell growth and death (4.109, $p = 0.008$), lysosome transport and catabolism (3.520, $p < 0.002$), peroxisome transport and catabolism (3.366, $p < 0.001$), ferroptosis (3.170, $p = 0.008$) and apoptosis (2.909, $p < 0.001$). Finally, within the organismal systems section, the intestinal microbial community in GD patients was found to participate in regulating the environmental adaptation, endocrine system and digestive system function, especially the adipocytokine signaling pathway (3.109, $p = 0.030$), thermogenesis (3.097, $p = 0.024$) and protein digestion and absorption (2.777, $p = 0.002$) (Figure 4).

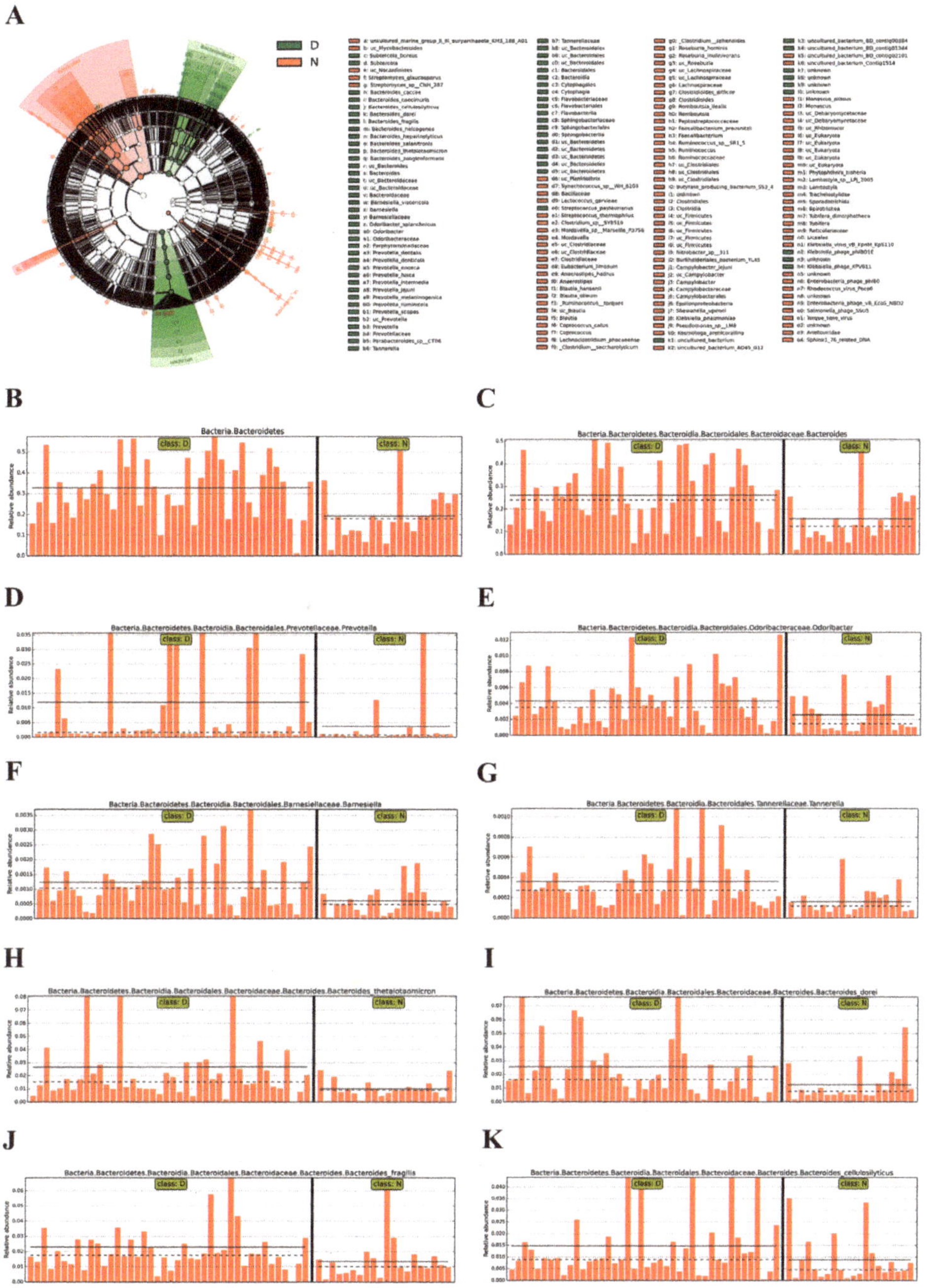

Figure 3. Analysis of the specific intestinal microbes in GD patients compared with those in healthy individuals with the LEfSe method. (**A**) The taxonomic rank shows the subordination of the species in turn from the inner circle to the outer circle. The node size corresponds to the average relative abundances of species. The node color indicates the species with significant dissimilarities between groups. The names of different species are identified using letters. (**B**–**K**) Intestinal microbes with the most significant difference in the patient group compared to those in healthy people. Note: N: healthy individuals, D: GD patients.

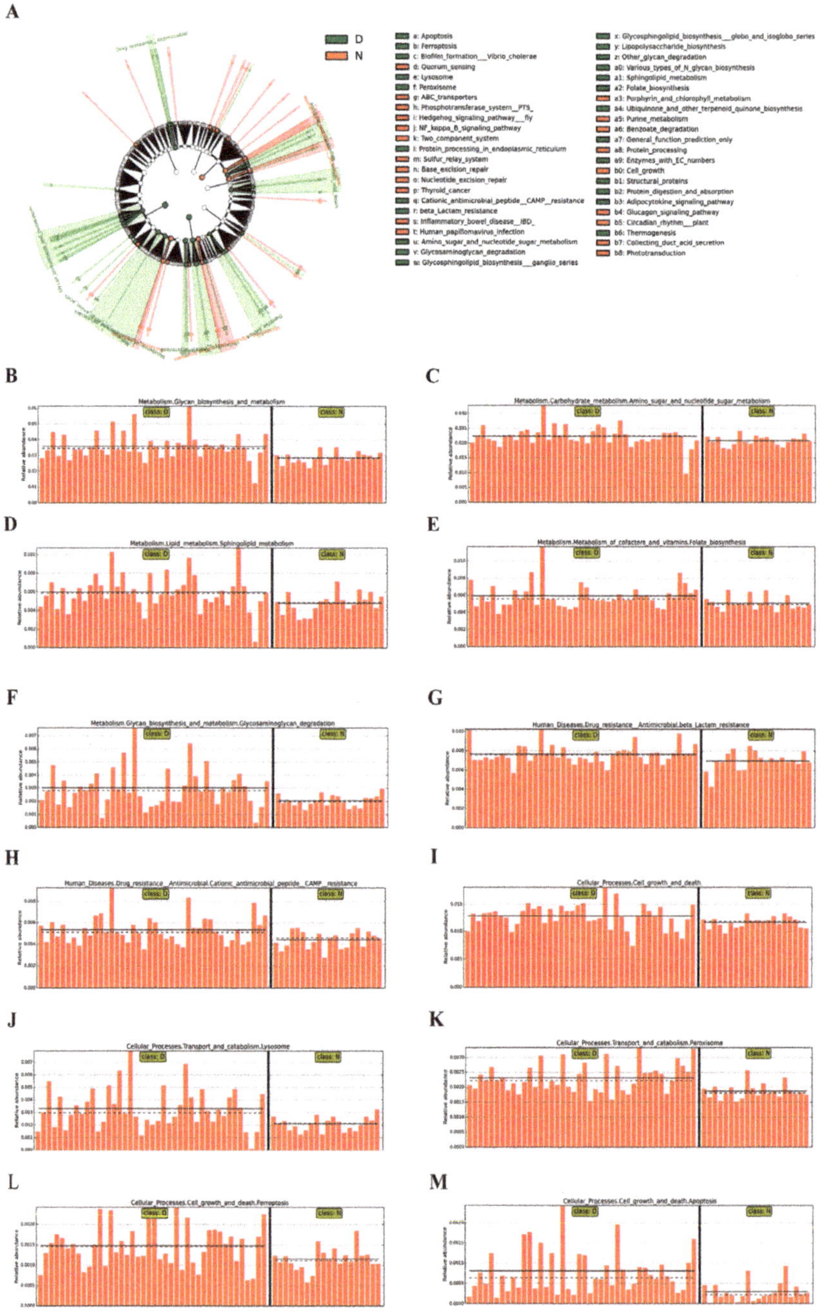

Figure 4. Analysis of the key function of intestinal microbiota in GD patients compared to that in healthy people with the LEfSe method. (**A**) The taxonomic rank shows the subordination of the functional taxa in turn from the inner circle to the outer circle. The node size corresponds to the average relative abundance of functional taxa. The node color indicates the functional taxa with significant dissimilarities between groups. The names of different functional taxa are identified using letters. (**B–M**) Microbial functions with the most significant differences in the patient group compared to those in healthy individuals. Note: N: healthy individuals, D: GD patients.

3.4. The Species and Functions with the Highest Discriminatory Power of Intestinal Microbiota in GD Patients

The random forest analysis was performed to figure out the species and functions with the highest discriminatory power of intestinal microbiota in GD patients [39]. Our results showed that *Sphingobacterium* sp. G1-14, uncultured *Agaricomycetes*, uncultured *Agaricales*, *Exiguobacterium* sp. 11–28, *Gymnopus* sp. VC-2017f, *Eubacterium ramulus*, *Faecalibacterium* sp., *Rhizomucor miehei*, *Acinetobacter nosocomialis* and *Enterobacter* sp. *Crenshaw* were the top 10 species in the patient group (Table 2). On the other hand, the secondary metabolites' biosynthesis, defense mechanisms, transcription, amino acid transport and metabolism, inorganic ion transport and metabolism, intracellular trafficking, secretion and vesicular transport, coenzyme transport and metabolism, cell cycle control, cell division and chromosome partitioning, energy production and conversion, post-translational modification and protein turnover were the top 10 biological functions of the gut microbes (Table 3).

Table 2. Species with the highest discriminatory power (top 10) of intestinal microbiota in GD patients.

Feature ID	Mean Decrease in Accuracy	Standard Deviation
k__*Bacteria*; p__*Bacteroidetes*; c__*Sphingobacteriia*; o__*Sphingobacteriales*; f__*Sphingobacteriaceae*; g__*Sphingobacterium*; s__*Sphingobacterium* sp. G1-14	0.001162928	0.000606256
k__*Eukaryota*; p__*Basidiomycota*; c__*Agaricomycetes*; o__uc_*Agaricomycetes*; f__uc_*Agaricomycetes*; g__uc_*Agaricomycetes*; s__uc_*Agaricomycetes*	0.001031263	0.000604338
k__*Eukaryota*; p__*Basidiomycota*; c__*Agaricomycetes*; o__*Agaricales*; f__uc_*Agaricales*; g__uc_*Agaricales*; s__uc_*Agaricales*	0.000936848	0.00046726
k__*Bacteria*; p__*Firmicutes*; c__*Bacilli*; o__*Bacillales*; f__unknown; g__*Exiguobacterium*; s__*Exiguobacterium* sp. 11–28	0.000832036	0.000560922
k__*Eukaryota*; p__*Basidiomycota*; c__*Agaricomycetes*; o__*Agaricales*; f__*Omphalotaceae*; g__*Gymnopus*; s__*Gymnopus* sp. VC-2017f	0.000810951	0.000455266
k__*Bacteria*; p__*Firmicutes*; c__*Clostridia*; o__*Clostridiales*; f__*Eubacteriaceae*; g__*Eubacterium*; s__*Eubacterium ramulus*	0.000759662	0.000347172
k__*Bacteria*; p__*Firmicutes*; c__*Clostridia*; o__*Clostridiales*; f__*Ruminococcaceae*; g__*Faecalibacterium*; s__*Faecalibacterium* sp.	0.000712143	0.000622133
k__*Eukaryota*; p__*Mucoromycota*; c__*Mucoromycetes*; o__*Mucorales*; f__*Lichtheimiaceae*; g__*Rhizomucor*; s__*Rhizomucor miehei*	0.000711614	0.000220115
k__*Bacteria*; p__*Proteobacteria*; c__*Gammaproteobacteria*; o__*Pseudomonadales*; f__*Moraxellaceae*; g__*Acinetobacter*; s__*Acinetobacter nosocomialis*	0.000686536	0.000425183
k__*Bacteria*; p__*Proteobacteria*; c__*Gammaproteobacteria*; o__*Enterobacterales*; f__*Enterobacteriaceae*; g__*Enterobacter*; s__*Enterobacter* sp. Crenshaw	0.000654157	0.000538885

Table 3. Microbial functions with the highest discriminatory power (top 10) of intestinal microbiota in GD patients.

Feature ID	Mean Decrease in Accuracy	Standard Deviation
S Function unknown; ENOG4107YKV	0.000523052	0.000482557
Q Secondary metabolites biosynthesis, transport and catabolism; ENOG4107VZP	0.000514268	0.000594528
S Function unknown; ENOG4106UH8	0.000445652	0.000245257
V Defense mechanisms; ENOG4107RKB	0.000408646	0.000340324
K Transcription; ENOG4105S4D	0.00038124	0.000329398
E Amino acid transport and metabolism; arCOG05229	0.000348469	0.000414534
S Function unknown; ENOG4108QVM	0.000348453	0.00046618
P Inorganic ion transport and metabolism; ENOG4105DH3	0.000347117	0.000180151
S Function unknown; ENOG4105V0F	0.000328789	0.000247238
S Function unknown; ENOG4108S9K	0.000307536	0.00033249

3.5. The Levels of Serum Biochemical Indicators Were Correlated with the Abundances of Intestinal Microbes in GD Patients

The serological detection is usually an adjunctive method for diagnosing cholelithiasis. In order to explore whether the serum biochemical indicators are related to the abundances of intestinal microbes in cholelithiasis subjects, the relevant information of such indicators including total bilirubin, direct bilirubin, total bile acid, alkaline phosphatase, γ-glutamyl transpeptidase, cystatin C, prealbumin, lactate dehydrogenase, glutamate dehydrogenase, etc., was collected. In addition, only the top 10 differential species screened out by LEfSe were subsumed for the analysis. A Spearman's rank correlation analysis showed that there was a positive correlation between the abundance of *Thetaiotaomicron* and the concentration of serum prealbumin (r = 0.483, p = 0.027). However, the concentration of serum total bilirubin was negatively correlated with the abundance of both *Dorei* (r = −0.395, p = 0.017) and *Cellulosilyticus* (r = −0.416, p = 0.012), and the abundance of *Fragilis* was negatively correlated with the concentration of serum cystatin C (r = −0.402, p = 0.027) (Table 4).

Table 4. The relationship between differential species and traditional biomarkers in GD patients.

	uc_*Bacteroide*		*Thetaiotaomicron*		*Dorei*		*Fragilis*		*Cellulosilyticus*	
	r	*p*-Value	*r*	*p*-Value	*r*	*p*-Value	*r*	*p*-Value	*r*	*p*-Value
Total bile acid	0.062	0.735	0.299	0.096	−0.041	0.822	0.208	0.253	0.169	0.356
Alkaline phosphatase	0.005	0.771	0.245	0.149	0.042	0.806	0.126	0.464	−0.080	0.645
γ-Glutamyl transpeptidase	−0.232	0.174	0.021	0.904	−0.067	0.700	0.040	0.819	−0.225	0.188
Direct bilirubin	−0.197	0.250	−0.021	0.903	−0.304	0.071	−0.113	0.513	−0.325	0.053
Total bilirubin	−0.256	0.131	−0.105	0.543	−0.395	0.017	−0.200	0.243	−0.416	0.012
Alpha-l-fucosidase	0.154	0.493	−0.098	0.665	0.296	0.181	−0.186	0.406	−0.197	0.379
Urea nitrogen	0.125	0.475	0.021	0.906	0.104	0.551	−0.156	0.370	0.086	0.624
Creatinine	0.151	0.386	0.282	0.101	0.180	0.301	−0.075	0.671	−0.044	0.803
Uric acid	0.030	0.863	0.248	0.151	0.047	0.788	−0.256	0.138	−0.116	0.506
Cystatin C	−0.264	0.158	−0.016	0.935	−0.307	0.099	−0.402	0.027	−0.065	0.734
Glutamate dehydrogenase	0.115	0.601	0.399	0.060	0.158	0.472	0.058	0.791	−0.001	0.995

Table 4. *Cont.*

	uc_*Bacteroide*		*Thetaiotaomicron*		*Dorei*		*Fragilis*		*Cellulosilyticus*	
	r	*p*-Value	*r*	*p*-Value	*r*	*p*-Value	*r*	*p*-Value	*r*	*p*-Value
Fibronectin	−0.290	0.203	−0.269	0.239	0.040	0.862	−0.113	0.626	0.047	0.841
Cholyglycine	0.015	0.937	0.238	0.198	−0.042	0.823	0.222	0.230	0.047	0.802
Total protein/albumin	0.301	0.066	0.162	0.331	0.102	0.544	0.150	0.368	0.014	0.934
Total protein	−0.024	0.889	−0.004	0.983	0.133	0.440	0.182	0.288	−0.089	0.606
Albumin	0.210	0.218	0.204	0.233	0.282	0.096	0.248	0.145	0.041	0.810
Globulin	−0.137	0.440	0.006	0.974	−0.056	0.755	0.053	0.767	−0.098	0.582
Prealbumin	0.077	0.741	0.483	0.027	0.288	0.205	0.336	0.136	−0.022	0.924
Alanine aminotransferase	0.024	0.887	0.096	0.572	0.113	0.507	−0.124	0.466	0.108	0.524
Aspartate aminotransferase	0.003	0.988	−0.068	0.688	−0.039	0.821	0.025	0.884	0.040	0.812
Lactate dehydrogenase	−0.108	0.642	−0.006	0.978	0.009	0.969	0.083	0.722	−0.029	0.900

4. Discussion

GD is recognized as a significant global health problem. At present, the prevalence of cholelithiasis keeps a constantly rising tendency, accompanied by the tremendous growing financial burden. It was reported that a great many intrinsic or extrinsic factors could contribute to GD [5,6]. The metabolic disturbances of cholesterol and bile acid are considered to be the key factors among them. However, the potential pathogenic mechanisms of gallstone formation still need to be illuminated.

To date, the microecosystem of the human intestinal tract has been widely studied. In recent years, some studies have explored the gut microbial community of GD patients with 16S rRNA amplicon sequencing [18,40]. However, the majority of them usually lay emphasis on the species composition or biological diversity of the microbiota. In our study, mNGS was used to describe the characteristics of cholelithic gut microbiota with GD patients. We not only focused on the composition and diversity of the microbes, but also explored their functions in the human intestinal ecosystem.

Additionally, we found that the intestinal tract of GD patients harbored a particular microbial community using bioinformatic analyses. In general, the intestinal microbiota were composed of four kinds of phyla including *Firmicutes, Bacteroidetes, Proteobacteria* and *Actinobacteria*, and one absolutely predominant genus *Bacteroides* and several species that shared analogous abundances like *Faecalibacterium prausnitzii, Escherichia coli, Bacteroides thetaiotaomicron*, etc. Such findings are similar to the studies of Keren et al. [19]. Interestingly, some researchers pointed out that the biliary microbiota in patients with gallbladder gallstones were represented by *Bacteroidetes, Firmicutes* and *Proteobacteria* at the phyla level and *Bacteroides* at the genera level, respectively, which indicated the biliary microbial distribution was almost in accordance with that in the intestine [41,42]. In view of a gut pathogen infection as one of the most significant factors to induce the occurrence and development of GD, we hypothesized that the microbes colonizing in gallbladders of GD patients might practically immigrate from the human intestinal tract. Obviously, there is a great deal of difference between the intestinal and biliary tract structures. Some microbes have to change their characteristics or metabolic activities so as to adapt to the new environment after the immigration. In this way, they might produce a few pathogenic or invasive metabolites, which can result in the disturbance of biliary functions.

Moreover, a random forest analysis was used to explore the intestinal species with the highest discriminatory power in GD patients. After sorting them according to the importance of the species, we found that *Sphingobacterium* sp. G1-14, *uncultured Agaricomycetes* and *uncultured Agaricales* were the three most vitally important microbes, which could be considered as the markers of the intestinal microbial community in GD patients. Additionally, the PCoA analysis distinguished the microbial similarity between two groups, showing a notably higher dispersion among the samples from GD patients. In particular, the microbial communities significantly differed from each other even among GD patients, which indicated that the composition of intestinal microbes in GD patients was quite various and complex. On the contrary, the microbes in the intestinal tract of healthy people were relatively stable and homogeneous.

Since the composition of intestinal microbiota was different between two groups, it was rather essential to figure out the exact microbes. Thus, the LEfSe method was applied for the further identification. In addition to the sequences matching the phylum *Bacteroidetes* and the genera *Bacteroides, Prevotella, Odoribacter*, etc., we observed that some particular species including *Bacteroides thetaiotaomicron, Bacteroides Fragilis, Bacteroides Cellulosilyticus*, etc., were remarkably more abundant in GD patients. Hence, we supposed that such species could be closely associated with the pathological conditions of cholelithiasis. For instance, *Bacteroides fragilis* belongs to bile-tolerant microbes as well as opportunistic pathogens. An opportunistic pathogen is an infectious pathogen that is normally commensal in the body but can colonize elsewhere and cause an infectious disease by taking advantage of the weakened immunity of the host or gut dysbacteriosis. *Bacteroides fragilis* can migrate from the gut to the biliary tract or gallbladder when the body suffers from impaired immunity or gut dysbacteriosis, which is caused by various internal and external factors. Thanks to its tolerance to bile, *Bacteroides fragilis* can stably inhabit in the biliary tract or gallbladder and may even induce the infection of the biliary system, promoting the formation of gallstones.

Furthermore, we also figured out that the glycan metabolism and the β-lactam resistance were two predominant functions of the intestinal microbiota in GD patients analyzed with the LEfSe method. *Bacteroides thetaiotaomicron* is a gut commensal that mainly degrades carbohydrates and promotes the absorption of bile and cholesterol, contributing to gut physiology. The overgrowth of *Bacteroides thetaiotaomicron* can undoubtedly affect the balance of intestinal bile metabolism, resulting in bile acid dysmetabolism. Although the mechanism of bile acids affecting glycometabolism in the development of cholelithiasis still remains unclear, there was evidence that bile acids could inhibit the transcription of gluconeogenesis-related genes in a Farnesoid-X-receptor–Small-Heterodimer-Partner (FXR-SHP)-dependent manner [43]. In addition, researchers showed that bile acids could stimulate the expression of TGR5 as its ligand, and further lead to the activation of adenylate cyclase and protein kinase A, thus regulating the carbohydrate metabolism [44]. To sum up, *Bacteroides thetaiotaomicron* might participate in the formation of gallstones due to its role in bile acid dysmetabolism. On the other hand, it has come to light that the β-lactams are the commonly used antibiotics for the treatment of gallstone disease caused by pathogenic bacteria infection. Thus, we predict that one of the most important reasons for the difficulty in eradicating GD is probably the antibiotic resistance resulting from intestinal microbial disorders.

In addition, the correlation between the abundances of differential intestinal microbes and serum biochemical markers in GD patients was far more important for investigation. We observed that there was a positive correlation between the abundance of *Thetaiotaomicron* and the concentration of serum prealbumin. Most GD patients often suffer from malnutrition and some of them may have abnormal serum prealbumin levels. *Thetaiotaomicron* can decompose polysaccharides so as to provide energy for the biological metabolism [45]. Theoretically, both the *Thetaiotaomicron* abundance and serum prealbumin level can reflect whether the body is in a normal physiological state to a certain extent. Apart from that, we also found that the concentration of serum total bilirubin was negatively correlated with the abundances of *Dorei* and *Cellulosilyticus*, while the abundance of *Fragilis* was negatively correlated with the serum cystatin C level. However, more studies should be conducted to reveal the underlying mechanism regarding how these correlations were formed. We suppose that such microbes may participate in the oxidation and epimerization of bile acids, thus disrupting the enterohepatic circulation and leading to the formation of gallstones.

Finally, although we recruited normal individuals and patients according to the enrollment criteria, the limited number of healthy controls might be a limitation of our present research. It would be better to recruit more healthy people to enrich our findings. In our further study, we will attempt to expand the number of healthy subjects to validate our results, which will achieve a far more comprehensive assessment of the intestinal microbial community in GD progression.

To sum up, our research elucidated the characteristics of the intestinal microbial community in GD patients and found the closely related species for them. Using a comparison with the healthy individuals, we discovered the differential intestinal microbes and the corresponding functions in cholelithiasis subjects. Meanwhile, we identified that the cholelithic intestinal microbiota were correlated with the traditional serum biochemical markers. All in all, our study opened up new strategies for drawing out the role of the intestinal microbial community in the progression of GD. Additionally, our results might reveal the underlying mechanisms of the occurrence or development of GD.

5. Conclusions

Our study revealed that the intestinal microbial community of GD patients was unique from that of healthy individuals. By means of the mNGS, we not only figured out the differential microbes of cholelithiasis but their functions as well. Moreover, the lithic species and corresponding functions with the highest discriminatory power were identified with a random forest analysis. Furthermore, the abundances of intestinal microbes were determined to be related to serum biochemical markers in GD patients. In conclusion, our study can broaden the insight into the potential mechanism of how gut microbes affect the progression of gallstones to some extent, which may provide potential targets for the prevention, diagnosis or treatment of GD.

Author Contributions: Data curation, W.J. and Y.M.; Methodology, S.W. (Su Wang); Project administration, Y.Z. and H.Z.; Resources, W.C., T.L. and Y.L.; Software, W.L., F.Y. and J.Z.; Supervision, S.W. (Shiwen Wang); Writing—review and editing, L.D. All authors have read and agreed to the published version of the manuscript.

Funding: This research was funded by the National Natural Science Foundation of China (No. 82272987, 82172933, 81902380), the Scientific Research Project of Shanghai Science and Technology Commission (No. 21ZR1421700), Shanghai Technological Innovation Action Projects (No. 21Y11900900), the Shanghai health and family planning commission youth project of scientific research subject (No. 20204Y0296), the Key Subject of Huadong Hospital (No. ZDXK2212), the Clinical Research Project of Huadong Hospital (No. HDLC2022007), the Shanghai Rising-Star Program (No. 23QA1403000) and the Medical Scientific Research Foundation of Guangdong Province (No. A2020567).

Institutional Review Board Statement: The study was conducted in accordance with the Declaration of Helsinki and approved by the Ethics Committee for Human Studies of Fudan University Huadong Hospital, Shanghai, China (Ethics Approval Number: 2018k045).

Informed Consent Statement: Written informed consent was obtained from the patients to publish this paper.

Data Availability Statement: All raw sequences were deposited in the NCBI Sequence Read Archive under accession number PRJNA999028.

Conflicts of Interest: The authors declare no conflict of interest. The funders had no role in the design of the study; in the collection, analyses or interpretation of data; in the writing of the manuscript; or in the decision to publish the results.

References

1. Gutt, C.; Schlafer, S.; Lammert, F. The treatment of gallstone disease. *Dtsch. Arztebl. Int.* **2020**, *117*, 148–158. [CrossRef] [PubMed]
2. Sun, H.; Warren, J.; Yip, J.; Ji, Y.; Hao, S.; Han, W.; Ding, Y. Factors influencing gallstone formation: A review of the literature. *Biomolecules* **2022**, *12*, 550. [CrossRef] [PubMed]
3. Perez-Palma, E.; Bustos, B.I.; Lal, D.; Buch, S.; Azocar, L.; Toliat, M.R.; Lieb, W.; Franke, A.; Hinz, S.; Burmeister, G.; et al. Copy number variants in lipid metabolism genes are associated with gallstones disease in men. *Eur. J. Hum. Genet.* **2020**, *28*, 264–273. [CrossRef] [PubMed]
4. Zhu, L.; Aili, A.; Zhang, C.; Saiding, A.; Abudureyimu, K. Prevalence of and risk factors for gallstones in Uighur and Han Chinese. *World J Gastroenterol.* **2014**, *20*, 14942–14949. [CrossRef] [PubMed]

5. Mallick, B.; Anand, A.C. Gallstone disease in cirrhosis-pathogenesis and management. *J. Clin. Exp. Hepatol.* **2022**, *12*, 551–559. [CrossRef] [PubMed]
6. Zhang, M.; Mao, M.; Zhang, C.; Hu, F.; Cui, P.; Li, G.; Shi, J.; Wang, X.; Shan, X. Blood lipid metabolism and the risk of gallstone disease: A multi-center study and meta-analysis. *Lipids Health Dis.* **2022**, *21*, 26. [CrossRef]
7. Jiang, Z.Y.; Parini, P.; Eggertsen, G.; Davis, M.A.; Hu, H.; Suo, G.J.; Zhang, S.D.; Rudel, L.L.; Han, T.Q.; Einarsson, C. Increased expression of lxr alpha, abcg5, abcg8, and sr-bi in the liver from normolipidemic, nonobese Chinese gallstone patients. *J. Lipid Res.* **2008**, *49*, 464–472. [CrossRef]
8. Wang, H.H.; Portincasa, P.; Mendez-Sanchez, N.; Uribe, M.; Wang, D.Q. Effect of ezetimibe on the prevention and dissolution of cholesterol gallstones. *Gastroenterology* **2008**, *134*, 2101–2110. [CrossRef]
9. Tilg, H.; Zmora, N.; Adolph, T.E.; Elinav, E. The intestinal microbiota fuelling metabolic inflammation. *Nat. Rev. Immunol.* **2020**, *20*, 40–54. [CrossRef]
10. Kc, D.; Sumner, R.; Lippmann, S. Gut microbiota and health. *Postgrad. Med.* **2020**, *132*, 274. [CrossRef]
11. Tang, W.; Li, D.Y.; Hazen, S.L. Dietary metabolism, the gut microbiome, and heart failure. *Nat. Rev. Cardiol.* **2019**, *16*, 137–154. [CrossRef] [PubMed]
12. Tang, W.H.; Kitai, T.; Hazen, S.L. Gut microbiota in cardiovascular health and disease. *Circ. Res.* **2017**, *120*, 1183–1196. [CrossRef] [PubMed]
13. Saltzman, E.T.; Palacios, T.; Thomsen, M.; Vitetta, L. Intestinal microbiome shifts, dysbiosis, inflammation, and non-alcoholic fatty liver disease. *Front. Microbiol.* **2018**, *9*, 61. [CrossRef] [PubMed]
14. Dai, Z.; Zhang, J.; Wu, Q.; Chen, J.; Liu, J.; Wang, L.; Chen, C.; Xu, J.; Zhang, H.; Shi, C.; et al. The role of microbiota in the development of colorectal cancer. *Int. J. Cancer* **2019**, *145*, 2032–2041. [CrossRef]
15. Ishii, W.; Komine-Aizawa, S.; Takano, C.; Fujita, Y.; Morioka, I.; Hayakawa, S. Relationship between the fecal microbiota and depression and anxiety in pediatric patients with orthostatic intolerance. *Prim. Care Companion CNS Disord.* **2019**, *21*, 25523. [CrossRef]
16. Fremont-Rahl, J.J.; Ge, Z.; Umana, C.; Whary, M.T.; Taylor, N.S.; Muthupalani, S.; Carey, M.C.; Fox, J.G.; Maurer, K.J. An analysis of the role of the indigenous microbiota in cholesterol gallstone pathogenesis. *PLoS ONE* **2013**, *8*, e70657. [CrossRef]
17. Wang, Q.; Jiao, L.; He, C.; Sun, H.; Cai, Q.; Han, T.; Hu, H. Alteration of gut microbiota in association with cholesterol gallstone formation in mice. *BMC Gastroenterol.* **2017**, *17*, 74. [CrossRef]
18. Wu, T.; Zhang, Z.; Liu, B.; Hou, D.; Liang, Y.; Zhang, J.; Shi, P. Gut microbiota dysbiosis and bacterial community assembly associated with cholesterol gallstones in large-scale study. *BMC Genom.* **2013**, *14*, 669. [CrossRef]
19. Keren, N.; Konikoff, F.M.; Paitan, Y.; Gabay, G.; Reshef, L.; Naftali, T.; Gophna, U. Interactions between the intestinal microbiota and bile acids in gallstones patients. *Environ. Microbiol. Rep.* **2015**, *7*, 874–880. [CrossRef]
20. Ridlon, J.M.; Kang, D.J.; Hylemon, P.B. Bile salt biotransformations by human intestinal bacteria. *J. Lipid Res.* **2006**, *47*, 241–259. [CrossRef]
21. Begley, M.; Gahan, C.G.; Hill, C. The interaction between bacteria and bile. *FEMS Microbiol. Rev.* **2005**, *29*, 625–651. [CrossRef] [PubMed]
22. Ramirez-Perez, O.; Cruz-Ramon, V.; Chinchilla-Lopez, P.; Mendez-Sanchez, N. The role of the gut microbiota in bile acid metabolism. *Ann. Hepatol.* **2017**, *16*, s15–s20. [CrossRef] [PubMed]
23. Guo, M.; Yao, J.; Yang, F.; Liu, W.; Bai, H.; Ma, J.; Ma, X.; Zhang, J.; Fang, Y.; Miao, Y.; et al. The composition of intestinal microbiota and its association with functional constipation of the elderly patients. *Future Microbiol.* **2020**, *15*, 163–175. [CrossRef] [PubMed]
24. Yang, F.; Jiang, Y.; Yang, L.; Qin, J.; Guo, M.; Lu, Y.; Chen, H.; Zhuang, Y.; Zhang, J.; Zhang, H.; et al. Molecular and conventional analysis of acute diarrheal isolates identifies epidemiological trends, antibiotic resistance and virulence profiles of common enteropathogens in shanghai. *Front. Microbiol.* **2018**, *9*, 164. [CrossRef]
25. Martin, M. Cutadapt removes adapter sequences from high-throughput sequencing reads. *EMBnet J.* **2011**, *17*, 10–12. [CrossRef]
26. Li, H.; Durbin, R. Fast and accurate short read alignment with burrows-wheeler transform. *Bioinformatics* **2009**, *25*, 1754–1760. [CrossRef]
27. Peng, Y.; Leung, H.C.; Yiu, S.M.; Chin, F.Y. Idba-ud: A de novo assembler for single-cell and metagenomic sequencing data with highly uneven depth. *Bioinformatics* **2012**, *28*, 1420–1428. [CrossRef]
28. Zhu, W.; Lomsadze, A.; Borodovsky, M. Ab initio gene identification in metagenomic sequences. *Nucleic Acids Res.* **2010**, *38*, e132. [CrossRef]
29. Fu, L.; Niu, B.; Zhu, Z.; Wu, S.; Li, W. Cd-hit: Accelerated for clustering the next-generation sequencing data. *Bioinformatics* **2012**, *28*, 3150–3152. [CrossRef]
30. Bray, J.R.; Curtis, J.T. An Ordination of the Upland Forest Communities of Southern Wisconsin. *Ecol. Monogr.* **1957**, *27*, 325–349. [CrossRef]
31. Ramette, A. Multivariate analyses in microbial ecology. *FEMS Microbiol. Ecol.* **2007**, *62*, 142–160. [CrossRef] [PubMed]
32. Buchfink, B.; Xie, C.; Huson, D.H. Fast and sensitive protein alignment using diamond. *Nat. Methods* **2015**, *12*, 59–60. [CrossRef] [PubMed]
33. Segata, N.; Izard, J.; Waldron, L.; Gevers, D.; Miropolsky, L.; Garrett, W.S.; Huttenhower, C. Metagenomic biomarker discovery and explanation. *Genome Biol.* **2011**, *12*, R60. [CrossRef] [PubMed]

34. Breiman, L. Random forests. *Mach. Learn.* **2001**, *45*, 5–32. [CrossRef]
35. Liaw, A.; Wiener, M. Classification and regression by random Forest. *R News* **2002**, *2*, 18–22.
36. Huson, D.H.; Auch, A.F.; Qi, J.; Schuster, S.C. Megan analysis of metagenomic data. *Genome Res.* **2007**, *17*, 377–386. [CrossRef]
37. Huson, D.H.; Mitra, S.; Ruscheweyh, H.J.; Weber, N.; Schuster, S.C. Integrative analysis of environmental sequences using megan4. *Genome Res.* **2011**, *21*, 1552–1560. [CrossRef]
38. Kanehisa, M.; Goto, S.; Kawashima, S.; Okuno, Y.; Hattori, M. The kegg resource for deciphering the genome. *Nucleic Acids Res.* **2004**, *32*, D277–D280. [CrossRef]
39. Yatsunenko, T.; Rey, F.E.; Manary, M.J.; Trehan, I.; Dominguez-Bello, M.G.; Contreras, M.; Magris, M.; Hidalgo, G.; Baldassano, R.N.; Anokhin, A.P.; et al. Human gut microbiome viewed across age and geography. *Nature* **2012**, *486*, 222–227. [CrossRef]
40. Wang, Q.; Hao, C.; Yao, W.; Zhu, D.; Lu, H.; Li, L.; Ma, B.; Sun, B.; Xue, D.; Zhang, W. Intestinal flora imbalance affects bile acid metabolism and is associated with gallstone formation. *BMC Gastroenterol.* **2020**, *20*, 59. [CrossRef]
41. Molinero, N.; Ruiz, L.; Milani, C.; Gutierrez-Diaz, I.; Sanchez, B.; Mangifesta, M.; Segura, J.; Cambero, I.; Campelo, A.B.; Garcia-Bernardo, C.M.; et al. The human gallbladder microbiome is related to the physiological state and the biliary metabolic profile. *Microbiome* **2019**, *7*, 100. [CrossRef] [PubMed]
42. Wang, Y.; Qi, M.; Qin, C.; Hong, J. Role of the biliary microbiome in gallstone disease. *Expert Rev. Gastroenterol. Hepatol.* **2018**, *12*, 1193–1205. [CrossRef] [PubMed]
43. Yamagata, K.; Daitoku, H.; Shimamoto, Y.; Matsuzaki, H.; Hirota, K.; Ishida, J.; Fukamizu, A. Bile acids regulate gluconeogenic gene expression via small heterodimer partner-mediated repression of hepatocyte nuclear factor 4 and foxo1. *J. Biol. Chem.* **2004**, *279*, 23158–23165. [CrossRef] [PubMed]
44. Staels, B.; Handelsman, Y.; Fonseca, V. Bile acid sequestrants for lipid and glucose control. *Curr. Diab. Rep.* **2010**, *10*, 70–77. [CrossRef] [PubMed]
45. Porter, N.T.; Luis, A.S.; Martens, E.C. Bacteroides thetaiotaomicron. *Trends Microbiol.* **2018**, *26*, 966–967. [CrossRef]

diagnostics

MDPI

Article

Diagnosis of Latent Tuberculosis Infection in Hemodialysis Patients: TST versus T-SPOT.TB

Umut Devrim Binay [1,*], Ali Veysel Kara [2], Faruk Karakeçili [1] and Orçun Barkay [1]

[1] Department of Infectious Diseases and Clinical Microbiology, Faculty of Medicine, Erzincan Binali Yıldırım University, 24100 Erzincan, Turkey; drfarukkarakecili@hotmail.com (F.K.); o.barkay1985@gmail.com (O.B.)
[2] Department of Nephrology, Faculty of Medicine, Erzincan Binali Yıldırım University, 24100 Erzincan, Turkey; aliveyselkara@hotmail.com
* Correspondence: umut.binay@erzincan.edu.tr or devrimbinay@hotmail.com

Abstract: Hemodialysis (HD) patients should be screened for latent tuberculosis (TB) infection. We aimed to determine the frequency of latent TB infection in HD patients and to compare the effectiveness of the tests used. The files of 56 HD patients followed between 1 January 2021 and 1 October 2022 were retrospectively analyzed. Demographic data, the presence of the Bacillus Calmette-Guerin (BCG) vaccine, whether or not the patients had previously received treatment for TB before, the status of encountering a patient with active TB of patients over 18 years of age, without active tuberculosis and who had a T-SPOT.TB test or a Tuberculin Skin Test (TST) were obtained from the patient files. The presence of previous TB in a posterior–anterior (PA) chest X-ray was obtained by evaluating PA chest X-rays taken routinely. Of the patients, 60.7% (n = 34) were male and their mean age was 60.18 $\pm$ 14.85 years. The mean duration of dialysis was 6.43 $\pm$ 6.03 years, and 76.8% (n = 43) had 2 BCG scars. The T-SPOT.TB test was positive in 32.1% (n = 18). Only 20 patients (35.7%) had a TST and all had negative results. While the mean age of those with positive T-SPOT.TB results was higher (p = 0.003), the time taken to enter HD was shorter (p = 0.029). T-SPOT.TB test positivity was higher in the group that had encountered active TB patients (p = 0.033). However, no significant difference was found between T-SPOT.TB results according to BCG vaccine, albumin, urea and lymphocyte levels. Although T-SPOT.TB test positivity was higher in patients with a previous TB finding in a PA chest X-ray, there was no statistically significant difference (p = 0.093). The applicability of the TST in the diagnosis of latent TB infection in HD patients is difficult and it is likely to give false-negative results. The T-SPOT.TB test is not affected by the BCG vaccine and immunosuppression. Therefore, using the T-SPOT.TB test would be a more appropriate and practical approach in the diagnosis of latent TB in HD patients.

Keywords: hemodialysis; latent tuberculosis; TST; T-SPOT.TB

Citation: Binay, U.D.; Kara, A.V.; Karakeçili, F.; Barkay, O. Diagnosis of Latent Tuberculosis Infection in Hemodialysis Patients: TST versus T-SPOT.TB. *Diagnostics* **2023**, *13*, 2369. https://doi.org/10.3390/diagnostics13142369

Academic Editor: Hsin-Yao Wang

Received: 23 May 2023
Revised: 7 July 2023
Accepted: 8 July 2023
Published: 14 July 2023

1. Introduction

Tuberculosis (TB) continues to be one of the main causes of death due to infectious diseases all over the world. The World Health Organization (WHO) has implemented the 'End tuberculosis' strategy and in relation to this, it recommends screening and treating latent TB infection (LTBI) [1]. According to the Turkish Ministry of Health's Tuberculosis Diagnosis and Treatment Guidelines, it is recommended that patients with a high risk of latent TB reactivation, such as hemodialysis (HD) patients, should be screened. Since the risk of transmission will be high in hemodialysis units, the development of tuberculosis disease in this patient group must be prevented [2]. When prior studies are examined, in the systematic reviews conducted by Alemu et al., LTBI and active tuberculosis infection were found to be more common in dialysis patients [3,4]. In the study of Xia et al., it was found that the rate of development of active tuberculosis was higher in hemodialysis patients with LTBI. In the same study, in which patients were followed up about three years, LTBI was also shown to be associated with major adverse cardiovascular events [5]. In the study of Park et al., it was shown that active tuberculosis is more common in dialysis patients and kidney transplant recipients compared to the general population and causes higher mortality rates [6]. In the study of Romanowski et al., it was found that active tuberculosis was seen less frequently in patients who were treated for LTBI [7].

Interferon Gamma Release Assays (IGRA) and the Tuberculin Skin Test (TST) are used in LTBI screening, and it is recommended that IGRA should be performed in immunocompromised groups such as hemodialysis patients when the TST is negative or cannot be performed. Among the IGRA tests, the T-SPOT.TB, QuantiFERON-TB Gold In Tube (QFT-GIT) or QuantiFERON-TB gold plus test are used [2,8–12]. When studies comparing the diagnostic tests are examined, there is no gold standard test. In the study of Akbar et al., the QuantiFERON-TB gold plus test was shown to be superior to the TST. However, the small sample size was determined as a limitation of the study [13]. On the other hand, in the study of Setyawati et al., the use of the TST was recommended in the diagnosis of LTBI [14]. However, although it is stated that IGRA tests are not affected by immunosuppression, studies in patients with chronic kidney disease have shown that, as the time of dialysis increases, IGRA tests are more likely to give false-negative results. In this context, it is recommended that patients with chronic kidney disease be screened for LTBI at an early stage [15–18]. Considering the systematic reviews carried out in recent years, it has been shown that IGRA tests are superior to the TST [11,19,20].

The aim of this study is to determine the frequency of latent TB infection in patients undergoing hemodialysis in our hospital and to compare the effectiveness of tests used in the diagnosis of latent TB infection. At the same time, the aim is to investigate the reasons for the inconsistency between the tests by determining the factors affecting the tests.

2. Materials and Methods

2.1. Study Design and Population

This study was planned as a retrospective, cross-sectional study and was conducted with the approval of Erzincan Binali Yildirim University Clinical Research Ethics Committee (Date: 10 November 2022/Decision No: 05/09).

Latent TB infection screening is routinely performed in the hemodialysis unit of our institution. Patients are regularly referred to a tuberculosis dispensary for a TST to be performed. The T-SPOT.TB test is performed simultaneously with a hemogram, biochemical examinations and a posterior–anterior (PA) chest X-ray taken during routine dialysis, for patients who cannot undergo a TST or whose results are negative.

So, the files of HD patients who were followed up in the hemodialysis unit of a tertiary research and training hospital between 1 January 2021 and 1 October 2022 were reviewed retrospectively. Demographic data of the patients (age, gender, comorbidities, duration of hemodialysis admission, etc.) and data on the presence of Bacillus Calmette-Guerin (BCG) vaccine, whether or not they had previously received treatment for active TB, and their prior encounters with a patient with active TB were obtained from patient files. The presence of previous TB in a PA chest X-ray was obtained by evaluating the PA chest X-rays taken routinely.

The inclusion criteria were:

1. To have regular hemodialysis;
2. To be over 18 years old;
3. To have T-SPOT.TB or TST results;
4. To not have a concurrent active TB diagnosis.

Accordingly, out of a total of 67 patients, 56 patients who met the inclusion criteria were included in the study. Since the number of patients who did not undergo a TST was high, a comparison of both tests could not be made. Therefore, the factors affecting the results of the T-SPOT.TB test and the TST were evaluated separately.

2.2. Methodology

After blood samples were taken using special tubes for the T-SPOT.TB test (Oxford Immunotec, Oxford, UK), T-Cell Xtend reagent was added to the blood samples and sent to the laboratory. Mononuclear cells were obtained by centrifugation from the blood taken for the T-SPOT.TB test. The resulting mononuclear cells were added to wells previously coated with IFN-γ antibodies. Then, the TB antigens ESAT-6 and CFP-10 and Phytohemagglutinin were added for positive control. The negative control was determined as the well without antigens. These wells were incubated overnight at 37 °C with 5% CO_2. After incubation, the wells were washed and secondary conjugated antibodies were added to measure the IFN-γ response. Spots that formed in the wells in which the IFN-γ response was observed were measured by an automated ELISPOT reader (AID systems, Strassberg, Germany). The result was considered positive if the test wells contained at least five more spot-forming cells than the average of the negative control wells [21].

The TST was applied intradermally to the upper inner 2/3 of the left forearm of the patients, in a hairless area away from the veins, with an insulin injector, with 0.1 mL of 5 TU PPD containing tuberculin solution. The transverse diameter of the formed induration was measured in mm after 48–72 h. Results with an induration diameter of 5 mm or more were considered positive [22].

The hemogram test of the patients was performed using the Sysmex XN-1000 Hematology System (Sysmex Corporation, Kobe, Japan); biochemical tests were performed with AU 5800 (Beckman Coulter, Brea, CA, USA).

2.3. Statistical Analysis

The NCSS (Number Cruncher Statistical System) 2007 (NCSS LLC, Kaysville, UT, USA) program was used for statistical analysis. Descriptive statistical methods (mean, standard deviation, median, frequency, ratio, minimum, maximum) were used while evaluating the study data. The conformity of quantitative data to normal distribution, the Shapiro–Wilk test and graphical evaluations were used.

Student's *t*-test was used for comparisons of normally distributed quantitative variables between two groups, and the Mann–Whitney U test was used for comparisons of non-normally distributed variables.

Pearson's chi-squared test, the Fisher–Freeman–Halton test and Fisher's exact test were used to compare qualitative data. Logistic regression analysis was used in multivariate evaluations of the risk factors affecting T-SPOT.TB positivity.

Significance was evaluated at the $p < 0.05$ level.

3. Results

The study was carried out at a research and training hospital between 1 January 2021 and 1 October 2022. It was carried out with 56 HD patients, of whom 39.3% ($n = 22$) were female and 60.7% ($n = 34$) were male. The ages of the patients ranged from 20 to 81, with a mean of 60.18 ± 14.85 years. The duration of HD ranged from 1 to 27 years, with a mean of 6.43 ± 6.03 years. In total, 66.1% ($n = 37$) of the cases had comorbidities. When the types of comorbidities were examined, it was observed that 32.4% ($n = 12$) had type 2 Diabetes Mellitus (DM), 78.4% ($n = 29$) had essential hypertension (HT) and 45.9% ($n = 17$) had other diseases.

Of the patients, 3.6% ($n = 2$) had a prior history of active TB. The patients stated that they had completed their treatment. The number of patients who had encountered active tuberculosis patients was 8.9% ($n = 5$).

In addition, 8.9% ($n = 5$) of the patients had no BCG vaccine scar, 14.3% ($n = 8$) had one scar and 76.8% ($n = 43$) had two scars (Table 1).

Table 1. Demographic Characteristics and Distribution of Laboratory and Imaging Results of the Patients.

		Min-Max (Median)	Mean ± Sd
Age (year)		20–81 (63)	60.18 ± 14.85
Time of dialysis (years)		1–27 (4)	6.43 ± 6.03
		n	%
Gender	Female	22	39.3
	Male	34	60.7
Presence of Comorbidity	Yes	37	66.1
	No	19	33.9
Type of comorbidities	Type 2 DM	12	32.4
	Hypertension	29	78.4
	Other *	17	45.9
History of active tuberculosis	Yes	2	3.6
	No	54	96.4
Encounter with active tuberculosis patient	Yes	5	8.9
	No	51	91.1
BCG scar	0	5	8.9
	1	8	14.3
	2	43	76.8
Leukocyte count (mm^3)		2800–25,400 (6250)	6992.86 ± 3842.15
Lymphocyte count (mm^3)		440–21,020 (1185)	1981.43 ± 3533.68
Albumin (g/dL)		2.1–41 (3.8)	17.42 ± 16.16
Urea (mg/dL)		85–238 (147.5)	149.18 ± 28.91
		n	%
Previous TB finding on PA chest X-ray	Yes	4	7.1
	No	52	92.9
T-SPOT.TB test	Negative	38	67.9
	Positive	18	32.1
TST	Negative	20	35.7
	Unknown	36	64.3

* Chronic Obstructive Pulmonary Disease, Alport Syndrome, Chronic Lymphoproliferative Leukemia, Coronary Artery Disease, Rheumatoid Arthritis.

Mean leukocyte counts were 6992.86 ± 3842.15/mm^3; mean lymphocyte counts were 1981.43 ± 3533.68/mm^3; mean albumin level was 17.42 ± 16.16 g/dL; and mean urea level was 149.18 ± 28.91 mg/dL.

Overall, 7.1% (n = 4) of the patients had previous tuberculosis findings on a chest X-ray.

The T-SPOT.TB test results were negative in 67.9% (n = 38) and positive in 32.1% (n = 18). A TST was performed in 35.7% (n = 20) of the patients and all of them were negative (Table 1).

3.1. Assessment of T-SPOT.TB Results

A statistically significant correlation was found between age and the T-SPOT.TB test result ($p = 0.003$; $p < 0.01$). The mean age of the group with positive results was found to be higher than the group with negative results.

A statistically significant correlation was found between the time on HD and the T-SPOT.TB test result ($p = 0.029$; $p < 0.05$). The HD time in the group with positive results was found to be shorter than in the group with negative results.

While the T-SPOT.TB test results did not show a statistically significant difference by gender ($p = 0.072$; $p > 0.05$), it is noteworthy that the rate of positive results in men was higher than that in women.

There was no statistically significant correlation between the presence of comorbidities and the T-SPOT.TB test results ($p > 0.05$).

A statistically significant correlation was found between encountering a patient with active tuberculosis and the T-SPOT.TB test results ($p = 0.033$; $p < 0.05$). The rate of positive results in the group that encountered a tuberculosis patient was higher than the group that had not.

No statistically significant correlation was found between the number of BCG scars and the T-SPOT.TB test results ($p > 0.05$) (Table 2).

Table 2. Relationship between Descriptive Characteristics and T-SPOT.TB Results.

		T-SPOT.TB Test		p
		Negative (n = 38)	**Positive (n = 18)**	
Age (year)	Min-Max (Median) Mean ± Sd	20–80 (57) 56.26 ± 15.08	38–81 (71) 68.44 ± 10.6	[a] 0.003 *
Time of dialysis (year)	Min-Max (Median) Mean ± Sd	1–27 (5) 7.45 ± 6.37	1–20 (3) 4.28 ± 4.71	[b] 0.029 *
Gender	Female Male	18 (81.8) 20 (58.8)	4 (18.2) 14 (41.2)	[c] 0.072
Presence of Comorbidity	Yes No	27 (73) 11 (57.9)	10 (27) 8 (42.1)	[c] 0.253
Type of comorbidities (n = 37)				
Type 2 DM	Yes No	8 (66.7) 19 (76)	4 (33.3) 6 (24)	[d] 0.696
Essential HT	Yes No	20 (69) 7 (87.5)	9 (31) 1 (12.5)	[d] 0.404
Other *	Yes No	13 (76.5) 14 (70)	4 (23.5) 6 (30)	[d] 0.725
Encounter with active tuberculosis patient	Yes No	1 (20) 37 (72.5)	4 (80) 14 (27.5)	[d] 0.033 *
BCG scar	0 1 2	3 (60) 6 (75) 29 (67.4)	2 (40) 2 (25) 14 (32.6)	[e] 1.000

[a] Student's t-Test; [b] Mann–Whitney U Test; [c] Pearson's Chi-Squared Test; [d] Fisher's Exact Test; [e] Fisher–Freeman–Halton Test; * Chronic Obstructive Pulmonary Disease, Alport Syndrome, Chronic Lymphoproliferative Leukemia, Coronary Artery Disease, Rheumatoid Arthritis.

No statistically significant correlation was found between leukocyte count, lymphocyte count, albumin level and urea level and the T-SPOT.TB test results ($p > 0.05$).

While no statistically significant correlation was found between previous TB findings on PA chest X-rays and the T-SPOT.TB test results ($p = 0.093$; $p > 0.05$), it is noteworthy that the rate of positive results was higher in the group with a previous TB finding in a PA chest X-ray (Table 3).

Table 3. Relationship between Laboratory and Imaging Results and T-SPOT.TB Test Results.

		T-SPOT.TB		p
		Negative (n = 38)	Positive (n = 18)	
Leukocyte (mm^3)	Min-Max (Median) Mean ± Sd	2800–13,300 (6350) 6602.63 ± 2108.09	4000–25,400 (5400) 7816.67 ± 6085.11	[b] 0.352
Lymphocyte (mm^3)	Min-Max (Median) Mean ± Sd	440–2710 (1165) 1322.11 ± 562.14	660–21,020 (1275) 3373.33 ± 6057.06	[b] 0.516
Albumin (g/dL)	Min-Max (Median) Mean ± Sd	2.9–41 (3.8) 16.46 ± 16.06	2.1–39 (17.9) 19.46 ± 16.65	[b] 0.853
Urea (mg/dL)	Min-Max (Median) Mean ± Sd	85–238 (152) 152.39 ± 31.85	103–180 (142.5) 142.39 ± 20.61	[a] 0.230
Previous TB finding on PA chest X-ray	Yes No	1 (25) 37 (71.2)	3 (75) 15 (28.8)	[d] 0.093

[a] Student's *t*-Test; [b] Mann–Whitney U Test; [d] Fisher's Exact Test.

When we evaluated the risk factors affecting the T-SPOT.TB test, such as age, gender, a previous TB finding on a PA chest X-ray, time of dialysis and encountering an active tuberculosis patient with Enter Logistic Regression Analysis, the model was found to be significant and the explanatory coefficient of the model (76.8%) was found to be at a good level. It is seen that the effect of a unit increase in age on T-SPOT.TB positivity increases the ODDS ratio 1.101 (95% CI: 1.016–1.192) times. The effect of encountering an active tuberculosis patient has an effect on T-SPOT.TB positivity with an ODDS value of 59.762 (95% CI:1.59–2233.42) times. The effects of gender, a previous TB finding on a PA chest X-ray and time of dialysis were not significant in the multivariate evaluation ($p > 0.05$) (Table 4).

Table 4. Logistic Regression Results of Factors Affecting T-SPOT.TB Test.

	p	ODDS	95% C.I.ODDS	
			Lower	Upper
Age	0.018 *	1.101	1.016	1.192
Gender (F)	0.128	3.937	0.674	23.003
Previous TB finding on PA chest X-ray (+)	0.311	3.766	0.290	48.857
Time of dialysis (year)	0.827	1.017	0.875	1.182
Encounter with active tuberculosis patient (+)	0.027 *	59.762	1.599	2233.422

* $p < 0.05$,

3.2. Results of Patients with Known History of TST

A TST was performed in 35.7% (n = 20) of the patients and it was found that all of them had negative results. Of these cases, 30% (n = 6) were female and 70% (n = 14) were male. Their ages ranged from 20 to 81 years, with a mean of 61.85 ± 17.1 years. The duration of HD ranged from 1 to 20 years, with a mean of 6.40 ± 6.08 years.

In total, 50% (n = 10) of the cases who underwent a TST had comorbidities. When the types of comorbidities were examined, it was observed that 20% (n = 2) had type 2 DM, 90% (n = 9) had essential hypertension and 50% (n = 5) had other diseases.

The rate of having had tuberculosis previously was found to be 5% (n = 1), while 20% (n = 4) of the patients who underwent a TST stated that they had previously encountered an active tuberculosis patient.

When the BCG scars of the tested participants were examined, 10% (n = 2) had no scar, 15% (n = 3) had one scar and 75% (n = 15) had two scars (Table 5).

Table 5. Distribution of the Descriptive Characteristics of the Patients who had TST.

N = 20		Min-Max (Median)	Mean ± Sd
Age (year)		20–81 (64)	61.85 ± 17.10
Time of dialysis (year)		1–20 (3.5)	6.40 ± 6.08
		n	%
Gender	Female	6	30
	Male	14	70
Presence of Comorbidity	Yes	10	50
	No	10	50
Type of comorbidities (n = 10)	Type 2 DM	2	20
	HT	9	90
	Other *	5	50
History of active tuberculosis	Yes	1	5
	No	19	95
Encounter with active tuberculosis patient	Yes	4	20
	No	16	80
BCG scar	0	2	10
	1	3	15
	2	15	75

* Chronic Obstructive Pulmonary Disease, Alport Syndrome, Chronic Lymphoproliferative Leukemia, Coronary Artery Disease, Rheumatoid Arthritis.

Mean leukocyte counts were 7000 ± 4336.87 mm3; mean lymphocyte counts were 2209 ± 3951.76 mm^3; the mean albumin level was 16.39 ± 16.41 g/dL; and the mean urea level was calculated as 141.95 ± 22.97 mg/dL. There was no significant difference between leukocyte and lymphocyte count according to the positive and negative T-SPOT.TB test.

In 10% (*n* = 2) of the patients who underwent a TST, previous TB was found in a PA chest X-ray.

The T-SPOT.TB test results of the patients who underwent a TST and all had negative results were found to be 20% (*n* = 4) negative and 80% (*n* = 16) positive (Table 6).

Table 6. Distribution of Laboratory and Imaging Results of the Patients who had TST.

N = 20			Min-Max (Median)	Mean ± Sd
Leukocyte (mm^3)			2800–21,900 (5400)	7000 ± 4336.87
Lymphocyte (mm^3)			660–18,850 (1285)	2209 ± 3951.76
Albumin (g/dL)			2.1–39 (3.7)	16.39 ± 16.41
Urea (mg/dL)			100–180 (142.5)	141.95 ± 22.97
			n	%
Previous TB finding on PA chest X-ray	Yes		2	10
	No		18	90
T-SPOT.TB test	Negative		4	20
	Positive		16	80
	T-SPOT.TB test			*p*
	Negative (n = 4)		Positive (n = 16)	
Leukocyte (mm^3)	2800–13,300 (6350) 7175.0 ± 4593.7		4200–21,900(5400) 6956.3 ± 4426.4	[b] 0.892
Lymphocyte (mm^3)	800–2210 (1285) 1395.0 ± 590.6		660–18,850 (1275) 2412.5 ± 4414.7	[b] 0.963

[b] Mann–Whitney U Test.

4. Discussion

The frequency of latent TB infection and the probability of TB reactivation in hemodialysis patients are higher than in the normal population [1,2,23–25]. Therefore, HD patients should be screened for latent TB infection [1,2]. The TST and IGRA are used in screening, and in a study investigating the frequency of latent TB infection in HD patients in low- and high-risk groups for latent TB infection, IGRA were shown to be superior to the TST [26]. In our study, the rate of latent TB infection was 32.1% and was similar to the study of Bandiara et al. that was conducted in HD patients (39.1%) [27]. In another study conducted in Thailand, the frequency of latent TB infection in dialysis patients was found to be 25% [28]. In the study of Lemrabott et al., 25% of latent TB infection was found in Senegal [29]. Similar rates of latent TB infection were found in the study of Putri et al. [17]. The frequency of latent TB infection in our study was as high as in Rheumatoid Arthritis and Ankylosing Spondylitis patients in the other immunosuppressive patient group [30].

The rate of latent TB infection in our study could be determined with the T-SPOT.TB test because only 35.7% (20) of the patients had a TST and all of them had negative results. Most of the patients (64.3%) refused to go to the tuberculosis dispensary for a TST. This shows that the applicability of the TST in hemodialysis patients is difficult. At the same time, in the study of Say et al., in which the QFT-GIT and TST were compared for the diagnosis of latent TB infection, there was no concordance between the two tests [31]. In the study of Southern et al., there was a high degree of discordance between IGRA and the TST in hemodialysis patients [15]. In a study conducted with HIV-infected individuals, another group of immunosuppressive patients, moderate concordance was found between T-SPOT.TB and the TST, and it was stated that the discordance might be due to false-positive and -negative results of the TST [32]. The disadvantages of the test are that the TST gives false positive results in the presence of the BCG vaccine and atypical mycobacterial infection, and false-negative results in the presence of immunosuppression [33,34]. In our study, T-SPOT.TB positivity was found in 16 (80%) of 20 patients whose TST results were negative. This result shows that the TST gives false-negative results. On the other hand, the expensiveness of IGRA is the disadvantage of the tests, while the advantages are that they are not affected by the presence of the BCG vaccine, atypical mycobacterial infection and immunosuppression [34,35]. In the study of Sargın et al., which was conducted in a rheumatologic patient group, the sensitivity and specificity of IGRA tests were shown to be superior to the TST [36]. In our study, no significant correlation was found between T-SPOT.TB test results according to BCG vaccine status, and this shows that the test is not affected by the BCG vaccine. The BCG vaccine is in the routine childhood vaccination schedule in our country and is administered at the end of the 2nd month [2]. It is important for our country that the T-SPOT.TB test is not affected by the BCG vaccine. Although the number of patients is small, the positive T-SPOT.TB test in patients with a TB finding on a PA chest X-ray indicates that the probability of a false-negative result is low. However, false-negative results should be investigated in HD patients, including in many patients with a history of microbiologically proven tuberculosis.

In our study, T-SPOT.TB test positivity was statistically higher in patients who had encountered active TB patients. In the study of Park et al., QFT GIT positivity, which is one of the IGRA tests, was higher in HD patients who had a history of TB [37]. In a study, T-SPOT.TB test positivity in patients with high risk factors, such as encountering an active TB patient, shows that the probability of developing active TB is higher [38]. In this case, it is important to initiate latent TB treatment without delay in high-risk patients with a positive T-SPOT.TB test.

It has been shown that advanced age, active smoking and close contact with someone who has previously had TB are among the risk factors for latent TB infection in HD patients. In the same study, it was stated that high albumin levels and short HD duration facilitate the detection of latent TB infection [39]. In a study conducted in Japan in hemodialysis patients, the frequency of LTBI was found to be higher, especially in people aged 60 and over [40] and in other studies conducted in China and Lebanon, advanced age was found among the risk factors for latent TB infection [5,41]. In our study, the high mean age of the patients with a positive T-SPOT.TB test and the shorter time to enter HD in patients with a positive T-SPOT.TB test support the literature. The incidence of TB in our country has been decreasing over the years, so that the incidence of TB, which was 29.8% in 2005, decreased to 14.4% in 2018 [42]. This may be the reason why the T-SPOT.TB test gives high positive results in older age groups. In our study, there was no significant difference between positive/negative results in terms of albumin, urea and lymphocyte levels, while the average albumin levels of patients with a T-SPOT.TB positive result were higher. However, the fact that there was no significant correlation between the T-SPOT.TB test results according to the urea levels and lymphocyte counts of the patients suggests that the test is not affected by immunosuppression.

The small number of patients and the fact that many patients did not have a TST are the limitations of the study.

In conclusion, HD patients should be screened for latent TB infection as soon as possible. Although it is recommended to perform a TST first in screening, the applicability of the test is not easy and the possibility of false-negative results is high, which limits its use. The most important advantage of the T-SPOT.TB test is that it is not affected by immunosuppression and it is studied with a single measurement from blood. Therefore, the use of the T-SPOT.TB test would be a more practical and accurate approach to screen for latent TB infection in HD patients.

Author Contributions: Concept and design: U.D.B., A.V.K., F.K. and O.B.; Data collection: U.D.B. and A.V.K.; Data analysis and interpretation: U.D.B., A.V.K., F.K. and O.B.; Draft of the article: U.D.B. and A.V.K.; Revision of the article: U.D.B., A.V.K., F.K. and O.B. All authors have read and agreed to the published version of the manuscript.

Funding: This research received no external funding.

Institutional Review Board Statement: The study was conducted in accordance with the Declaration of Helsinki, and approved by the Erzincan Binali Yildirim University Clinical Research Ethics Committee (Date: 10 November 2022/Decision No: 05/09).

Informed Consent Statement: Since it is a retrospective study, patient consent was not obtained.

Data Availability Statement: Data will be shared upon request.

Conflicts of Interest: The authors declare no conflict of interest.

References

1. World Health Organization. *WHO Operational Handbook on Tuberculosis (Module 1—Prevention): Tuberculosis Preventive Treatment*; World Health Organization: Geneva, Switzerland, 2020.
2. Er, A.G.; Süer, A.İ.; Yurteri, A.Ş.; Babalık, A.; Yıldırım, A.; Öztomurcuk, D.; İnce, E.; Kabasakal, E.; Çakır, E.; İlhan, F.; et al. *Tüberküloz Tanı ve Tedavi Rehberi*, 2nd ed.; Artı6 Medya Tanıtım Matbaa Ltd. Şti.: Ankara, Turkey, 2019; pp. 1–344. ISBN 978-975-590-717-8.
3. Alemu, A.; Bitew, Z.W.; Diriba, G.; Seid, G.; Moga, S.; Abdella, S.; Gashu, E.; Eshetu, K.; Tollera, G.; Dangisso, M.H.; et al. The prevalence of latent tuberculosis infection in patients with chronic kidney disease: A systematic review and meta-analysis. *Heliyon* **2023**, *9*, e17181. [CrossRef]
4. Alemu, A.; Bitew, Z.W.; Diriba, G.; Seid, G.; Eshetu, K.; Chekol, M.T.; Berhe, N.; Gumi, B. Tuberculosis incidence in patients with chronic kidney disease: A systematic review and meta-analysis. *Int. J. Infect. Dis.* **2022**, *122*, 188–201. [CrossRef]
5. Xia, Y.; Fan, Q.; Zhang, J.; Jiang, L.; Huang, X.; Xiong, Z.; Xiong, Z. Risk factors and prognosis for latent tuberculosis infection in dialysis patients: A retrospective cohort study at a single tertiary care center. *Semin. Dial.* **2023**, 1–6. [CrossRef] [PubMed]
6. Park, S.; Park, S.; Kim, J.E.; Yu, M.Y.; Kim, Y.C.; Kim, D.K.; Joo, K.W.; Kim, Y.S.; Han, K.; Lee, H. Risk of active tuberculosis infection in kidney transplantation recipients: A matched comparative nationwide cohort study. *Am J Transplan.* **2021**, *21*, 3629–3639. [CrossRef] [PubMed]
7. Romanowski, K.; Rose, C.; Cook, V.J.; Sekirov, I.; Morshed, M.; Djurdjev, O.; Levin, A.; Johnston, J.C. Effectiveness of Latent TB Screening and Treatment in People Initiating Dialysis in British Columbia, Canada. *Can. J. Kidney Health Dis.* **2020**, *7*, 2054358120937104. [CrossRef] [PubMed]

8. Grant, J.; Jastrzebski, J.; Johnston, J.; Stefanovic, A.; Jastrabesky, J.; Elwood, K.; Roscoe, D.; Balshaw, R.; Bryce, E. Interferon-gamma release assays are a better tuberculosis screening test for hemodialysis patients: A study and review of the literature. *Can. J. Infect. Dis. Med. Microbiol.* **2012**, *23*, 114–116. [CrossRef]
9. Carranza, C.; Pedraza-Sanchez, S.; de Oyarzabal-Mendez, E.; Torres, M. Diagnosis for latent tuberculosis infection: New alternatives. *Front. Immunol.* **2020**, *11*, 2006. [CrossRef]
10. Jonas, D.E.; Riley, S.R.; Lee, L.C.; Coffey, C.P.; Wang, S.H.; Asher, G.N.; Berry, A.M.; Williams, N.; Balio, C.; Voisin, C.E.; et al. Screening for latent tuberculosis infection in adults: Updated evidence report and systematic review for the US Preventive Services Task Force. *JAMA* **2023**, *329*, 1495–1509. [CrossRef]
11. Zhou, G.; Luo, Q.; Luo, S.; Teng, Z.; Ji, Z.; Yang, J.; Wang, F.; Wen, S.; Ding, Z.; Li, L.; et al. Interferon-γ release assays or tuberculin skin test for detection and management of latent tuberculosis infection: A systematic review and meta-analysis. *Lancet Infect. Dis.* **2020**, *20*, 1457–1469. [CrossRef]
12. Ho, C.S.; Feng, P.J.I.; Narita, M.; Stout, J.E.; Chen, M.; Pascopella, L.; Garfein, R.; Reves, R.; Katz, D.J.; Flood, J.; et al. Comparison of three tests for latent tuberculosis infection in high-risk people in the USA: An observational cohort study. *Lancet Infect. Dis.* **2022**, *22*, 85–96. [CrossRef]
13. Akbar, A.A.; Islam, M.N.; Rahman, M. Comparison of Mantoux test with quantiFERON-TB gold plus assay for detection of tuberculosis infection among chronic kidney disease patients in a tertiary care hospital in Dhaka city. *Bangladesh Med. Coll. J.* **2021**, *26*, 24–29.
14. Setyawati, A.; Reviono, R.; Putranto, W. The Compability Level of Tuberculin Skin Test and T-SPOT. TB, Sensitivity and Spesifisity of T-SPOT. TB in Detecting Latent Tuberculosis in Hemodialysis Patients. *J. Respirol. Indones.* **2021**, *41*, 19–27. [CrossRef]
15. Southern, J.; Sridhar, S.; Tsou, C.Y.; Hopkins, S.; Collier, S.; Nikolayevskyy, V.; Lozewicz, S.; Lalvani, A.; Abubakar, I.; Lipman, M. Discordance in latent tuberculosis (TB) test results in patients with end-stage renal disease. *Public Health* **2019**, *166*, 34–39. [CrossRef] [PubMed]
16. Wang, P.H.; Lin, S.Y.; Lee, S.S.; Lin, S.W.; Lee, C.Y.; Wei, Y.F.; Shu, C.C.; Wang, J.Y.; Yu, C.J. CD4 response of QuantiFERON-TB Gold Plus for positive consistency of latent tuberculosis infection in patients on dialysis. *Sci. Rep.* **2020**, *10*, 21367. [CrossRef] [PubMed]
17. Putri, D.U.; Chen, C.L.; Wang, C.H.; Sue, Y.M.; Tseng, P.C.; Lin, C.F.; Tsai, C.W.; Liu, Y.J.; Lee, C.H. Hemodialysis acutely altered interferon-gamma release assay test result and immune cell profile. *J. Microbiol. Immunol. Infect.* **2022**, *55*, 332–335. [CrossRef]
18. Park, H.; Kang, Y.-J.; Kim, Y.N.; Park, S.-B.; Lim, J.; Park, J.Y.; Kang, Y.A.; Lee, H.; Kim, J.; Kim, S. Predictors for False-Negative Interferon-Gamma Release Assay Results in Hemodialysis Patients with Latent Tuberculosis Infection. *Diagnostics* **2023**, *13*, 88. [CrossRef]
19. Nasiri, M.J.; Pormohammad, A.; Goudarzi, H.; Mardani, M.; Zamani, S.; Migliori, G.B.; Sotgiu, G. Latent tuberculosis infection in transplant candidates: A systematic review and meta-analysis on TST and IGRA. *Infection* **2019**, *47*, 353–361. [CrossRef]
20. Zhou, G.; Luo, Q.; Luo, S.; He, J.; Chen, N.; Zhang, Y.; Yang, R.; Qiu, Y.; Li, S.; Ping, Q.; et al. Positive rates of interferon-γ release assay and tuberculin skin test in detection of latent tuberculosis infection: A systematic review and meta-analysis of 200, 000 head-to-head comparative tests. *Clin. Immunol.* **2022**, *245*, 109132. [CrossRef]
21. Soysal, A.; Torun, T.; Efe, S.; Gencer, H.; Tahaoglu, K.; Bakir, M. Evaluation of cut-off values of interferon-gamma- based assays in the diagnosis of M. *tuberculosis infection. Int. J. Tuberc. Lung Dis.* **2008**, *12*, 50–56.
22. Kılınç, O. Tüberkülin Deri Testi (TDT), Yorumu Ve Son Gelişmeler. In Proceedings of the 21. Yüzyılda Tüberküloz Sempozyumu ve II. Tüberküloz Laboratuvar Tanı Yöntemleri Kursu, Samsun, Turkey, 11–14 June 2003; pp. 203–207.
23. Kiazyk, S.; Ball, T.B. Latent tuberculosis infection: An overview. *Can. Commun. Dis. Rep.* **2017**, *43*, 62–66. [CrossRef]
24. Moran, E.; Baharani, J.; Dedicoat, M.; Robinson, E.; Smith, G.; Bhomra, P.; Thien, O.S.; Ryan, R. Risk factors associated with the development of active tuberculosis among patients with advanced chronic kidney disease. *J. Infect.* **2018**, *77*, 291–295. [CrossRef]
25. Dobler, C.C.; McDonald, S.P.; Marks, G.B. Risk of tuberculosis in dialysis patients: A nationwide cohort study. *PLoS ONE* **2011**, *6*, e29563. [CrossRef] [PubMed]
26. Chung, W.K.; Zheng, Z.L.; Sung, J.Y.; Kim, S.; Lee, H.H.; Choi, S.J.; Yang, J. Validity of interferon-γ-release assays for the diagnosis of latent tuberculosis in haemodialysis patients. *Clin. Microbiol. Infect.* **2010**, *16*, 960–965. [CrossRef] [PubMed]
27. Bandiara, R.; Indrasari, A.; Rengganis, A.D.; Sukesi, L.; Afiatin, A.; Santoso, P. Risk factors of latent tuberculosis among chronic kidney disease with routine haemodialysis patients. *J. Clin. Tuberc. Other Mycobact. Dis.* **2022**, *27*, 100302. [CrossRef]
28. Hayuk, P.; Boongird, S.; Pornsuriyasak, P.; Bruminhent, J. Interferon-gamma release assays for diagnosis of latent TB infection in chronic kidney diseases and dialysis patients. *Front. Cell. Infect. Microbiol.* **2022**, *12*, 1046373. [CrossRef] [PubMed]
29. Lemrabott, A.T.; Faye, M.; Faye, M.; Kane, Y.; Cisse, M.M. Contribution of an Interferon Gamma Released Assay to the Detection of Latent Tuberculosis in Chronic Dialysis Patients in Sub-Saharan Africa. *J. Nephrol. Ther.* **2019**, *9*, 2161-0959. [CrossRef]
30. Doğru, G.; Şahin, M. Romatoid Artrit ve Ankilozan Spondilit Hastalarında Anti-TNF Alfa Tedavi Öncesi Latent Tüberküloz Taramasında Tüberkülin Deri Testi ve İnterferon Gama Salınım Testinin Karşılaştırılması. *Süleyman Demirel Üniversitesi Sağlık Bilim. Derg.* **2021**, *12*, 70–76.
31. Say, İ.; Küçük, B.; Orak, F.; Aral, M.; Doğaner, A. Latent Tüberküloz Enfeksiyonu Araştırılan Hastalarda QuantiFERON-TB GOLD Testi ile Tüberkülin Deri Testinin Karşılaştırılması. *Türk Mikrobiyoloji Cemiy. Derg.* **2021**, *51*, 271–275.
32. Binay, U.D.; Fincanci, M.; Fersan, E.; Karakecili, F. Comparison of Tuberculin Skin Test (TST) and T-SPOT. TB Tests for Diagnosis of Latent Tuberculosis Infection (LTBI) in HIV-infected Patients. *Mikrobiyol. Bul.* **2019**, *53*, 388–400. [CrossRef]

33. Richardson, R.M. The diagnosis of tuberculosis in dialysis patients. *Semin. Dial.* **2012**, *25*, 419–422. [CrossRef]
34. Zhang, X.; Chen, P.; Xu, G. Update of the mechanism and characteristics of tuberculosis in chronic kidney disease. *Wien. Klin. Wochenschr.* **2022**, *134*, 501–510. [CrossRef]
35. Wardani, H.R.; Wicaksi, D. Detection of Latent Tuberculosis Infection in Haemodialysis Patients: A Systematic Review. *Unej E-Proceeding* **2021**, *S.I.*, 55–62.
36. Sargın, G.; Şentürk, T.; Ceylan, E.; Telli, M.; Çildağ, S.; Doğan, H. TST, QuantiFERON-TB Gold test and T-SPOT. TB test for detecting latent tuberculosis infection in patients with rheumatic disease prior to anti-TNF therapy. *Tuberk. Toraks* **2018**, *66*, 136–143. [CrossRef] [PubMed]
37. Park, J.Y.; Park, S.B.; Park, H.; Kim, J.; Kim, Y.N.; Kim, S. Cytokine and Chemokine mRNA Expressions after Mycobacterium tuberculosis-Specific Antigen Stimulation in Whole Blood from Hemodialysis Patients with Latent Tuberculosis Infection. *Diagnostics* **2021**, *11*, 595. [CrossRef] [PubMed]
38. Abubakar, I.; Drobniewski, F.; Southern, J.; Sitch, A.J.; Jackson, C.; Lipman, M.; Deeks, J.J.; Griffiths, C.; Bothamley, G.; Lynn, W.; et al. Prognostic value of interferon-γ release assays and tuberculin skin test in predicting the development of active tuberculosis (UK PREDICT TB): A prospective cohort study. *Lancet Infect. Dis.* **2018**, *18*, 1077–1087. [CrossRef]
39. Shu, C.C.; Wu, V.C.; Yang, F.J.; Pan, S.C.; Lai, T.S.; Wang, J.Y.; Wang, J.T.; Lee, L.N. Predictors and prevalence of latent tuberculosis infection in patients receiving long-term hemodialysis and peritoneal dialysis. *PLoS ONE* **2012**, *7*, e42592. [CrossRef]
40. Ogawa, Y.; Harada, M.; Hashimoto, K.; Kamijo, Y. Prevalence of latent tuberculosis infection and its risk factors in Japanese hemodialysis patients. *Clin. Exp. Nephrol.* **2021**, *25*, 1255–1265. [CrossRef]
41. Ismail, M.B.; Zarriaa, N.; Osman, M.; Helfawi, S.; Kabbara, N.; Chatah, A.N.; Kamaleddine, A.; Alameddine, R.; Dabboussi, F.; Hamze, M. Prevalence of Latent Tuberculosis Infection among Patients Undergoing Regular Hemodialysis in Disenfranchised Communities: A Multicenter Study during COVID-19 Pandemic. *Medicina* **2023**, *59*, 654. [CrossRef]
42. Yıllara GöRe Toplam Tb Olgu Sayısı, Toplam Olgu Hızı Ve İNsiDans HızI, 2005–2018. Available online: https://hsgmdestek.saglik.gov.tr/depo/birimler/tuberkuloz_db/dosya/Istatistikler/Yeni/2-Yllara_Gore_Toplam_TB_Olgu_Hz_ve_TB_Insidans_2005-2018.pdf (accessed on 2 July 2023).

diagnostics MDPI

Article

Performance Evaluation of VIDAS® Diagnostic Assays Detecting Anti-Chikungunya Virus IgM and IgG Antibodies: An International Study

Geovana M. Pereira [1,†], Erika R. Manuli [1,2,3,†], Laurie Coulon [4], Marina F. Côrtes [1], Mariana S. Ramundo [1], Loïc Dromenq [4], Audrey Larue-Triolet [4], Frédérique Raymond [4], Carole Tourneur [4], Carolina dos Santos Lázari [5], Patricia Brasil [6], Ana Maria Bispo de Filippis [7], Glaucia Paranhos-Baccalà [1,4], Alice Banz [4] and Ester C. Sabino [1,2,3,*]

1 Instituto de Medicina Tropical, Faculdade de Medicina da Universidade de São Paulo, São Paulo 05403-000, Brazil; geovanapereira16@gmail.com (G.M.P.); erikamanuli@gmail.com (E.R.M.); marinafarrel23@gmail.com (M.F.C.); marianasevero@gmail.com (M.S.R.); glaucia.baccala@biomerieux.com (G.P.-B.)
2 Faculdade de Medicina da Universidade Municipal de São Caetano do Sul, São Paulo 09521-160, Brazil
3 Laboratório de Investigação Médica/Parasitologia LIM/46, Hospital das Clínicas da Faculdade de Medicina da Universidade de São Paulo, São Paulo 05403-010, Brazil
4 bioMérieux, 69280 Marcy l'Etoile, France; lauriecoulon11@gmail.com (L.C.); loic.dromenq@biomerieux.com (L.D.); audrey.larue@me.com (A.L.-T.); frederique.raymond@biomerieux.com (F.R.); carole.tourneur@biomerieux.com (C.T.); alice.banz@biomerieux.com (A.B.)
5 Hospital das Clínicas da Faculdade de Medicina da Universidade de São Paulo, São Paulo 05403-010, Brazil; carolina.lazari@hc.fm.usp.br
6 Instituto Nacional de Infectologia Evandro Chagas, Fundação Oswaldo Cruz, Fiocruz, Rio de Janeiro 21040-360, Brazil; patricia.brasil33@gmail.com
7 Laboratório de Arbovírus e Vírus Hemorrágicos, Instituto Oswaldo Cruz/Fiocruz, Rio de Janeiro 21040-360, Brazil; ana.bispo@ioc.fiocruz.br
* Correspondence: sabinoec@gmail.com
† These authors contributed equally to this work.

Citation: Pereira, G.M.; Manuli, E.R.; Coulon, L.; Côrtes, M.F.; Ramundo, M.S.; Dromenq, L.; Larue-Triolet, A.; Raymond, F.; Tourneur, C.; Lázari, C.d.S.; et al. Performance Evaluation of VIDAS® Diagnostic Assays Detecting Anti-Chikungunya Virus IgM and IgG Antibodies: An International Study. *Diagnostics* **2023**, *13*, 2306. https://doi.org/10.3390/diagnostics13132306

Academic Editor: Hsin-Yao Wang

Received: 25 April 2023
Revised: 26 June 2023
Accepted: 30 June 2023
Published: 7 July 2023

Abstract: Chikungunya (CHIK) is a debilitating mosquito-borne disease with an epidemiology and early clinical symptoms similar to those of other arboviruses-triggered diseases such as dengue or Zika. Accurate and rapid diagnosis of CHIK virus (CHIKV) infection is therefore challenging. This international study evaluated the performance of the automated VIDAS® anti-CHIKV IgM and IgG assays compared to that of manual competitor IgM and IgG ELISA for the detection of anti-CHIKV IgM and IgG antibodies in 660 patients with suspected CHIKV infection. Positive and negative agreements of the VIDAS® CHIKV assays with ELISA ranged from 97.5% to 100.0%. The sensitivity of the VIDAS® CHIKV assays evaluated in patients with a proven CHIKV infection confirmed reported kinetics of anti-CHIKV IgM and IgG response, with a positive detection of 88.2–100.0% for IgM $\geq$ 5 days post symptom onset and of 100.0% for IgG $\geq$ 11 days post symptom onset. Our study also demonstrated the superiority of ELISA and VIDAS® assays over rapid diagnostic IgM/IgG tests. The analytical performance of VIDAS® anti-CHIKV IgM and IgG assays was excellent, with a high precision (coefficients of variation $\leq$ 7.4%) and high specificity (cross-reactivity rate $\leq$ 2.9%). This study demonstrates the suitability of the automated VIDAS® anti-CHIKV IgM and IgG assays to diagnose CHIKV infections and supports its applicability for epidemiological surveillance and differential diagnosis in regions endemic for CHIKV.

Keywords: chikungunya virus; CHIKV; VIDAS; enzyme-linked immunosorbent assay; ELISA; IgM; IgG; capture immunoassay; enzyme-linked fluorescent assay; ELFA

1. Introduction

Chikungunya (CHIK) is a debilitating disease caused by the chikungunya virus (CHIKV) and transmitted to humans by *Aedes* spp. mosquitoes [1]. CHIKV was first identified in 1952 in Tanzania [2] and has now spread to over 100 countries across Africa, Asia, Europe, and the Americas, with multiple outbreaks affecting millions of people [1,3–6]. This alarming increase in CHIKV spread is likely of multifactorial origin, including virus and vector adaptation to changes in the environment and human behaviour, and enhanced global dissemination due to increased urbanisation and international travel [1,7]. Phylogenetic studies identified four main CHIKV genotypes, namely the (i) 'East Central South African' (ECSA), (ii) 'West African' (WA), (iii) 'Asian', and (iv) the recently emerged, ECSA-diverged 'India Ocean' lineage (IOL) [1,3,5,6]. Although studies directly comparing the virulence of these geographic genotypes are scarce, a few investigations have suggested that CHIKV lineages present differences in their transmission cycles and that some genotypes might be preferentially associated with a higher prevalence of self-reported long-term chronic CHIKV symptoms [1,3,6].

Like dengue virus (DENV) and Zika virus (ZIKV), CHIKV is a single-stranded RNA arbovirus with similar epidemiology and transmission cycles [8]. Accordingly, co-circulation of these arboviruses in overlapping endemic regions and co-infection cases have been described [7–11]. Moreover, following infection by these arboviruses, clinical symptoms at disease onset are often similar and clinically non-specific, including fever, headache, myalgia, arthralgia, and maculopapular rash [7,8,12,13]. This raises the challenge of CHIKV diagnosis and emphasises the need for efficient strategies of epidemiological surveillance and differential diagnosis [7,8,10,11,13,14].

Following CHIKV infection, the incubation period ranges from 1 to 12 days. The early acute phase of infection is usually characterised by a sudden onset of high fever (in 85% of patients), correlating with the presence of elevated CHIK viral load in the blood. The onset of fever is followed by intense polyarthralgia, which can last two to three weeks, and a rash (in 40–75% of patients). In the post-acute phase (>3 weeks to 3 months), clinical manifestations, notably joint pain, persist in more than half of the patients. When symptoms have not subsided after 3 months, the patient enters the chronic phase of the disease (>3 months to several years, affecting 40–80% of patients). The chronic disease can progress to (i) cure without sequelae, upon treatment or spontaneously, (ii) further persistence of joint and/or other symptoms, or (iii) aggravation because of exacerbation of inflammatory and/or degenerative processes [1,5,6,15,16].

In addition to these typical clinical manifestations, atypical features and complications might occur, such as neurologic disorders, notably in infected individuals with comorbidities, and according to age (the elderly and infants) [1,7,12]. Altogether, despite a low mortality rate, the morbidity associated with CHIKV infection is high, and CHIK illness can be severe and durably debilitating [1].

No specific antiviral therapy exists for acute CHIKV infection, and patient management relies mainly on supportive care to treat pain and inflammatory symptoms [1,7,12,16,17]. Despite sharing similar clinical manifestations at illness onset, which is associated with a risk of misdiagnosis, the course of disease following infection by distinct arboviruses such as CHIKV, DENV, and ZIKV varies greatly. Therefore, a reliable and accurate early diagnosis is essential to ensure proper patient management, while adopting timely preventive measures and implementing suitable epidemiologic surveillance [7,8,10,11,13,14].

Current recommendations [13,15,17,18] for the confirmation of CHIKV infection in a suspected case (i.e., with the characteristic triad of fever, rash, and joint manifestations) are based on the kinetics of CHIKV viremia and of the host immune response, with the detection of CHIKV RNA by means of real-time reverse transcription-polymerase chain reaction (rRT-PCR) within the first week ($\leq$7 days) of symptom onset, and detection of anti-CHIKV immunoglobulin M (IgM) and/or IgG thereafter (>7 days). rRT-PCR alone is usually recommended between day 0 and 5 post symptom onset, rRT-PCR and anti-CHIKV IgM serology between day 5 and 7, and serology only after day 7. A positive rRT-PCR is confirmatory of an acute CHIKV infection, while a positive anti-CHIKV IgM test is presumptive of a CHIKV infection. Seroconversion or a 4-fold rise in anti-CHIKV IgG measured in paired serum samples collected in the acute and post-acute (convalescent) phases (two to three weeks apart) also indicates an active CHIKV infection. Given that CHIKV-specific IgG can be detected several years after the initial infection, seroconversion/antibody rise also allows us to rule out a past infection. In the chronic phase, as for the post-acute phase, CHIKV serology should confirm the diagnosis together with a biological evaluation of inflammatory rheumatism. Finally, in the case of negative rRT-PCR and serology in acute samples, serology should be repeated on convalescent-phase samples to definitively rule out CHIKV diagnosis [1,5–7,13,15,17–20].

rRT-PCR assays, both as singleplex (CHIKV RNA) or multiplex (e.g., differential screening of CHIKV, DENV, and ZIKV RNAs), have proven to be highly sensitive and specific, although no molecular gold standard exists to date [5,10,14,19]. rRT-PCR tests present, however, the potential caveat that not all existing assays detect all known CHIKV genotypes [6,19], an issue not shared by existing anti-CHIKV antibody detection tests due to the demonstrated cross-reactivity against heterogenous CHIKV genotypes [6,21]. Numerous serological tests detecting CHIKV-specific IgM and IgG antibodies have been developed and commercialised [5,6,10,11,19,20,22–24]. Enzyme-linked immunosorbent assays (ELISA) have demonstrated acceptable performance for the detection of anti-CHIKV IgM and IgG. In comparison, rapid diagnostic tests (RDT) showed very low sensitivity and specificity for the detection of CHIKV-specific IgM and IgG antibodies [5,6,10–12,19,20,22–24]. Despite demonstrating good performance, ELISAs are manual and time-consuming (about 1.5–2 h per test) methods, which might represent a burden for testing laboratories at times of epidemic outbreaks. The implementation of an automated system allowing rapid execution and interpretation of results would be of clear benefit.

VIDAS® anti-CHIKV IgM and IgG assays are fully automated CE-marked enzyme-linked fluorescence assays (ELFA) intended as an aid in the diagnosis of patients with clinical symptoms consistent with CHIKV infection. VIDAS® anti-CHIKV IgM and IgG assays are qualitative immunocapture assays detecting CHIKV-specific IgM and IgG antibodies, respectively. They can be tested in parallel or independently, are rapid (40 min to result), easy to use, and easy to interpret (positive or negative) with no equivocal zone. The performance of these automated assays has not yet been directly compared to that of conventional manual assays. The aim of this international study was to evaluate for the first time the clinical performance of the VIDAS® anti-CHIKV IgM and IgG assays in samples from patients with a suspected CHIKV infection, enrolled from multiple CHIK-endemic regions of the world (Asia, Latin America). The clinical performance of the VIDAS® anti-CHIKV assays was compared to that of existing manual competitor ELISA and RDT assays.

2. Materials and Methods

2.1. Patients and Samples

A total of 660 sera were collected at three sites in patients with a suspected CHIKV infection and from several CHIKV-endemic regions, including Asia (India) and Latin America (Brazil, Colombia, Dominican Republic, Honduras, Peru) (Table 1). Retrospective and prospective cohorts of samples collected between January 2016 and September 2021 were used for this study. For retrospective biobanked samples, a suspicion of CHIKV infection was established based on the documented presence of one or more of the following symptoms at the time of sampling: fever, joint pain or arthritis, tenosynovitis, bursitis, headache, back pain, rash, myalgia, cutaneous pruritus, polyadenopathy, oedema of the face and extremities. For prospective samples, a suspicion of CHIKV infection was established during a routine medical procedure based on the presence of fever and joint pain or arthritis within 3 months of sampling, associated with one or more of the following symptoms: headache, back pain, rash, myalgia, cutaneous pruritus, polyadenopathy, oedema of the face and extremities.

Table 1. Study samples.

Site	Collection Site	Samples	Collection Time	Testing Site
1	National Institute of Infectious Diseases-Fiocruz, Rio de Janeiro, Brazil	Retrospective, follow-up cohort	18 April 2019–1 November 2019	Tropical Medicine Institute, Faculty of Medicine of the University of São Paulo, Brazil
2	Biospecimen Solutions Pvt Ltd., Sampigehalli, Bangalore, Karnataka, India	Prospective cohort	24 July 2021–20 September 2021	Clinical Affairs Laboratory, bioMérieux, Marcy l'Etoile, France
3	Colombia, Dominican Republic, Honduras, and Peru	Retrospective cohort [1]	28 January 2016–8 September 2020	Clinical Affairs Laboratory, bioMérieux, Marcy l'Etoile, France

[1] Samples purchased from Boca Biolistics (Pompano Beach, FL, USA), Trans-Hit Bio/Azenta Life Sciences (Chelmsford, MA, USA), and ABO Pharmaceuticals (San Diego, CA, USA).

All collected sera ($\geq$1.0 to 1.5 mL) were aliquoted to allow testing with the different assays on the same freeze/thaw cycle. Aliquots were stored frozen at −80 °C until testing. When applicable (collection sites 2 and 3), frozen samples or aliquots were transported to the testing site under controlled conditions.

Samples were tested at two central laboratories: the Tropical Medicine Institute of the University of São Paulo, Brazil for retrospective longitudinal samples collected in Brazil (site 1; Table 1), and the Clinical Affairs Laboratory of bioMérieux, Marcy l'Etoile, France for samples collected prospectively in India (site 2; Table 1) and for retrospective biobanked samples collected in Latin America and purchased from commercial providers (site 3; Table 1).

This study was conducted in adherence to the Declaration of Helsinki and approved by the institutional ethics committee (CEP) of the Faculty of Medicine of the University of São Paulo, Brazil (approval number 4.692.542, dated 5 May 2021), and by the independent ethics committee Namaste Integrated Services, Lanka, Varanasi, India (approval number BS-IND-001, dated 7 August 2021). Purchased samples were collected and approved for use for research purposes by the respective commercial providers (Boca Biolistics, Pompano Beach, FL, USA; Trans-Hit Bio/Azenta Life Sciences, Burlington, MA, USA; ABO Pharmaceuticals, San Diego, CA, USA). All participants, or a parent or legal guardian in the case of children, provided informed consent before the start of the study.

Precision experiments were conducted using characterised negative and positive samples (bioMérieux collection). Negative samples were provided by the French blood bank (Etablissement Français du Sang [EFS], La Plaine Saint-Denis, France). Each volunteer donor signed a written informed consent form for the use of blood for research purposes. EFS obtained authorisation from the French Ministry of Research to collect and transfer samples to partners (Ministère de l'Enseignement Supérieur, de la Recherche et de l'Innovation, reference AC-2017-2958).

Cross-reactivity experiments were performed using native samples collected from patients with other potentially interfering infections who tested positive for antibodies against the respective pathogens (bioMérieux collection).

2.2. Study Design and Definitions

The aim of this performance evaluation study was to compare the performance of the automated VIDAS® anti-CHIKV IgM and IgG assays with that of manual competitor ELISA for the detection of anti-CHIKV IgM and IgG antibodies in patients with a suspected CHIKV infection.

Three distinct analyses were performed. First, an agreement analysis was conducted on the whole cohort, comparing the results of the VIDAS® CHIKV IgM and IgG assays to those of competitor ELISA, which was used as a comparative method (Table 2). To consolidate the detection of anti-CHIKV IgM antibodies, two competitor IgM ELISA methods were used (Table 2). This choice was motivated by the acknowledged non-negligible rate of false-positive and false-negative results of IgM serology assays in general [25,26], and of CHIKV IgM serology assays in particular [23,27]. To limit the bias that could be introduced in the agreement analysis by false-positive and/or false-negative results of the comparative method, the results of two well-validated commercial IgM ELISAs were taken into consideration. An IgM result by the competitor ELISA was defined as positive when both IgM ELISA tests were positive, and negative when both IgM ELISA tests were negative (Table 3). Discordant results were excluded from the analysis (Figure 1).

Table 2. Competitor ELISA used for the agreement analysis with the VIDAS® CHIKV IgM and IgG assays.

Competitor ELISA	Name of Assay	Manufacturer
IgM [1]	CHIKjj Detect™ IgM ELISA (CHKM-R)	InBios International, Seattle, WA, USA
	NovaLisa Chikungunya Virus IgM μ-capture, ELISA Kit (NOVCHIM0590)	NovaTec Immundiagnostica, Dietzenbach, Germany
IgG	Chikungunya virus (CHIKV) (EI 293a-9601 G)	Euroimmun, Lübeck, Germany

[1] The results of both IgM ELISAs were used to interpret the competitor IgM ELISA results (considered positive when both were positive, negative when both were negative, and undetermined when at least one was discordant). Sensitivity and specificity of the respective competitor ELISA, as reported in the package insert by the respective manufacturers, were: 100% sensitivity and specificity for both IgM ELISA, >96.8% sensitivity and 98.0% specificity for the IgG ELISA.

Table 3. Definitions of samples used for agreement analysis (PPA, NPA) according to results of competitor ELISA.

Sample Definition	IgM Competitor ELISA Results [1]		IgG Competitor ELISA Result [2]	CHIKV IgM Agreement Study	CHIKV IgG Agreement Study
	InBios	NovaTec	Euroimmun		
IgM+/IgG−	positive	positive	negative	PPA	N/A
IgM+/IgG+	positive	positive	positive	PPA	PPA
IgM−/IgG+	negative	negative	positive	N/A	PPA
IgM−/IgG−	negative	negative	negative	NPA [3]	NPA [3]

[1] Anti-CHIKV IgM competitor ELISA, as described in Table 2; both IgM assays must be concordant (negative or positive); samples with discordant competitor IgM ELISA results were excluded from the analysis (see Figure 1). [2] Anti-CHIKV IgG competitor ELISA, as described in Table 2. [3] Only samples negative for both IgM and IgG were included in the NPA analyses. Abbreviations: N/A, not applicable (samples excluded from the respective NPA analyses); NPA, negative percent agreement; PPA, positive percent agreement.

Positive percent agreement (PPA) analyses for anti-CHIKV IgM assays were conducted on samples positive with the competitor IgM ELISA (regardless of the IgG status). Similarly, PPA analyses for anti-CHIKV IgG assays were conducted on samples positive with the competitor IgG ELISA (regardless of the IgM status) (Table 3). For a more robust negative agreement (NPA) analysis, only samples negative for both IgM and IgG (with competitor ELISA) were included in the test comparison (Table 3). Only one sample per patient was included in the agreement analysis. In the case of multiple samples per patient, the first sample available chronologically was analysed.

This agreement analysis on the whole population was completed by an agreement analysis on the same samples but according to the time from symptom onset. The five periods investigated were defined according to the documented time intervals post symptom onset: 0–6 days, 7–10 days, 11–21 days, 22 days–3 months, and >3 months.

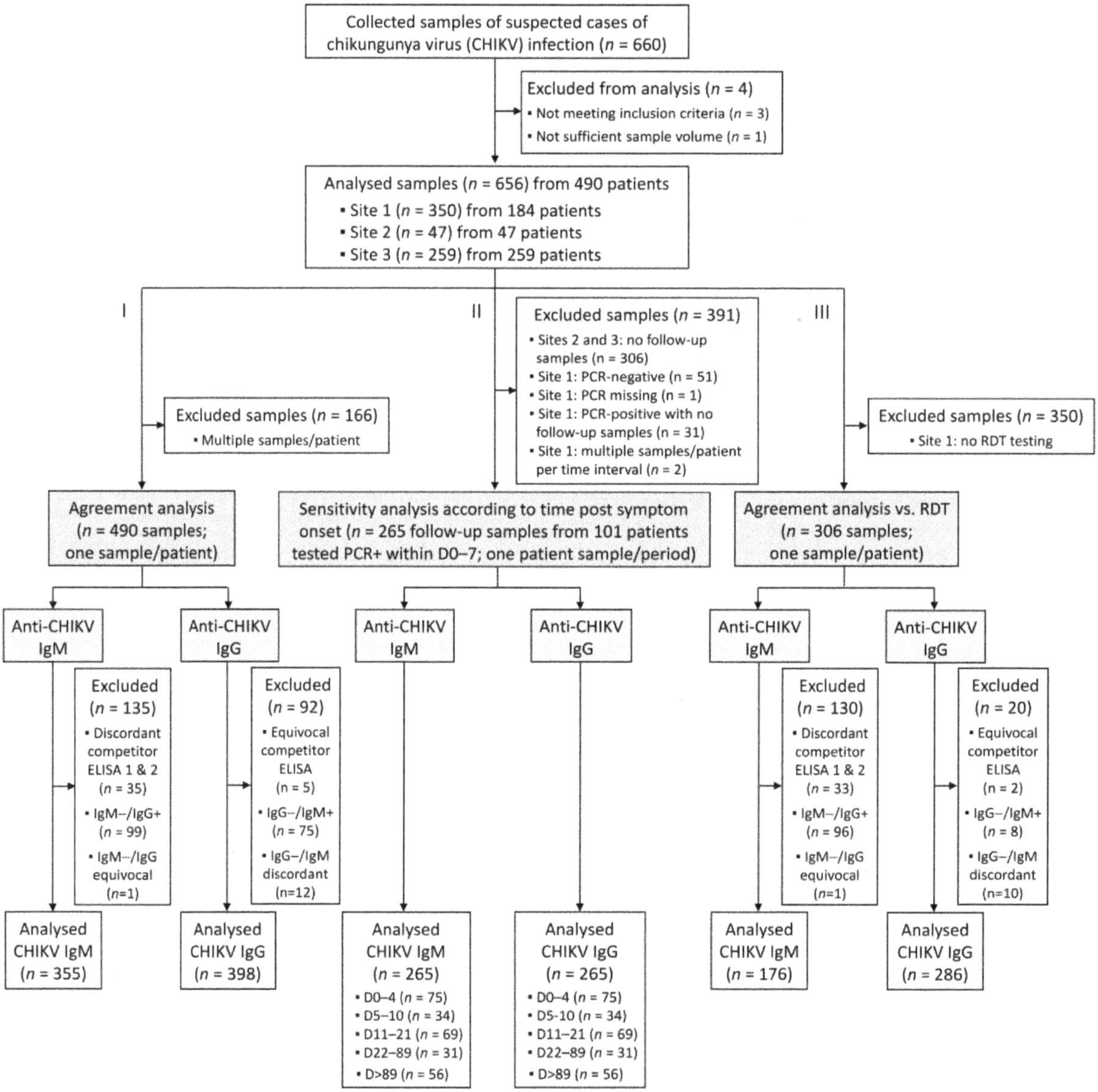

Figure 1. Study flow diagram. Three analyses were conducted: (**I**) an agreement analysis assessed the performance of the VIDAS® CHIKV IgM and IgG assays in comparison to commercial competitor ELISA; (**II**) the sensitivity of the VIDAS® CHIKV IgM and IgG assays was evaluated in patients with a confirmed CHIKV infection (defined as an rRT-PCR-positive within 7 days of symptom onset); (**III**) the agreements of VIDAS® CHIKV IgM and IgG assays or of RDT IgM/IgG with competitor ELISA were evaluated on a common set of samples and compared to each other.

A second analysis was conducted on the follow-up retrospective samples collected at site 1 (Brazil; Table 1) to evaluate the sensitivity of the VIDAS® anti-CHIKV IgM and IgG assays at different time points following a confirmed CHIKV infection. A CHIKV infection was defined as confirmed when positive for CHIKV RNA by rRT-PCR, set as the gold standard. Patients with a positive rRT-PCR at $\leq$7 days post symptom onset and at least one follow-up sample were included in this analysis (Figure 1). Five periods following symptom onset were investigated according to the documented days post symptom onset: 0–4 days, 5–10 days, 11–21 days (acute phase of CHIKV infection), 22–89 days (post-acute phase of CHIKV infection), and >89 days (chronic phase of CHIKV infection). Only one sample per patient per period was included in the analysis. In the case of multiple samples per patient per period, the first sample collected chronologically was used. The sensitivity of the VIDAS® IgM and IgG assays was defined as the percentage of positive test results in patients confirmed positive for CHIKV infection.

A third analysis was conducted on backup samples from sites 2 and 3 (Table 1) to evaluate the performance of VIDAS® anti-CHIKV IgM and IgG assays vs. that of an RDT (Standard Q Chikungunya IgM/IgG, SD Biosensor, Gurugram, Haryana, India). To that aim, the concordance of the VIDAS® anti-CHIKV IgM and IgG assays to competitor ELISA was compared to the concordance of the RDT to the same competitor ELISA (as a comparative method). This agreement sub-analysis was conducted following the same rules as those of the agreement analysis applied to the whole cohort (see above and Tables 2 and 3). One sample per patient was included in the analysis (Figure 1). Clinical agreement (PPA, NPA) of each method (VIDAS® or RDT) with competitor ELISA was assessed independently and compared with a statistical method.

2.3. *VIDAS® Assays*

VIDAS® Anti-CHIKUNGUNYA IgM (CHKM; 423229) and VIDAS® Anti-CHIKUNGUNYA IgG (CHKG; 423230) (bioMérieux SA, Marcy-l'Étoile, France) are automated qualitative two-step immunocapture assays combined with enzyme-linked fluorescent assay (ELFA) detection, developed for the VIDAS® family of instruments. They are intended as an aid in the diagnosis of patients with clinical symptoms consistent with CHIKV infection. The Solid Phase Receptacle (SPR®) serves as the solid phase as well as the pipetting device. Reagents for the assay are ready-to-use and pre-dispensed in the sealed reagent strip. All steps are performed automatically by the instrument and completed within approximately 40 min. The reagents used for assay development and for this performance evaluation study are identical to those included in the commercialised CE-marked assays.

For the VIDAS® Anti-CHIKUNGUNYA IgM assay (hereafter referred to as the VIDAS® anti-CHIKV IgM assay), total IgM is captured by a monoclonal antibody specific for human IgM coated on the interior of the SPR. In the second step, anti-CHIKV IgM is specifically detected by a CHIKV-specific antigen and anti-CHIKV antibodies conjugated to alkaline phosphatase.

For the VIDAS® Anti-CHIKUNGUNYA IgG assay (hereafter referred to as the VIDAS® anti-CHIKV IgG assay), anti-CHIKV IgG is captured by the CHIKV-specific antigen coated on the interior of the SPR. In the second step, the captured anti-CHIKV IgG is detected by an antibody specific for human IgG conjugated to alkaline phosphatase.

The CHIKV-specific antigen used in both VIDAS® anti-CHIKV assays is a virus-like particle (VLP) produced by transient transfection of HEK293 cells with a eukaryotic expression plasmid encoding the CHIKV capsid and envelope structural polyproteins C-E3-E2-6K-E1 (from strain 37997 of the West African lineage) [28,29]. CHIKV VLPs are composed of 240 copies of capsid proteins surrounded by the host cell plasma membrane and an outermost layer of 240 heterodimers of the immunogenic envelope proteins E1-E2, assembled into 80 glycoprotein spikes [28,29]. CHIKV-specific VLPs secreted in the culture medium were purified by ion exchange chromatography and on a multimodal resin using proprietary protocols.

During the final detection step of both VIDAS® anti-CHIKV immunoassays, the substrate (4-Methyl-umbelliferyl phosphate) is cycled in and out of the SPR. The conjugate enzyme catalyzes the hydrolysis of the substrate into a fluorescent product (4-Methyl-umbelliferone). Fluorescence is measured at 450 nm and a relative fluorescence value (RFV) is generated (background reading subtracted from the final fluorescence reading). The results are automatically calculated by the instrument, according to a standard (S1), and an index value (i) is obtained (where $i = RFV_{sample}/RFV_{S1}$). The test is interpreted as negative when $i < 1.0$ and positive when $i \geq 1.0$. The positivity cut-off values for the VIDAS® CHIKM and CHKG assays were determined based on the area under the receiver operating characteristic (ROC) curve and Youden index analyses, using clinically characterised positive and negative human samples.

For the study, VIDAS® anti-CHIKV IgM and IgG assays were performed and interpreted according to the instructions for use (056847-01 and 055960-01, respectively). VIDAS® assays were repeated in the event of invalid calibration, established human error, or absence of results delivered by the device. Only valid repeated results were taken into account for data analysis. Two lots of VIDAS® anti-CHIKV IgM and IgG assays were used, and the same lots were used at both testing sites (Brazil and France; Table 1). At the testing site in Brazil (Table 1), samples were evaluated on one VIDAS® instrument and in parallel by ELISA on a Mustikan FC reader (ThermoFisher Scientific, Waltham, MA, USA) between 4 October 2021, and 18 October 2021. At the testing site in France (Table 1), two VIDAS instruments were employed, one for the VIDAS® anti-CHIKV IgM assays and one for the VIDAS® anti-CHIKV IgG assays. Samples were evaluated in parallel on VIDAS® and by ELISA on an ELISA reader BioTek 800TS (Agilent, Santa Clara, CA, USA) between 26 July 2021, and 7 October 2021.

2.4. Competitor Enzyme-Linked Immunosorbent Assays (ELISAs)

Competitor ELISAs (Table 2) were conducted and interpreted according to the manufacturers' recommendations. Competitor ELISA tests were repeated in the event of established human error or in the absence of results delivered by the ELISA reader. Only valid repeated results were taken into account for data analysis.

IgM ELISA (InBios) was interpreted as negative for result values (Immune Status Ratio [ISR]) < 0.9, positive for ISR > 1.1, and equivocal for ISR of 0.9–1.1. IgM ELISA (NovaTec) was interpreted as negative for result values (NovaTec Units [NTU]) < 9, positive for NTU > 11, and equivocal for NTU of 9–11. Equivocal IgM assays were repeated in duplicate (inBios) or singlicate (NovaTec). The repeated result (mean of duplicate for InBios, singlicate value for NovaTec) was interpreted as either negative (<1.0 for InBios, ≤ 11 for NovaTec) or positive (≥ 1.0 for InBios, >11 for NovaTec). Thus, the final interpretation of IgM competitor ELISA was either negative or positive. Discordant IgM ELISA test results were excluded from the analysis (Figure 1).

IgG ELISA (Euroimmun) was interpreted as negative for result values (Ratio) < 0.8, positive for a ratio ≥ 1.1, and equivocal for a ratio of 0.8 to <1.1. Equivocal IgG ELISA test results were excluded from the analysis (Figure 1).

2.5. Rapid Diagnostic Test (RDT)

The Standard Q Chikungunya IgM/IgG Rapid Kit (SD Biosensor, Gurugram, Haryana, India) was applied to backup samples of sites 2 and 3 (Table 1). The test was performed and interpreted according to the manufacturer's instructions. In case of an invalid RDT result, the test was repeated. In the event of a repeated invalid test result, the test was confirmed as invalid and excluded from the analysis. Only valid repeated results were taken into account for data analysis.

2.6. Real-Time RT-PCR Assays

At the collection and testing site in Brazil (Table 1), rRT-PCR was performed on samples with a time from symptom onset ≤ 7 days using the ZDC kit (Zika, dengue, and chikungunya) from Bio-Manguinhos, a unit of Fiocruz (Institute of Technology in Immunobiologicals) approved by the National Agency for Health Surveillance ANVISA (register number 80142170032). Samples with a positive rRT-PCR result and with at least one follow-up sample were included in the sensitivity analysis.

At the testing site in France for samples collected at sites 2 and 3 (Table 1), rRT-PCR was performed on samples with a time from symptom onset ≤ 14 days for information purposes only, using the CE-approved RealStar Chikungunya RT-PCR Kit 2.0 (Altona diagnostics GmbH, Hamburg, Germany). The testing was outsourced to BIOMEX GmbH (Heidelberg, Germany).

2.7. Precision Experiments

Precision experiments were conducted at bioMérieux (Marcy l'Etoile, France). Assay precision was evaluated according to the CLSI EP05-A3 guideline [30] using characterised high negative, low positive, and moderate positive human serum samples, as determined by VIDAS® anti-CHIKV IgM and IgG assays. Samples were prepared from negative native EFS samples spiked with a high positive native sample to obtain the expected index value levels. Samples were stored at −20 °C/−30 °C until use.

Within-run precision (repeatability) and within-laboratory precision (between-lot reproducibility) of the VIDAS® anti-CHIKV IgM and IgG assays were determined on samples run in triplicate twice a day for 10 days (equivalent to a 20-day precision), using two lots of VIDAS® assays on one VIDAS® instrument calibrated every second day, thus generating 120 measurements per sample. A visual data integrity check was performed to identify possible outliers. Visually discordant results were confirmed to be statistical outliers using the Generalized Extreme Studentized Deviate (ESD) test with a 1% α risk. In case of confirmed outliers, data analysis was performed on both the full dataset and on the dataset without statistical outliers. Only statistical outliers with an impact on the precision estimates were considered outliers. Variance was expressed as standard deviation (SD) and coefficient of variation (CV).

2.8. Cross-Reactivity Experiments

The analytical specificity of the VIDAS® anti-CHIKV IgM and IgG assays was evaluated at bioMérieux (Marcy l'Etoile, France) on samples containing potentially interfering antibodies directed against other pathogens. Cross-reactivity experiments were performed using native samples collected from patients who tested positive for antibodies against related or unrelated pathogens, as follows. Samples used for evaluating the cross-reactivity with VIDAS® anti-CHIKV IgM were positive for pathogen-specific IgM, except for HAV, HBV, HCV, HIV, IAV/IBV, and *Plasmodium falciparum* samples, which were positive for pathogen-specific total antibodies. Samples used for evaluating the cross-reactivity with anti-CHIKV IgG were positive for pathogen-specific IgG, except for HAV, HBV, HCV, HIV, IAV/IBV, YFV, and *Plasmodium falciparum* samples, which were positive for pathogen-specific total antibodies.

In addition, samples tested with VIDAS® anti-CHIKV IgM were previously characterized as negative using a competitor anti-CHIKV IgM ELISA (Euroimmun Anti-Chikungunya Virus ELISA (IgM), Inbios CHIKjj Detect™ IgM ELISA or NovaLisa® Chikungunya Virus IgM µ-capture). Samples tested with VIDAS® anti-CHIKV IgG were previously characterized as negative using the Euroimmun Anti-Chikungunya Virus ELISA (IgG).

All samples were stored at −80 °C until use, except for samples of SARS-CoV-2-infected patients, which were stored at −30 °C. Samples were tested in singlicate, using one kit lot each (IgM, IgG) on either five VIDAS® instruments (IgM) or two VIDAS® instruments (IgG). A total of 210 and 205 samples with other potentially interfering infections were tested on the VIDAS® anti-CHIKV IgM and IgG assays, respectively.

2.9. Statistical Analyses

Agreement analyses were conducted between the VIDAS® assays and competitor ELISA used as a comparative method. Agreement analyses (PPA, NPA, and overall percent agreement) were performed in adherence to the CLSI EP12-A2 guideline [31]. The 95% confidence intervals (95% CI) were computed, either as Wilson Score Confidence Interval if the percentage agreement was in the range]5%, 95%[or as Exact Binomial Confidence Interval otherwise, using the SAS Enterprise Guide 7.12 software.

The sensitivity of the VIDAS® IgM and IgG assays was evaluated by determining the percentage of positive VIDAS® results on follow-up samples of patients with a CHIKV rRT-PCR-positive status established between day 0 and 7 post symptom onset. The respective 95% CIs were computed as above. The sensitivity of the competitor IgM and IgG ELISA was evaluated in parallel and compared to that of the VIDAS® assays in a pairwise comparison using a McNemar's test with Bonferroni correction (correction for three tests for IgM assays, and for two tests for IgG assays).

Agreement of the VIDAS® and RDT assays with competitor ELISA was compared according to the CLSI EP12-A2 guidelines [31], using the 95% CI of the differences of these two concordance values; if 0 belonged to the 95% CI then both concordance values were not considered significantly different, while if 0 was outside the 95% CI then both concordance values were considered significantly different.

The assay precision was assessed in adherence to the CLSI EP05-A3 guideline [30] by a component-of-variance analysis for nested design (Restricted Maximum Likelihood) using the SAS Enterprise Guide 7.12 software.

VIDAS® CHIK IgM and IgG index values of longitudinal study samples used for the sensitivity analysis (i.e., in patients with a confirmed CHIKV infection) were displayed as Tukey box plots according to the time post symptom onset, using GraphPad Prism 5.04 (GraphPad Software, San Diego, CA, USA).

3. Results

3.1. Patients' Characteristics

A total of 660 serum samples were collected, of which 656 were analysed (Figure 1). The 656 included samples were from 490 patients with suspected CHIKV infection, as described in Table 4. The whole study population was composed of 340 (69.4%) females and presented a median (range) age of 37 (15–92) years (Table 4). Out of the 490 included patients, 184 (37.5%) were from Brazil, 165 (33.7%) from Colombia, 72 (14.7%) from Peru, 47 (9.6%) from India, 16 (3.3%) from the Dominican Republic, and 6 (1.2%) from Honduras (Table 4).

Table 4. Patients' and samples' characteristics.

Characteristics	Total	Site 1	Site 2	Site 3
Centre	-	Brazil	India	France
Study population, *N* (%)	490 (100.0%)	184 (37.5%)	47 (9.6%)	259 (52.9%) [1]
Age in years, median (range)	37.0 (15–92)	41.0 (19–83)	43.0 (20–83)	33.0 (15–92)
Sex, *N* (%)				
Female	340 (69.4%)	124 (67.4%)	19 (40.4%)	197 (76.1%)
Male	150 (30.6%)	60 (32.6%)	28 (59.6%)	62 (23.9%)
Study samples, *N* (%)	656 (100.0%)	350 (53.3%)	47 (7.2%)	259 (39.5%)

[1] Out of the 259 purchased samples, 165 (63.7%) were from Colombia, 72 (27.8%) from Peru, 16 (6.2%) from the Dominican Republic, and 6 (2.3%) from Honduras.

A total of 490 samples were included in the agreement analysis comparing the VIDAS® anti-CHIKV IgM and IgG assays to competitor ELISA (Figure 1, analysis I), 265 follow-up samples of patients confirmed positive for CHIKV infection were included in the sensitivity analysis (Table S1 and Figure 1, analysis II), and 306 samples were part of the agreement sub-analysis comparing VIDAS® assays to ELISA vs. RDT to ELISA (Figure 1, analysis III).

3.2. Clinical Performance of the VIDAS® Anti-CHIKV IgM and IgG Assays

3.2.1. Clinical Sensitivity

The sensitivity of the VIDAS® assays was evaluated in patients confirmed positive for CHIKV infection (as determined by a positive CHIKV rRT-PCR at ≤7 days post symptom onset; Table S1). Clinical sensitivity was defined as the percentage of positive test results and was evaluated at different time intervals following the onset of symptoms. Sensitivity of the competitor ELISA was evaluated in parallel (Table 5 and Figure S1).

Table 5. Percentage of positive test results with VIDAS® assays and competitor ELISA in patients confirmed positive for CHIKV infection according to the time post symptom onset (n = 265 samples from 101 patients; see Figure 1 and Table 4).

Assay		Time from Symptom Onset				
		Acute Phase			Post-Acute Phase	Chronic Phase
		0–4 Days (n = 75)	**5–10 Days (n = 34)**	**11–21 Days (n = 69)**	**22–89 Days (n = 31)**	**>89 Days (n = 56)**
VIDAS® CHIKV IgM	n/N [1] (%) [95% CI]	11/75 (14.7%) [8.4–24.4]	30/34 (88.2%) [73.4–95.3]	69/69 (100.0%) [94.8–100.0]	30/31 (96.8%) [83.3–99.9]	53/56 (94.6%) [85.4–98.2]
InBios ELISA IgM	n/N [1] (%) [95% CI]	12/75 (16.0%) [9.4–25.9]	31/34 (91.2%) [77.0–97.0]	69/69 (100.0%) [94.8–100.0]	29/31 (93.5%) [79.3–98.2]	55/56 (98.2%) [90.4–100.0]
NovaTec ELISA IgM	n/N [1] (%) [95% CI]	18/75 (24.0%) [15.8–34.8]	31/34 (91.2%) [77.0–97.0]	69/69 (100.0%) [94.8–100.0]	31/31 (100.0%) [88.8–100.0]	56/56 (100.0%) [93.6–100.0]
VIDAS® CHIKV IgG	n/N [1] (%) [95% CI]	2/75 (2.7%) [0.3–9.3]	9/34 (26.5%) [14.6–43.1]	69/69 (100.0%) [94.8–100.0]	31/31 (100.0%) [88.8–100.0]	56/56 (100.0%) [93.6–100.0]
Euroimmun ELISA IgG	n/N [1] (%) [95% CI]	1/75 (1.3%) [0.0–7.2]	6/33 (18.2%) [2] [8.6–34.4]	69/69 (100.0%) [94.8–100.0]	31/31 (100.0%) [88.8–100.0]	56/56 (100.0%) [93.6–100.0]

[1] n/N is the ratio of the number of samples positive for the respective immunoassays to the number of rRT-PCR-positive samples. [2] One sample with an equivocal result with the Euroimmun IgG ELISA assay was excluded from the calculation. An exact McNemar's test with Bonferroni correction showed a significant difference in sensitivity between the VIDAS® CHIK IgM and the NovaTec ELISA IgM assays for the 0–4 days samples (p = 0.047). All other pairwise comparisons of the 0–4 days (IgM, IgG) and 5–10 days (IgG) samples were not statistically significant. The percentage of positive test results according to the time post symptom onset shown in this Table are depicted in Figure S1. Abbreviations: CHIK, chikungunya; CI, confidence interval.

All evaluated anti-CHIKV IgM assays demonstrated high sensitivity (88.2–100.0%) from day 5 post symptom onset, while all anti-CHIKV IgG assays showed 100.0% sensitivity from day 11 post symptom onset (Table 5 and Figure S1). Anti-CHIKV IgM and IgG assays presented a lower sensitivity at earlier time points after the onset of symptoms (≤24.0% for CHIKV IgM assays at 0–4 days, and ≤26.5% for CHIKV IgG assays at 0–10 days; Table 5 and Figure S1), as predicted from the reported kinetics of antibody response following a CHIKV infection [5,6,19,20].

Altogether, over the whole evaluated period, few differences in sensitivity were observed between the compared assays, with differences of 1.9% (5/265) between VIDAS® CHIKV IgM and inBios IgM ELISA, 4.5% (12/265) between VIDAS® CHIKV IgM and NovaTec IGM ELISA, and 1.5% (4/265) between VIDAS® CHIKV IgG and Euroimmun IgG ELISA (Table 5). Pairwise differences in sensitivity were evaluated in case of apparent differences in proportions at earlier time points (0–4 days for IgM assays, 0–4 days and 5–10 days for IgG assays; Table 5) using an exact McNemar's test with Bonferroni correction. All pairwise differences in sensitivity were not statistically significant (p = 1.000 for VIDAS® CHIKV IgM vs. InBios IgM ELISA at 0–4 days, p = 0.094 for NovaTec IgM ELISA vs. InBios IgM ELISA at 0–4 days, p = 1.000 for VIDAS® CHIKV IgG vs. Euroimmun IgG ELISA at both 0–4 and 5–10 days), except for the comparison of VIDAS® CHIKV IgM vs. NovaTec IgM ELISA at 0–4 days (p = 0.047). However, a closer evaluation of the result values of the 12 apparent discordant VIDAS® CHIKV IgM test results vs. NovaTec IgM ELISA (corresponding to samples negative for VIDAS® and positive for NovaTec ELISA; Table 5) revealed low positive test results for the NovaTec IgM ELISA (with a median [IQR] of 14.4 [13.6–14.9], close to the positivity cutoff of 11.0), indicating no major discordance between test results, and thus no great differences in sensitivity.

In agreement with these qualitative test results, index values of the VIDAS® CHIKV IgM and IgG assays showed the expected kinetics of the antibody response [5,6,19,20], with significant detection of anti-CHIKV IgM from day 5 after onset of symptoms, peaking at 11–21 days, subsiding afterward (Figure 2a and Table S2), while anti-CHIKV IgG strongly increased from day 11 after onset of symptoms and remained high over the evaluated period (Figure 2b and Table S2).

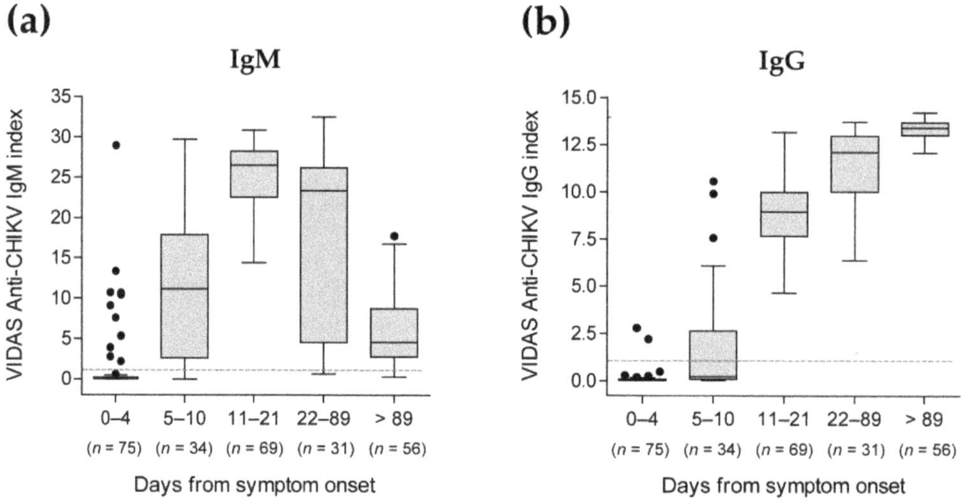

Figure 2. Distribution of VIDAS® CHIKV IgM (**a**) and IgG (**b**) index values in patients confirmed positive for CHIKV infection according to the time post symptom onset. VIDAS® CHIKV IgM and IgG index values of 265 samples from 101 CHIKV-positive patients (as determined by rRT-PCR within 7 days of symptom onset) are displayed as Tukey box plots according to the time from symptom onset. No more than one patient's sample is included per period. The dashed horizontal line shows the positivity cut-off of both assays (i = 1.0). The median and interquartile range of the respective index values are shown in Table S2.

3.2.2. Concordance of the VIDAS® CHIKV IgM and IgG Assays with Competitor ELISA in the Total Study Population

Agreement analysis comparing the performance of the VIDAS® CHIKV IgM and IgG assays to that of the competitor ELISA demonstrated very high positive and negative percent agreements (PPA and NPA between 97.5% and 100.0%; Table 6). The PPA (95% CI) of the comparison of anti-CHIKV IgM assays was the lowest, with 97.5% (93.8–99.3%).

Table 6. Concordance of the VIDAS® CHIKV assays with the respective competitor ELISA (n = 355 for anti-IgM assays, n = 398 for anti-IgG assays; see Figure 1).

VIDAS® CHIKV Assay		Positive Percent Agreement (PPA)	Negative Percent Agreement (NPA)	Overall Percent Agreement (OPA)
IgM	n/N [1] (%) [95% CI]	157/161 (97.5%) [93.8–99.3]	194/194 (100.0%) [98.1–100.0]	351/355 (98.9%) [97.1–99.7]
IgG	n/N [1] (%) [95% CI]	203/204 (99.5%) [97.3–100.0]	193/194 (99.5%) [97.2–100.0]	396/398 (99.5%) [98.2–99.9]

[1] n/N is the ratio of the number of samples for which VIDAS® assays are in agreement (positive, negative, and overall) with the competitor ELISA (comparative method) to the number of samples that tested either positive or negative (and overall) with the competitor ELISA. Positive and negative agreement with competitor ELISA was calculated according to the rules described in Table 3. Abbreviations: CI, confidence interval.

Altogether, very few test results were discordant between the VIDAS® CHIKV assays and the comparative methods, with 4/355 (1.1%) discordant anti-CHIKV IgM assays and 2/398 (0.5%) anti-CHIKV IgG assays (Table 6). For IgM assays, evaluation of the four discordant samples (negative for VIDAS® CHIKV IgM and positive for the competitor IgM ELISA; Table 6) revealed inBios IgM test results close to the positivity cutoff of 1.0 and NovaTec IgM test results that were moderately positive (median [IQR] of 17.95 [14.96–21.81]). These four discordant samples were collected early after symptom onset (0–6 days; Table S3). For IgG assays, the two discordant samples (one in the PPA analysis and one in the NPA analysis; Table 6) revealed test results close to the respective positivity cutoff, thus not strongly discordant. As for IgM assays, the one discordant PPA result (negative for VIDAS® CHIKV IgG and positive for the competitor IgG ELISA) was from a sample collected within 0–6 days of symptom onset (Table S3), when the antibody response starts to mount (see Figure 2). The one discordant NPA result in the anti-CHIKV IgG assay comparison (positive for VIDAS® CHIKV IgG and negative for the competitor IgG ELISA) was collected in the post-acute phase (22 days–3 months post symptom onset; Table S3).

3.2.3. Comparison of Assay Concordance of the VIDAS® CHIKV Assays and RDT with Competitor ELISA

An agreement sub-analysis was conducted aiming to compare on common samples the agreement of VIDAS® assays with the competitor ELISA to that of lateral flow RDT with the same competitor ELISA (Figure 1). In this sub-cohort, VIDAS® CHIKV IgM and IgG assays showed PPA and NPA with the competitor ELISA close to 100.0% (ranging from 99.2% to 100.0%; Table 7). By contrast, the PPA of RDT IgM/IgG with the competitor ELISA was moderate (68.4% and 67.4% for IgM and IgG, respectively), together with an NPA of 100.0% (Table 7).

Table 7. Concordance of the VIDAS® CHIKV assays and of the RDT IgM/IgG assay with competitor ELISA (n = 176 for IgM, n = 286 for IgG; see Figure 1).

Assay		Positive Percent Agreement (PPA)	Negative Percent Agreement (NPA)	Overall Percent Agreement (OPA)
VIDAS® CHIKVIgM	n/N [1] (%) [95% CI]	19/19 (100.0%) [82.4–100.0]	157/157 (100.0%) [97.7–100.0]	176/176 (100.0%) [97.9–100.0]
RDT IgM/IgG [2]	n/N [1] (%) [95% CI]	13/19 (68.4%) [46.0–84.6]	157/157 (100.0%) [97.7–100.0]	170/176 (96.6%) [92.7–98.7]
VIDAS® CHIKVIgG	n/N [1] (%) [95% CI]	128/129 (99.2%) [95.8–100.0]	156/157 (99.4%) [96.5–100.0]	284/286 (99.3%) [97.5–100.0]
RDT IgM/IgG [2]	n/N [1] (%) [95% CI]	87/129 (67.4%) [59.0–74.9]	157/157 (100.0%) [97.7–100.0]	244/286 (85.3%) [80.7–88.9]

[1] n/N is the ratio of the number of samples for which VIDAS® or RDT assays are in agreement (positive, negative, and overall) with the competitor ELISA (reference test) to the number of samples that tested either positive or negative (and overall) with the competitor ELISA. [2] Standard Q Chikungunya IgM/IgG (SD Biosensor). Positive and negative agreement with competitor ELISA was calculated according to the rules described in Table 3. Abbreviations: CI, confidence interval; RDT, rapid diagnostic test.

Differences in agreement to ELISA of the VIDAS® and RDT assays were tested using the 95% CI of the differences of both concordance values, as described in the Materials and Methods (Section 2.9). For anti-CHIKV IgM assays, the NPA of VIDAS® and RDT assays were both in perfect concordance with the comparative method (100.0%; Table 7). By contrast, the difference (95% CI) of the PPA of the VIDAS® and RDT assays was 31.6% (7.61–53.99), indicating that the PPA of VIDAS® CHIKV IgM to ELISA was significantly higher than that of the RDT IgM. Similarly, for anti-CHIKV IgG assays, the difference (95% CI) of the NPA of the VIDAS® and RDT assays was −0.6% (−3.50–1.77), inferring that the NPA of VIDAS® CHIKV IgG to ELISA was not significantly different from that of RDT IgG. As for IgM assays, the PPA of VIDAS® CHIKV IgG (99.2%) was significantly higher than that of the RDT IgG (67.4%), with a difference (95% CI) in the PPA of VIDAS® and RDT assays of 31.8% (23.54–40.31). Therefore, while the NPA of the VIDAS® anti-CHIKV IgM and IgG assays were comparable to that of the rapid test STANDARD™ Q IgM/IgG (both close to 100.0%), the PPA of VIDAS® anti-CHIKV IgM and IgG assays were significantly higher than that of the RDT.

A closer evaluation of the discordant RDT test results in the PPA analysis (i.e., negative for RDT and positive for the competitor ELISA) showed that the 6/19 (31.6%) samples with negative RDT IgM results (Table 7) were moderately positive with the NovaTec IgM ELISA (median NTU of 24.6), the inBios IgM ELISA (median ISR of 7.7), and the VIDAS® CHIKV IgM (median index of 14.3). Similarly, 42/129 (32.6%) samples with negative RDT IgG results (Table 7) were moderately positive with the Euroimmun IgG ELISA (median ratio of 4.28), and 41/42 of those were moderately positive with the VIDAS® CHIKV IgG (median index of 14.2). Altogether, these results demonstrate that the RDT IgM/IgG assay is less sensitive than ELISA, but also less sensitive than the VIDAS® CHIKV assays.

3.3. *Analytical Performance of the VIDAS® CHIKV IgM and IgG Assays*

3.3.1. Assay Precision

The assay precision of the VIDAS® anti-CHIKV IgM and IgG assays was evaluated on high negative, low positive, and moderate positive samples. No outliers were identified and a total of 120 measurements were included in the precision calculation. The coefficient of variation (CV) across both assays did not exceed 5.0% for repeatability (within-run precision) and 7.4% for within-laboratory (between-lot) precision (Table 8).

Table 8. Precision of the VIDAS® CHIKV IgM and IgG assays.

VIDAS® CHIKV Assay	Sample	Measurements (*N*)	Mean Index	Repeatability (Within-Run Precision)		Within-Laboratory Precision [1]	
				SD	CV (%)	SD	CV (%)
IgM	High negative	120	0.84	0.02	2.2	0.04	5.1
	Low positive	120	1.39	0.03	2.5	0.06	4.6
	Moderate positive	120	3.68	0.07	1.9	0.11	3.0
IgG	High negative	120	0.92	0.05	5.0	0.07	7.4
	Low positive	120	1.32	0.06	4.6	0.07	5.6
	Moderate positive	120	5.82	0.22	3.7	0.34	5.9

[1] Between-lot reproducibility. Abbreviations: SD, standard deviation; CV, coefficient of variation.

3.3.2. Assay Cross-Reactivity

The analytical specificity of the VIDAS® anti-CHIKV IgM and IgG assays was evaluated using samples from patients with other proven infections and who had tested positive for the respective pathogen-specific IgM, IgG, or total antibodies, and tested negative with the respective competitor ELISA. The potentially interfering pathogens evaluated were those responsible for febrile infections that could be misdiagnosed as CHIKV, such as other alphaviruses (Barmah Forest virus, Ross River virus), flaviviruses (dengue virus, West Nile virus, yellow fever virus, Zika virus, Japanese encephalitis virus), or other pathogens (*Plasmodium falciparum*, leptospira, severe acute respiratory syndrome coronavirus 2 [SARS-CoV-2], …). Cross-reactivity was measured as the proportion of positive VIDAS® anti-CHIKV IgM and IgG test results among these samples (Table 9).

Overall cross-reactivity with the VIDAS® anti-CHIKV IgM and IgG assays was very low (1/210 [0.5%] for VIDAS® anti-CHIKV IgM and 6/205 [2.9%] for VIDAS® anti-CHIKV IgG; Table 9). The VIDAS® anti-CHIKV IgM assay showed one cross-reactivity with a native sample positive for *Toxoplasma gondii*-specific IgM. The VIDAS® anti-CHIKV IgG assay was cross-reactive with one native sample positive for herpes simplex virus (HSV)-specific IgG, and with five samples positive for IgG against mosquito-borne viruses, including West Nile virus (two cross-reactive samples out of ten tested) and Ross River virus (three cross-reactive samples out of ten tested). No VIDAS® anti-CHIKV IgG cross-reactivity was observed with IgG-positive samples of patients infected with other flaviviruses such as dengue, yellow fever, and Zika viruses. Similarly, the VIDAS® anti-CHIKV IgM assay showed no cross-reactivity with samples of patients who tested IgM-positive for any of the investigated alphaviruses (Barmah Forest virus, Ross River virus) and flaviviruses (dengue virus, West Nile virus, yellow fever virus, Zika virus, Japanese encephalitis virus). Moreover, VIDAS® anti-CHIKV IgM and IgG assays demonstrated no cross-reactivity with samples positive for SARS-CoV-2 IgM and IgG antibodies, respectively (Table 9).

Table 9. Cross-reactivity of human native samples from patients with other infections potentially interfering with the VIDAS® CHIKV IgM and IgG assays.

Potentially Interfering Infections	Proportion of Cross-Reactions with VIDAS® CHIKV Assays	
	IgM	**IgG**
Herpes simplex virus (HSV1/2)	0/10	1/10
Varicella zoster virus (VZV)	0/10	0/10
Cytomegalovirus (CMV)	0/11	0/10
Epstein-Barr virus (EBV)	0/9	0/10
Influenza virus (IAV/IBV)	0/12	0/12
Hepatitis A virus (HAV)	0/10	0/10
Hepatitis B virus (HBV)	0/10	0/10
Hepatitis C Virus (HCV)	0/10	0/10
Parvovirus B19	0/6	0/10
Human immunodeficiency virus (HIV)	0/10	0/10
Borrelia burgdorferi	0/10	0/10
Plasmodium falciparum	0/10	0/10
Toxoplasma gondii	1/12	0/10
Leptospira	0/11	0/10
Dengue virus (DENV)	0/10	0/10
West Nile virus (WNV)	0/10	2/10
Yellow fever virus (YFV)	0/10	0/10
Zika virus (ZIKV)	0/11	0/10
Japanese encephalitis virus (JEV)	0/5	n.d.
Barmah Forest virus (BFV)	0/2	0/3
Ross River virus (RRV)	0/10	3/10
Severe acute respiratory syndrome coronavirus 2 (SARS-CoV-2)	0/11	0/10
Total, *n/N* (%)	**1/210 (0.48%)**	**6/205 (2.93%)**

Abbreviation: n.d., not determined.

4. Discussion

This international study assessed the clinical performance of the automated VIDAS® anti-CHIKV IgM and IgG assays in comparison to a manual competitor ELISA used as a comparative method and evaluated assay sensitivity in patients with a confirmed CHIKV infection.

In this first performance evaluation study, VIDAS® anti-CHIKV IgM and IgG results were comparable to those of competitor IgM and IgG ELISAs, with positive and negative agreements between 97.5% and 100.0%. Given that existing commercial anti-CHIKV IgM and IgG ELISA are recognised for their ability to accurately detect anti-CHIKV antibodies [5,6,10,11,19,20,22–24], our study, therefore, demonstrates the good clinical performance of the VIDAS® anti-CHIKV IgM and IgG assays. Our study also confirmed the superior performance of ELISA over RDT, in accordance with the existing literature [5,6,10,11,19,20,22–24]. Moreover, the significant difference between the PPA of VIDAS® and RDT assays (each compared to competitor ELISA) demonstrates for the first time the superior performance of VIDAS® anti-CHIKV assays over that of RDT. On the other hand, both VIDAS® and RDT assays showed NPA near or equal to 100.0%, suggesting a clinical specificity comparable to that of ELISA.

Sensitivity of the VIDAS® anti-CHIKV IgM and IgG assays, assessed as the percentage of positive test results in patients with a proven CHIKV infection, confirmed reports from the literature as to the kinetics of the anti-CHIKV antibody response [5,6,19,20], with >88% IgM detection at ≥5 days and 100% IgG detection at ≥11 days after symptom onset. Our results, therefore, support the current guidelines for CHIKV infection diagnosis, recommending the detection of CHIKV RNA by real-time RT-PCR within the first week of symptom onset, and detection of anti-CHIKV IgM and/or IgG thereafter [13,15,17,18].

In addition to their strong clinical performance, VIDAS® anti-CHIKV IgM and IgG assays demonstrated excellent analytical performance with high precision (CV < 8%) and analytical specificity (cross-reactivities < 3%). Few cross-reactivities were identified using samples of patients with related or unrelated infections. Nonetheless, five samples that were positive for IgG against mosquito-borne arboviruses (2/10 West Nile virus and 3/10 Ross River virus), but negative with the competitor IgG ELISA, were positive with the VIDAS® anti-CHIKV IgG assay. Cross-reactivity with samples of patients with a past alphavirus infection, such as Ross River virus, was expected given the close homology of alphaviruses [32–34] and previous reports of immune cross-reactivities between sera of patients infected with CHIKV and other alphaviruses, including O'nyong-nyong, Mayaro, and Ross River viruses [27,34–37]. These potentially cross-reactive viruses, together with CHIKV, are endemic in partly overlapping regions and are responsible for diseases presenting similar symptoms [1,38,39]. This emphasizes the potential risk of misdiagnosis, even with good-performing assays, and the importance of conducting differential diagnosis and combining rRT-PCR, IgM, and/or IgG testing, depending on the time after symptom onset, to confirm a CHIKV infection, as recommended [13,15,17,18].

The major strengths of this study include the enrolment of a large number of samples (n = 660) covering multiple endemic regions of the world, including Asia (India) and Latin America (Brazil, Colombia, Peru, Dominican Republic, Honduras), the large number of samples included in the cross-reactivity analysis, the parallel evaluation of samples with VIDAS® and competitor assays, and the use of a unique rRT-PCR test in one central lab for the confirmation of a CHIKV infection for the sensitivity analysis.

Our study presents, nevertheless, a few limitations. First, the choice of considering two competitor IgM ELISAs as comparators to the VIDAS® anti-CHIKV IgM assay led to the exclusion of 35 samples (out of 490 [7.1%]) from the IgM analysis (because of discordance between the two competitor IgM ELISAs), which might have introduced a bias in the analysis. In the absence of a gold standard anti-CHIKV IgM assay, this strategy, however, allowed a more robust agreement analysis of the VIDAS® anti-CHIKV IgM assay. A second possible limitation is the selection of samples negative for both IgM and IgG (with competitor ELISAs) for NPA analyses, which led to the exclusion of 187 'mismatched' IgM/IgG samples and might have introduced a bias in the analysis. This is, however, unlikely, since an analysis including all samples yielded comparable results. Third, given the heterogeneity in the number of recruited samples per site (ranging from 47 to 350; Table 4), no analysis per site was conducted. However, a preliminary analysis indicated comparable performance of the VIDAS® anti-CHIKV assays per site and in the pooled cohort. A future multicentre study enrolling sufficient participants per site should fill this gap. Finally, although we tested the potential cross-reactivity of the VIDAS® anti-CHIKV assays with some alphaviruses (Ross River virus, Barmah Forest virus), the difficulty to acquire alphavirus-specific sera prevented us from testing further cross-reactivities with other related alphaviruses, notably O'nyong-nyong and Mayaro viruses, known to cross-react in competitor ELISA assays [27,34–37]. Additional investigations will be needed to address this question.

5. Conclusions

This international performance evaluation study, conducted on a large number of samples representative of several chikungunya-endemic regions, demonstrated the excellent analytical and clinical performances of the VIDAS® anti-CHIKV assays for the detection of CHIKV-specific IgM and IgG following CHIKV infection. The VIDAS® anti-CHIKV assays, therefore, fulfil the requirements of the current guidelines for the diagnosis of a CHIKV infection. Furthermore, they present the advantage over conventional ELISA to be executed and interpreted automatically within 40 min, which is a clear clinical and epidemiological benefit in CHIKV endemic regions and at the time of outbreaks. They also offer more testing flexibility over ELISA (single testing vs. batch testing), and are as easy to perform as RDT, while offering a higher clinical performance than these rapid tests.

Supplementary Materials: The following supporting information can be downloaded at: https://www.mdpi.com/article/10.3390/diagnostics13132306/s1, Table S1: Description of the follow-up samples of patients confirmed positive for CHIKV infection and included in the sensitivity analysis (Figure 1, analysis II); Table S2: Median and interquartile range (IQR) of VIDAS®CHIK IgM and IgG results depicted in Figure 2, according to the time from symptom onset ($n = 265$); Table S3: Concordance of the VIDAS®CHIKV assays with the respective competitor ELISA according to the time from symptom onset ($n = 355$ samples for anti-IgM assays, $n = 398$ samples for anti-IgG assays [Figure 1]; see Table 6 for the concordance in the whole study population); Figure S1: Sensitivity of the VIDAS and competitor ELISA CHIK IgM (a) and IgG (b) assays.

Author Contributions: Conceptualization, L.C., A.L.-T., C.d.S.L., G.P.-B., A.B. and E.C.S.; methodology, L.C., A.L.-T., C.T. and A.B.; software, L.D.; validation, G.M.P., E.R.M., L.C., C.T. and A.B.; formal analysis, A.L.-T.; investigation, G.M.P., M.F.C., C.T., P.B., A.M.B.d.F. and A.B.; resources, G.M.P., E.R.M., F.R., C.d.S.L., P.B., A.M.B.d.F., G.P.-B. and E.C.S.; data curation, G.M.P., M.S.R., L.D., C.T. and A.B.; writing—review and editing, G.M.P., E.R.M., L.C., M.F.C., M.S.R., L.D., A.L.-T., F.R., C.T., A.B. and E.C.S.; visualization, A.L.-T.; supervision, L.C., C.T., A.B. and E.C.S.; project administration, L.C., C.T., A.B. and E.R.M. All authors have read and agreed to the published version of the manuscript.

Funding: This study was funded by bioMérieux and received no external funding. The APC was funded by bioMérieux.

Institutional Review Board Statement: The study was conducted in accordance with the Declaration of Helsinki, and approved by institutional ethics committee (CEP) of the Faculty of Medicine of the University of São Paulo, Brazil (approval number 4.692.542, dated 5 May 2021), and by the independent ethics committee Namaste Integrated Services, Lanka, Varanasi, India (approval number BS-IND-001, dated 7 August 2021).

Informed Consent Statement: Informed consent was obtained from all subjects involved in the study.

Data Availability Statement: The data presented in this study are available within the article and Supplementary Material.

Acknowledgments: Development of the VIDAS® Anti-CHIKUNGUNYA IgM and VIDAS® Anti-CHIKUNGUNYA IgG assays was made possible through the contribution of technology and methods developed at the Vaccine Research Center (VRC), National Institute of Allergy and Infectious Diseases (NIAID), and National Institute of Health (NIH) (Maryland, USA). The authors are grateful to the collaborators at bioMérieux (Marcy L'Etoile, France) for their contribution to VLP culture and purification development (Guillaume Gerez), VLP characterization (Jérôme Martinez, Guillaume Gerez), VIDAS® Anti-CHIKV IgM and IgG assay development, optimisation and production (Evelyne Blein, Aude Lantz, Solenne Farcy, Lisa Prophète, Brigitte Riou), selection and provision of samples (Mathilde Sanvert, Marie-Paule Troubat), VIDAS® Anti-CHIKV IgM and IgG assay performance (Florence Sénot), VIDAS® Anti-CHIKV IgM and IgG assay analytical validation (Adeline Faussurier, Mathilde Fumagalli), statistical analysis (Ludovic Brossault), and publication coordination and discussions (Irena Iankova, Nadège Goutagny, Fanette Ravel, Françoise Gay-Andrieu). The authors thank Biospecimen Solutions Pvt Ltd. (Sampigehalli, Bangalore, Karnataka, India) for the prospective collection and transfer of human sera to bioMérieux (Marcy L'Etoile, France). The authors also thank Anne Rascle of AR Medical Writing (Regensburg, Germany) for providing medical writing support, which was funded by bioMérieux (Marcy L'Etoile, France) in accordance with Good Publication Practice (GPP3) guidelines (http://www.ismpp.org/gpp3; accessed on 20 March 2023).

Conflicts of Interest: L.C., L.D., A.L.-T., F.R., C.T., G.P.-B. and A.B. are or were employees of bioMérieux. This study was funded by bioMérieux. The funder was involved in the design and execution of the study, in the data analysis and interpretation, in the decision to publish the results, and in the writing of the manuscript.

References

1. Vairo, F.; Haider, N.; Kock, R.; Ntoumi, F.; Ippolito, G.; Zumla, A. Chikungunya: Epidemiology, Pathogenesis, Clinical Features, Management, and Prevention. *Infect. Dis. Clin. N. Am.* **2019**, *33*, 1003–1025. [CrossRef]
2. Robinson, M.C. An Epidemic of Virus Disease in Southern Province, Tanganyika Territory, in 1952–1953—I: Clinical Features. *Trans R. Soc. Trop. Med. Hyg.* **1955**, *49*, 28–32. [CrossRef]
3. Deeba, F.; Haider, M.S.H.; Ahmed, A.; Tazeen, A.; Faizan, M.I.; Salam, N.; Hussain, T.; Alamery, S.F.; Parveen, S. Global Transmission and Evolutionary Dynamics of the Chikungunya Virus. *Epidemiol. Infect.* **2020**, *148*, e63. [CrossRef] [PubMed]
4. Leparc-Goffart, I.; Nougairede, A.; Cassadou, S.; Prat, C.; de Lamballerie, X. Chikungunya in the Americas. *Lancet* **2014**, *383*, 514. [CrossRef] [PubMed]
5. Natrajan, M.S.; Rojas, A.; Waggoner, J.J. Beyond Fever and Pain: Diagnostic Methods for Chikungunya Virus. *J. Clin. Microbiol.* **2019**, *57*, e00350-19. [CrossRef]
6. Álvarez-Argüelles, M.E.; Alba, S.R.; Pérez, M.R.; Riveiro, J.A.B.; García, S.M.; Álvarez-Argüelles, M.E.; Alba, S.R.; Pérez, M.R.; Riveiro, J.A.B.; García, S.M. *Diagnosis and Molecular Characterization of Chikungunya Virus Infections*; IntechOpen: London, UK, 2019; ISBN 978-1-78923-890-7.
7. Silva, J.V.J.; Ludwig-Begall, L.F.; Oliveira-Filho, E.F.; de Oliveira, R.A.S.; Durães-Carvalho, R.; Lopes, T.R.R.; Silva, D.E.A.; Gil, L.H.V.G. A Scoping Review of Chikungunya Virus Infection: Epidemiology, Clinical Characteristics, Viral Co-Circulation Complications, and Control. *Acta Trop.* **2018**, *188*, 213–224. [CrossRef]
8. Paixão, E.S.; Teixeira, M.G.; Rodrigues, L.C. Zika, Chikungunya and Dengue: The Causes and Threats of New and Re-Emerging Arboviral Diseases. *BMJ Glob. Health* **2018**, *3*, e000530. [CrossRef]
9. Furuya-Kanamori, L.; Liang, S.; Milinovich, G.; Soares Magalhaes, R.J.; Clements, A.C.A.; Hu, W.; Brasil, P.; Frentiu, F.D.; Dunning, R.; Yakob, L. Co-Distribution and Co-Infection of Chikungunya and Dengue Viruses. *BMC Infect. Dis.* **2016**, *16*, 84. [CrossRef]
10. Mota, M.L.; Dos Santos Souza Marinho, R.; Duro, R.L.S.; Hunter, J.; de Menezes, I.R.A.; de Lima Silva, J.M.F.; Pereira, G.L.T.; Sabino, E.C.; Grumach, A.; Diaz, R.S.; et al. Serological and Molecular Epidemiology of the Dengue, Zika and Chikungunya Viruses in a Risk Area in Brazil. *BMC Infect. Dis.* **2021**, *21*, 704. [CrossRef] [PubMed]
11. Ohst, C.; Saschenbrecker, S.; Stiba, K.; Steinhagen, K.; Probst, C.; Radzimski, C.; Lattwein, E.; Komorowski, L.; Stöcker, W.; Schlumberger, W. Reliable Serological Testing for the Diagnosis of Emerging Infectious Diseases. *Adv. Exp. Med. Biol.* **2018**, *1062*, 19–43. [CrossRef]
12. Vu, D.M.; Jungkind, D.; LaBeaud, A.D. Chikungunya Virus. *Clin. Lab. Med.* **2017**, *37*, 371–382. [CrossRef] [PubMed]
13. Pan American Health Organization. Tool for the Diagnosis and Care of Patients with Suspected Arboviral Diseases. Available online: https://iris.paho.org/bitstream/handle/10665.2/33895/9789275119365_eng.pdf?sequence=1&isAllowed=y (accessed on 15 October 2022).
14. Ribeiro, M.O.; Godoy, D.T.; Fontana-Maurell, M.; Costa, E.M.; Andrade, E.F.; Rocha, D.R.; Ferreira, A.G.P.; Brindeiro, R.; Tanuri, A.; Alvarez, P. Analytical and Clinical Performance of Molecular Assay Used by the Brazilian Public Laboratory Network to Detect and Discriminate Zika, Dengue and Chikungunya Viruses in Blood. *Braz. J. Infect. Dis.* **2021**, *25*, 101542. [CrossRef]
15. Simon, F.; Javelle, E.; Cabie, A.; Bouquillard, E.; Troisgros, O.; Gentile, G.; Leparc-Goffart, I.; Hoen, B.; Gandjbakhch, F.; Rene-Corail, P.; et al. French Guidelines for the Management of Chikungunya (Acute and Persistent Presentations). November 2014. *Med. Mal. Infect.* **2015**, *45*, 243–263. [CrossRef] [PubMed]
16. Cunha, R.V.; da Trinta, K.S. Chikungunya Virus: Clinical Aspects and Treatment—A Review. *Mem. Inst. Oswaldo Cruz* **2017**, *112*, 523–531. [CrossRef]
17. World Health Organization. Guidelines on Clinical Management of Chikungunya Fever. Available online: https://www.who.int/publications-detail-redirect/guidelines-on-clinical-management-of-chikungunya-fever (accessed on 12 October 2022).
18. Centers for Disease Control and Prevention. Diagnostic Testing | Chikungunya Virus | CDC. Available online: https://www.cdc.gov/chikungunya/hc/diagnostic.html (accessed on 13 October 2022).
19. Johnson, B.W.; Russell, B.J.; Goodman, C.H. Laboratory Diagnosis of Chikungunya Virus Infections and Commercial Sources for Diagnostic Assays. *J. Infect. Dis.* **2016**, *214*, S471–S474. [CrossRef] [PubMed]
20. Andrew, A.; Navien, T.N.; Yeoh, T.S.; Citartan, M.; Mangantig, E.; Sum, M.S.H.; Ch'ng, E.S.; Tang, T.-H. Diagnostic Accuracy of Serological Tests for the Diagnosis of Chikungunya Virus Infection: A Systematic Review and Meta-Analysis. *PLoS Negl. Trop. Dis.* **2022**, *16*, e0010152. [CrossRef]
21. Chua, C.-L.; Sam, I.-C.; Merits, A.; Chan, Y.-F. Antigenic Variation of East/Central/South African and Asian Chikungunya Virus Genotypes in Neutralization by Immune Sera. *PLoS Negl. Trop. Dis.* **2016**, *10*, e0004960. [CrossRef]

22. Mascarenhas, M.; Garasia, S.; Berthiaume, P.; Corrin, T.; Greig, J.; Ng, V.; Young, I.; Waddell, L. A Scoping Review of Published Literature on Chikungunya Virus. *PLoS ONE* **2018**, *13*, e0207554. [CrossRef]
23. Johnson, B.W.; Goodman, C.H.; Holloway, K.; de Salazar, P.M.; Valadere, A.M.; Drebot, M.A. Evaluation of Commercially Available Chikungunya Virus Immunoglobulin M Detection Assays. *Am. J. Trop. Med. Hyg.* **2016**, *95*, 182–192. [CrossRef]
24. Kikuti, M.; Tauro, L.B.; Moreira, P.S.S.; Nascimento, L.C.J.; Portilho, M.M.; Soares, G.C.; Weaver, S.C.; Reis, M.G.; Kitron, U.; Ribeiro, G.S. Evaluation of Two Commercially Available Chikungunya Virus IgM Enzyme-Linked Immunoassays (ELISA) in a Setting of Concomitant Transmission of Chikungunya, Dengue and Zika Viruses. *Int. J. Infect. Dis.* **2020**, *91*, 38–43. [CrossRef]
25. Woods, C.R. False-Positive Results for Immunoglobulin M Serologic Results: Explanations and Examples. *J. Pediatr. Infect. Dis. Soc.* **2013**, *2*, 87–90. [CrossRef]
26. Landry, M.L. Immunoglobulin M for Acute Infection: True or False? *Clin. Vaccine Immunol.* **2016**, *23*, 540–545. [CrossRef]
27. Prat, C.M.; Flusin, O.; Panella, A.; Tenebray, B.; Lanciotti, R.; Leparc-Goffart, I. Evaluation of Commercially Available Serologic Diagnostic Tests for Chikungunya Virus. *Emerg. Infect. Dis.* **2014**, *20*, 2129–2132. [CrossRef]
28. Akahata, W.; Yang, Z.-Y.; Andersen, H.; Sun, S.; Holdaway, H.A.; Kong, W.-P.; Lewis, M.G.; Higgs, S.; Rossmann, M.G.; Rao, S.; et al. A Virus-like Particle Vaccine for Epidemic Chikungunya Virus Protects Nonhuman Primates against Infection. *Nat. Med.* **2010**, *16*, 334–338. [CrossRef] [PubMed]
29. Yap, M.L.; Klose, T.; Urakami, A.; Hasan, S.S.; Akahata, W.; Rossmann, M.G. Structural Studies of Chikungunya Virus Maturation. *Proc. Natl. Acad. Sci. USA* **2017**, *114*, 13703–13707. [CrossRef]
30. Clinical & Laboratory Standards Institute. *EP05-A3: Evaluating Quantitative Measurement Precision*, 3rd ed.; Clinical and Laboratory Standards Institute: Wayne, PA, USA, 2014. Available online: https://clsi.org/standards/products/method-evaluation/documents/ep05/ (accessed on 27 October 2021).
31. Clinical & Laboratory Standards Institute. *EP12-A2: User Protocol for Evaluation of Qualitative Test Performance*, 2nd ed.; Clinical and Laboratory Standards Institute: Wayne, PA, USA, 2008. Available online: https://clsi.org/standards/products/method-evaluation/documents/ep12/ (accessed on 12 October 2022).
32. Khan, A.H.; Morita, K.; Parquet, M.D.C.; Hasebe, F.; Mathenge, E.G.M.; Igarashi, A. Complete Nucleotide Sequence of Chikungunya Virus and Evidence for an Internal Polyadenylation Site. *J. Gen. Virol.* **2002**, *83*, 3075–3084. [CrossRef]
33. Lwande, O.W.; Obanda, V.; Bucht, G.; Mosomtai, G.; Otieno, V.; Ahlm, C.; Evander, M. Global Emergence of Alphaviruses That Cause Arthritis in Humans. *Infect. Ecol. Epidemiol.* **2015**, *5*, 29853. [CrossRef] [PubMed]
34. Henss, L.; Yue, C.; Kandler, J.; Faddy, H.M.; Simmons, G.; Panning, M.; Lewis-Ximenez, L.L.; Baylis, S.A.; Schnierle, B.S. Establishment of an Alphavirus-Specific Neutralization Assay to Distinguish Infections with Different Members of the Semliki Forest Complex. *Viruses* **2019**, *11*, 82. [CrossRef]
35. Smith, J.L.; Pugh, C.L.; Cisney, E.D.; Keasey, S.L.; Guevara, C.; Ampuero, J.S.; Comach, G.; Gomez, D.; Ochoa-Diaz, M.; Hontz, R.D.; et al. Human Antibody Responses to Emerging Mayaro Virus and Cocirculating Alphavirus Infections Examined by Using Structural Proteins from Nine New and Old World Lineages. *mSphere* **2018**, *3*, e00003-18. [CrossRef] [PubMed]
36. Partidos, C.D.; Paykel, J.; Weger, J.; Borland, E.M.; Powers, A.M.; Seymour, R.; Weaver, S.C.; Stinchcomb, D.T.; Osorio, J.E. Cross-Protective Immunity against o'nyong-Nyong Virus Afforded by a Novel Recombinant Chikungunya Vaccine. *Vaccine* **2012**, *30*, 4638–4643. [CrossRef]
37. Kam, Y.-W.; Pok, K.-Y.; Eng, K.E.; Tan, L.-K.; Kaur, S.; Lee, W.W.L.; Leo, Y.-S.; Ng, L.-C.; Ng, L.F.P. Sero-Prevalence and Cross-Reactivity of Chikungunya Virus Specific Anti-E2EP3 Antibodies in Arbovirus-Infected Patients. *PLoS Negl. Trop. Dis.* **2015**, *9*, e3445. [CrossRef] [PubMed]
38. Flies, E.J.; Lau, C.L.; Carver, S.; Weinstein, P. Another Emerging Mosquito-Borne Disease? Endemic Ross River Virus Transmission in the Absence of Marsupial Reservoirs. *BioScience* **2018**, *68*, 288–293. [CrossRef]
39. Paz, S. Climate Change Impacts on West Nile Virus Transmission in a Global Context. *Philos. Trans. R. Soc. Lond. B Biol. Sci.* **2015**, *370*, 20130561. [CrossRef] [PubMed]

diagnostics

MDPI

Article

Evaluation of the Performance Characteristics of a New POC Multiplex PCR Assay for the Diagnosis of Viral and Bacterial Neuromeningeal Infections

Hervé Le Bars [1], Neil Madany [2], Claudie Lamoureux [1,3], Clémence Beauruelle [1,3], Sophie Vallet [2,3], Christopher Payan [2,3] and Léa Pilorgé [2,*]

[1] Unity of Bacteriology, Department of Bacteriology-Virology-Parasitology-Mycology-Hygiene, Pole of Biology-Pathology, University Hospital of Brest, F-29200 Brest, France
[2] Unity of Virology, Department of Bacteriology-Virology-Parasitology-Mycology-Hygiene, Pole of Biology-Pathology, University Hospital of Brest, F-29200 Brest, France
[3] Univ Brest, Inserm, EFS, UMR 1078, GGB CEDEX, F-29200 Brest, France
* Correspondence: lea.pilorge@chu-brest.fr; Tel.: +33-298-347-191; Fax: +33-298-347-193

Abstract: Point-of-care syndromic PCR (POC SPCR) assays are useful tools for the rapid detection of the most common causative agents of community-acquired infections responsible for meningitis and encephalitis infections. We evaluated the performance characteristics of the new QIAstat-Dx® Meningitis/Encephalitis panel (QS) compared to the laboratory reference methods and the POC SPCR Biofire® FilmArray® Meningitis Encephalitis Panel (FA). Viral (Enterovirus, Parechovirus, HSV-1, HSV-2, HHV-6, VZV) and bacterial (*E. coli* K1, *H. influenzae*, *L. monocytogenes*, encapsulated *N. meningitidis*, *M. pneumoniae*, *S. agalactiae*, *S. pneumoniae*, *S. pyogenes*) pathogens were suspended at low concentrations and tested with the POC SPCR systems. The reproducibility, analytical specificity, carryover contamination, interferences and clinical samples were evaluated. All samples tested positive with both QS and FA except for those containing the lowest concentrations of Enterovirus-D68-B3, Echovirus-30 and *S. agalactiae* which were only detected by FA. In terms of analytical specificity, we observed 3 false positive results out of 48 QS tests versus 1 out of 37 FA tests. For the other studied criteria, both QS and FA performed as expected. Our results suggest that the performance characteristics of QS are close to those of FA. A prospective multicenter study would be useful to complete the performances evaluation of QS.

Keywords: point of care; syndromic; PCR; cerebrospinal fluid; meningitis; encephalitis; bacteria; virus

Citation: Le Bars, H.; Madany, N.; Lamoureux, C.; Beauruelle, C.; Vallet, S.; Payan, C.; Pilorgé, L. Evaluation of the Performance Characteristics of a New POC Multiplex PCR Assay for the Diagnosis of Viral and Bacterial Neuromeningeal Infections. *Diagnostics* **2023**, *13*, 1110. https://doi.org/10.3390/diagnostics13061110

Academic Editor: Hsin-Yao Wang

Received: 18 November 2022
Revised: 5 March 2023
Accepted: 7 March 2023
Published: 15 March 2023

1. Introduction

Point-of-care syndromic PCR (POC SPCR) assays are useful tools for the detection of the most common causative agents of community acquired infectious meningitis/encephalitis in cerebrospinal fluid (CSF) within less than 2 h. Such a rapid diagnosis is of clinical importance to improve the medical care of the patients suffering from these life-threatening infections [1,2]. Indeed, a rapid initiation of appropriate treatment based on the causative pathogen (e.g., amoxycillin and gentamicin in cases of *Listeria*) is necessary to improve patient outcomes [3]. POC SPCR may be complementary of direct microbiological examination following Gram staining which is less sensitive in cases with low bacterial inoculum and/or antibiotic intake prior to lumbar puncture [3]. Furthermore, in those cases of prior antibiotic intake to lumbar puncture, POC SPCR may be the only way to identify the causative agent since the sensitivity of culture greatly decreases in these cases [3]. POC SPCR may also enable to give a rapid diagnosis of viral meningitis (Enterovirus, Parechovirus) therefore reducing inappropriate antibiotic use [4]. In addition, POC SPCR assays target a large number of pathogens in 200 μL of CSF, thus enabling to spare some of this precious biological matrix. Finally, diagnosis algorithms may be useful to determine when POC SPCR should be used in the laboratory in order to optimize their clinical relevance [5].

In 2022, the new POC SPCR QIAstat-Dx® Meningitis/Encephalitis panel (QS) assay, run-on the QIAstat-Dx analyzer system, allows detection of 15 bacteria, virus and fungal that cause meningitis/encephalitis became available.

In this investigation, we evaluated the performance characteristics of this panel compared to the laboratory reference methods and the previously commercialized POC SPCR BioFire® FilmArray® Meningitis Encephalitis Panel (FA), for the detection of viral and bacterial nucleic acids in CSF. Fungal pathogens were not evaluated in this study.

2. Materials and Methods

2.1. POC Syndromic PCR Meningitis/Encephalitis Panel

The QS panel (Qiagen, Germany) has the capacity to detect 15 pathogens including 6 viral targets (Herpes simplex HSV-1, HSV-2, Varicella-zoster VZV, enterovirus (EV), parechovirus (PeV), herpesvirus human 6 (HHV-6)), 8 bacterial targets (*Escherichia coli K1* (*Ec*), *Haemophilus influenzae* (*Hi*), *Listeria monocytogenes* (*Lm*), encapsulated *Neisseria meningitidis* (*Nm*), *Streptococcus agalactiae* (GBS), *Streptococcus pneumoniae* (*Sp*), *Streptococcus pyogenes* (GAS) and *Mycoplasma pneumoniae* (*Mp*)), 2 fungal pathogens (*Cryptococcus gattii*/*Cryptococcus neoformans* both detected but not differentiated) and an internal control (IC). QS provides semi-quantitative results by providing access to amplification curves and cycle threshold (Ct) values for all pathogens and the internal control. The FA panel (bioMérieux, Marcy l'Etoile, France) is an FDA-cleared test since 2015. FA contains 14 targets and are the same as those found on QS except for *Streptococcus pyogenes* and *Mycoplasma pneumoniae* which are not included. On the other hand, cytomegalovirus is an additional target present in FA and not found in QS. Reported results with FA are only qualitative. It takes around 1 h to obtain test results for both POC SPCR assays.

2.2. CSF Pool Preparation

We used a pool of CSF samples from 100 patients. Each of these CSF samples had the following features: less than 10 leukocytes and 10 red blood cells per μL and no bacterial growth. The pool was also tested to confirm the absence of HSV-1, HSV-2, VZV, HHV-6 and *Mp* DNA and EV and PeV RNA with specific real-time PCR assays (R-GENE®, bioMérieux, France). This negative CSF pool was then spiked with virus or bacteria to evaluate the different parameters of the study. The pool dilution in the matrix containing the virus (Universal transport medium UTM) or bacteria (Phosphate buffered solution PBS) was 10% maximum. Spiked CSF aliquots were then kept at −80 °C until analysis.

2.3. Virus

We used 4 strains of EV: Enterovirus-A71-C1 (EV-A71-C1), Enterovirus-D68-B3 (Ev-D68-B3), Echovirus-30 (E-30), Echovirus-6 (E-6), and 2 strains of PeV: parechovirus 1 (PeV-1) and 3 (PeV-3). EV-A71-C1, E-30 and PeV-1 were kindly provided by the National Reference Center for enteroviruses (National Reference Center for enteroviruses, Lyon, France). The other EV and PeV strains correspond to external quality controls provided by the international external quality assessment organization Quality Control for Molecular Diagnostics (QCMD). We used clinical strains of HSV-1, HSV-2 and VZV isolated in our laboratory and the World Health Organization international standard for HHV-6B (NIBSC code 15/266).

2.4. Bacteria

The bacterial strains used in this study and their origin are described in Table 1. They were either standard reference strains from ATCC and DSMZ or clinical strain isolated in the teaching hospital of Brest (France) and further confirmed by the French national reference centers. *Mycoplasma pneumoniae* M129 was obtained from the laboratory of bacteriology of the university hospital of Bordeaux (France).

Table 1. Bacterial strains used in the study.

Species	Origin Description
Escherichia coli K1	Clinical strain isolated from CSF
Haemophilus influenzae Type e	Clinical strain isolated from CSF
Listeria monocytogenes Type 4b	Clinical strain isolated from blood culture
Neisseria meningitidis Serotype B	Clinical strain isolated from CSF
Mycoplasma pneumoniae	M129
Streptococcus agalactiae ST17 clone	Clinical strain isolated from CSF
Streptococcus mitis	DSM 12643
Streptococcus oralis	DSM 20627
Streptococcus pneumoniae	ATCC 49619
Streptococcus pseudopneumoniae	DSM 18670
Streptococcus pyogenes Serotype M77	Clinical strain isolated from blood culture

2.5. Assessed Parameters

2.5.1. Detection of Low Viral and *Mycoplasma pneumoniae* Loads

Our reference method was a specific real-time PCR assay (R-GENE®, bioMérieux) for HSV-1, HSV-2, VZV, HHV-6, EV, PeV and *Mp*. Ten-fold serial dilutions were prepared in CSF pool for each virus and *Mp* and aliquots of each dilution were stored at −80 °C. Then, one aliquot of each dilution was thawed at room temperature, nucleic acids were extracted with the eMAG® (bioMérieux, France) and the eluate was tested 5 times with R-GENE® PCR assays. The lowest concentration of viral or *Mp* nucleic acids amplified with R-GENE® PCR assay in 5 cases out of the 5 replicates was chosen for testing once with QS and FA, using a new thawed aliquot. If the QS and FA result was positive, no further testing was performed. If QS or FA result was negative, the previous diluted sample, i.e., 10 times more concentrated, was tested once. In case of a negative result at this dilution, no further testing was performed. In case of positivity, 5 new replicates were tested at the lowest concentration of viral nucleic acids amplified in 100% of cases with the R-GENE® PCR assay. A schematic diagram of this strategy is shown in Figure 1.

2.5.2. Detection of Low Bacterial Concentrations

We evaluated the detection of low bacterial concentrations with QS and FA by testing samples prepared by spiking the CSF pool with CFU/mL quantified suspensions of bacteria to reach the limit of detection (LoD) announced by the manufacturer of the already commercialized FA (1000 CFU/mL for *Escherichia coli, Haemophilus influenzae, Listeria monocytogenes, Streptococcus agalactiae* and 100 CFU/mL for encapsulated *Neisseria meningitidis* and *Streptococcus pneumoniae*). For *Streptococcus pyogenes*, which is only included in the QS panel, a 1000 CFU/mL suspension was analyzed.

2.5.3. False Positive Results

We observed that no pathogen was detected with QS and FA in addition to the spiked pathogen in the CSF pool. We also tested high concentrated (106 CFU/mL) suspensions of three closely related species of *Streptococcus pneumoniae*: *Streptococcus mitis, Streptococcus oralis* and *Streptococcus pseudopneumoniae* (Table 1).

2.5.4. Reproducibility and Carryover Contamination

We spiked the CSF pool with HSV-1, PeV-1, *Nm* and *Sp* (Ct values between 28 and 32). Reproducibility was evaluated by performing 3 QS and 3 FA assays with this spiked CSF pool. Carryover contamination was studied by testing 2 cartridges of non-spiked CSF pool between them.

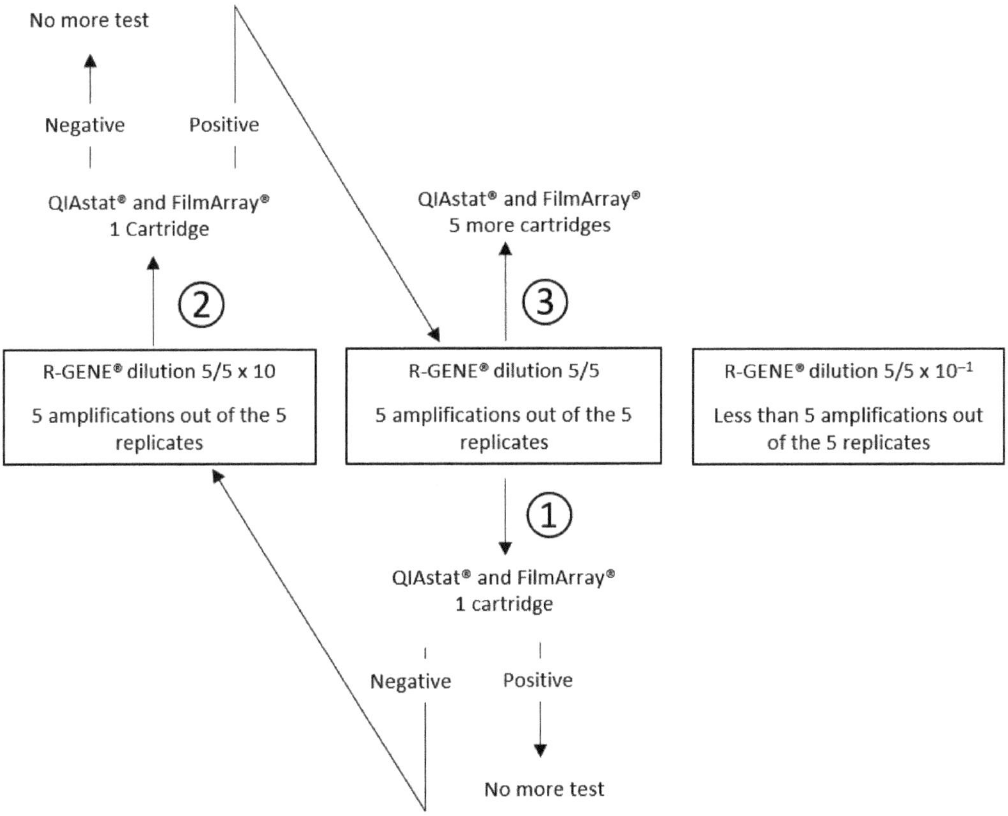

Figure 1. Strategy for assessing the detection of low viral and *Mp* loads, from step 1 to 3, using CSF diluted pool with positive results with R-GENE® in 5 replicates and tested by two point-of-care syndromic PCR QIAstat Dx® (QS) and FilmArray® (FA).

2.5.5. Interferences

We spiked the CSF pool with HSV-1 alone, or both HSV-1 and a potentially interfering agent: 10% of whole blood, 5 g/L of bovine serum albumin (Ambion®) or 1500 leukocytes/µL. Whole blood was tested with a specific real-time PCR assay (R-GENE®) to confirm the absence of HSV-1, HSV-2, VZV and HHV-6 DNA. The leukocytes were isolated from a urine sample. For the QS assay, we considered interference if the HSV-1 Ct value in the CSF pool with an interfering agent was more than 3 compared to the HSV-1 Ct value in the CSF pool without an interfering agent. For the FA assay, which does not provide Ct values, we considered interference if HSV-1 result in the CSF pool with interfering agent was negative.

2.5.6. Clinical CSF Samples

We tested QS and FA retrospectively with 3 clinical CSF samples known to be positive for HSV-2 (Ct value at 37.2 with BioGX® Viral Meningitis HSV/VZV assay), VZV (Ct value at 33.7 with R-GENE® PCR assay) and PeV (Ct value at 34.3 with R-GENE® PCR assay) and 2 clinical CSF samples which had previously grown *Nm* or *Sp*. For HSV and VZV, these fluids had been stored at −80 °C. For bacteria, CSF samples had been stored at 4 °C and tested less than 48 h after collection.

3. Results

3.1. Detection of Low Viral and Mycoplasma pneumoniae Loads

R-GENE® PCR assays, QS and FA results and Ct values when available are described in Table 2. The dilution chosen to be tested with QS and FA in the first place is the 1/10 dilution because it was the lowest one that generates 5 out of 5 positive results with R-GENE® PCR assays.

Table 2. Detections of low viral and *Mp* loads with R-GENE® PCR assays, QS and FA.

Target	Dilution	Detected by R-GENE®	R-GENE® Median Ct Value	R-GENE® Median Titer (copies/mL)	Detected by FA	Detected by QS	QS Ct Value
EV-A71-C1	1	5/5	34.99	ND	ND	1/1	36.0
	1/10	5/5	37.7	ND	1/1	3/6	38.5/38.7/38.5
	1/100	3/5	38.22	ND	ND	ND	ND
EV-D68-B3	1	5/5	32.71	ND	1/1	0/1	ND
	1/10	5/5	35.57	ND	5/6	0/1	ND
	1/100	4/5	40	ND	ND	ND	ND
E-30	1	5/5	34.52	ND	ND	1/1	37.5
	1/10	5/5	37.49	ND	1/1	0/6	ND
	1/100	3/5	40	ND	ND	ND	ND
E-6	1/10	5/5	38.58	ND	1/1	1/1	38.5
	1/100	3/5	40	ND	ND	ND	ND
PeV-1	1/10	5/5	38.41	ND	1/1	1/1	33.4
	1/100	3/5	40	ND	ND	ND	ND
PeV-3	1/10	5/5	37.52	ND	1/1	1/1	35.0
	1/100	3/5	40	ND	ND	ND	ND
HSV-1	1/10	5/5	36.41	1280	1/1	1/1	35.4
	1/100	2/5	39.03	<250	ND	ND	ND
HSV-2	1/10	5/5	35.39	277	1/1	1/1	36.5
	1/100	3/5	37.61	<100	ND	ND	ND
HHV-6	1/10	5/5	35.83	534	1/1	1/1	37.2
	1/100	1/5	39.28	<200	ND	ND	ND
VZV	1/10	5/5	37.25	<300	1/1	1/1	35.6
	1/100	3/5	40	<300	ND	ND	ND
Mp	1/10	5/5	36.21	ND	ND	1/1	34.8
	1/100	2/5	39.32	ND	ND	ND	ND

Ct: cycle threshold; EV: Enterovirus; E: Echovirus; PeV: Parechovirus; HSV: Herpes simplex virus; HHV-6: Human herpesvirus 6; VZV: Varicella-zoster virus; *Mp*: *Mycoplasma pneumoniae*. ND: Not determined.

Of the 10 viral targets tested once at 1/10 dilution with QS, all were positive except 3 EV strains. Of these 3 strains, E-30 was positive without dilution and positive in 3 of the 5 new replicates at 1/10 dilution. EV-A71-C1 was only positive without dilution and EV-D68-B3 was not positive at either 1/10 or without dilution. FA detected all viral targets at 1/10 dilution except for EV-D68-B3 which was positive without dilution and positive in 5 of 5 new replicates at 1/10 dilution.

3.2. Detection of Low Bacterial Concentrations

For each bacterial target, suspensions at the FA announced LoD were tested. They were all detected by both QS and FA except for GBS which was only detected by FA. With QS, 3000 CFU/mL was the lowest concentration of GBS which tested positive (Table 3).

Table 3. Results of the detection of low bacterial concentrations with QS and FA.

Bacterial Target	Concentration (CFU/mL)	Detected by QS	QS Ct Value	Detected by FA
E. coli (Ec)	1000	1/1	34.7	1/1
L. monocytogenes (Lm)	1000	1/1	36	1/1
H. influenzae (Hi)	1000	1/1	30	1/1
N. meningitidis (Nm)	100	1/1	34.1	1/1
S. pneumoniae (Sp)	100	1/1	35.6	1/1
	200	1/1	34.7	1/1
	1000	0/1	ND	1/1
S. agalactiae (GBS)	1750	0/1	ND	ND
	3000	1/1	35.9	ND
S. pyogenes (GAS)	1000	1/1	38.2	ND

ND: Not determined.

3.3. Analytical Specificity

We performed 48 QS assays and 37 FA assays. False positive results for QS and FA are described in Table 4.

Table 4. QS and FA false positive results.

	Assays (*n*)	False Positive Assays (*n*)
QS	48	3
FA	37	1

We found four false positive results. In the CSF pool spiked with 200 CFU/mL of *Sp*, HSV-1 was unexpectedly detected by both QS (Ct 35.6) and FA. Furthermore, QS unexpectedly detected *Hi* (Ct 37.5) in the CSF pool spiked with *Lm* and HHV-6 (Ct 37.3) in the HSV-1 spiked CSF pool with 10% whole blood used in the interference's tests.

No cross reactivity was observed on FA and QS between *Streptococcus mitis, Streptococcus oralis, Streptococcus pseudopneumoniae* and the detection of *Streptococcus pneumoniae.*

3.4. Reproducibility and Carryover Contamination

The four pathogen targets were 100% positive with both POC SPCR assays for the three cartridges. QS Ct values were very close to each other (below 1 Ct). The two cartridges tested with the negative CSF pool did not detect any viral or bacterial targets.

3.5. Interferences

HSV-1 DNA was detected by both QS and FA POC SPCR assays in all four cases and the addition of potentially interfering agents did not significantly shift the QS Ct values (below 3 Ct, from 0.3 to 1 Ct).

3.6. Clinical CSF Samples

The five viral and bacterial targets (HSV-2, VZV, PeV, *Nm, Sp*) detected in the clinical CSF samples were all found positive with QS and FA (Table 5).

Table 5. Clinical CSF samples results with QS and FA.

	Routinely-Used PCR Ct Value	Detected by QS	QS Ct Value	Detected by FA
CSF + *N. meningitidis*	ND	1/1	31.3	1/1
CSF + *S. pneumoniae*	ND	1/1	19.8	1/1
CSF + HSV-2	37.2	1/1	36.5	1/1
CSF + VZV	33.7	1/1	33.0	1/1
CSF + PeV	34.3	1/1	31.9	1/1

ND: Not determined.

3.7. Internal Control Reproducibility

The maximum differences of the internal control Ct values in 2 series of 5 cartridges loaded with the same sample were 3 (E-30 at 1/10 dilution) and 3.8 (EV-A71-C1 at 1/10 dilution).

4. Discussion

This study was designed to provide the first analytical assessment of the POC SPCR assay QIAstat Dx® (QS) which has recently been developed by Qiagen for the detection of pathogens that potentially cause central nervous system (CNS) infections.

For HSV-1, HSV-2, VZV, HHV-6, PeV-1, PeV-3, E-6 and *Mycoplasma pneumoniae*, both QS and FA correctly detected the lowest loads included in the study. Prior studies noticed low HSV-1, HSV-2 and VZV DNA concentrations in CSF in cases of encephalitis and meningitis [6–10]. A cut-off of approximately 200 copies/mL is considered to be necessary for accurate diagnostics [11]. In our study, DNA quantification of HSV-1, HSV-2, and VZV in 1/10 dilutions CSF was 1280 copies/mL, 277 copies/mL and <300 copies/mL with R-GENE® PCR assays, respectively. These concentrations are close to the 200 copies/mL cut-off. As a comparison, the 95% LoD of the R-GENE® PCR assays have been determined at 250 copies/mL, 100 copies/mL and 300 copies/mL for HSV-1, HSV-2 and VZV, respectively (bioMérieux's manufacturing data). Those for FA were recently recalculated by bioMérieux's research and development department and evaluated at 500 copies/mL for HSV-1 and HSV-2, and 1000 copies/mL for VZV (bioMérieux's manufacturing data). A recent report with the analysis of 1334 pediatric and 336 adult CSF samples tested with FA describes a sensitivity of 75% for HSV-1 compared to a virus-specific PCR [12]. Of note, QS 95% LoD were expressed in TCID50/mL (supplier's technical data sheets), so they were not appropriate for molecular biology. Use of an absolute quantification tool to calibrate the quantification standards, such as digital PCR [13] and comparison of replicates results on limit dilutions would allow for a reliable determination of the LoD and relative sensitivity of the two POC SPCR assays. For EV detection PCR assays, the challenge is to include as many genotypes as possible [14]. Indeed, the sensitivity of EV PCR assays depends on the genotypes [15]. Moreover, CSF viral loads vary according to the genotype [16]. In our study, QS did not detect the lowest loads of E-30 and EV-D68-B3 in contrast to the R-GENE® PCR assay and FA. As EV-D68 genotype is mostly detected in peripheral samples and not in CSF samples in case of neuromeningeal symptoms [17], this may not constitute an important pitfall. However, additional testing including a larger number of genotypes would be necessary for a more accurate assessment of EV inclusivity. The study of Schnuriger et al. describes a FA sensitivity of 89% for enterovirus detection compared to a virus-specific PCR [12].

Concerning the Detection of low bacterial concentrations, all the analyzed samples were correctly detected by both QS and FA except GBS. The sample containing 1000 CFU/mL of GBS tested positive with FA only. These results are consistent with the LoD announced by both manufacturers. Previous studies have found false negative results to be very uncommon with FA [18] meaning that in the vast majority of bacterial meningitis, the bacterial loads are higher than FA's LoD. The LoD announced for both QS and FA are lower for *Sp* and *Nm* than for other targets, which is clinically relevant since *Sp* and *Nm* are the two main species isolated as causative agents of community-acquired bacterial meningitis in France, representing more than 70% of the cases [3]. For GBS, our results suggest a slightly better detection of low concentrations with FA since it was solely able to detect 1000 CFU/mL. However, a 3000 CFU/mL suspension of GBS tested positive with QS which does not seem very far from FA and such a tiny difference may not be clinically relevant for the detection of most GBS meningitis cases since most CSF samples contains more than 1000 CFU/mL in clinical cases [19].

Concerning cross reactivity between close species, *Streptococcus mitis*, *Streptococcus oralis* and *Streptococcus pseudopneumoniae* were not detected as *S. pneumoniae* as it is specified in the producer's data. QS and FA producer's data both report cross reactivity between

Haemophilus haemolyticus and *Haemophilus influenzae*. Given our results and the producers' data, the specificity of these two POC SPCR seems equivalent.

Among all CSF samples tests performed with QS (n = 48) and FA (n = 37), 3 false positive results were obtained with QS and 1 with FA, corresponding to a specificity of 93.8% and 97.3%, respectively. The QS false positives results for *Hi* with a 37.5 Ct value and HSV-1 with a 35.6 Ct value and the FA false positive result for HSV-1 would probably be due to contaminations during handling. Indeed, suspensions of *Hi* and HSV-1 had been prepared near the POC SPCR assays preparation site shortly before. These results are a reminder of the vulnerability of POC SPCR assays to contaminations, due to their implementation in a not dedicated area to molecular biology [20,21]. A reserved cabinet was used for the following assays. The QS uses a one-step cartridge and FA a two-step. Thus, a one-step may help to reduce sample contamination and hence false positive results. The QS false positive result for HHV-6 with a 37.3 Ct value may be due to the presence a very small amount of HHV-6 DNA in the whole blood added for the interference test, below the positivity threshold of the R-GENE® PCR assay, or a false positive due to the use of RUO cartridges. In fact, the production lines of RUO cartridges would be less controlled than those of CE-IVD ones. In daily practice, the availability of Ct values in the QS system, indicating a high Ct value can likely be alerted of possible false positive results. This is an important advantage over FA, which provides only qualitative results. Of note, the QS raw data is not available and replaced by curves improved by the manufacturer. Previous studies of POC PCR have shown the interest of having access to the raw curves [22]. The 2 viral targets (HSV-1 and PeV) and the 2 bacterial targets (*Nm* and *Sp*) were tested positive with 3 cartridges of the 2 SPCR POC assays. QS Ct values were very close (Ct value variation below 2) which is in favor of a high reproducibility of this POC SPCR assay. Surprisingly, internal control Ct values obtained with series of cartridges loaded with same content were sometimes significantly scattered (Ct value variation below 2). This can be inconvenient to evaluate a mild inhibition, which could mask a low positive viral or bacterial target. The potentially interfering substances tested (leukocytes, whole blood, proteins) did not significantly impact the HSV-1 Ct values compared to the reference Ct value. This suggests a robustness of the QS POC SPCR assay towards interfering substances found in CSF samples. FA results were in agreement with what was expected for reproducibility and absence of interferences, but a detailed analysis could not be performed on these qualitative results (no Ct values available).

Only QS allows for the detection of GAS Meningitis which are uncommon among cases of meningitis [3,23].

The main strength of this study is to provide a detailed analysis of the performance characteristics of QS for the detection of both viruses and bacteria, thus giving a global vision of QS performance from a point of view independent of that of the manufacturer. This work has several limitations such as the small number of clinical samples included due to the limited number of cartridges available for this study. The absence of *Cryptococcus neoformans/gattii* among the included strains is another limitation of this work which should be completed by the study of QS performances for the detection of these pathogenic yeasts. As it has been done before with FA, further prospective and retrospective studies are needed to accurately study the clinical performances of QS for the diagnosis of meningitis/encephalitis infections.

Nosocomial bacterial meningitis are common events in hospitals within a neurosurgical unit, but they are mostly due to bacterial species which are different from those causing community-acquired meningitis [24] and therefore neither QS nor FA are prepared for their diagnosis. Such a "nosocomial" panel which would include most of the corresponding species could be a really forthcoming tool for physicians in this context.

5. Conclusions

QIAstat-Dx® Meningitis/Encephalitis panel gave the expected results in terms of assays reproducibility, carryover contamination and interferences as well as with the clinical CSF samples included in this study. Concerning the low concentration samples, the QIAstat-Dx® Meningitis/Encephalitis panel correctly detected all the targets except for *S. agalactiae* (detected at 3000 CFU/mL instead of 1000 CFU/mL), Enterovirus-D68-B3 (not detected) but this may not be of clinical significance, and Echovirus-30 (not detected at the 1/10 dilution). It will be interesting to follow the data concerning these pathogens in future clinical studies with QIAstat-Dx® system and QIAstat-Dx® Meningitis/Encephalitis panel for the diagnosis of meningitis/encephalitis infections. Overall, our results suggest a good performance of QS which could constitute a suitable tool for laboratories provided that it is used with caution to reduce the rate of false positive results. Defining a diagnosis algorithm may also optimize its usefulness. This recently developed POC SPCR assay has the advantage of availability of Ct values and amplification curves from a one-step cartridge and also proposes original and interesting targets (*M. pneumoniae* and *S. pyogenes*) for the bacterial panel.

Author Contributions: Conceptualization: L.P. and H.L.B.; methodology: L.P. and H.L.B.; validation: L.P. and H.L.B. and S.V.; formal analysis: N.M.; data curation: C.L.; writing—original draft preparation: L.P., H.L.B. and N.M.; writing—review and editing: C.P., C.L. and C.B.; visualization: C.L. and C.P.; supervision: L.P., H.L.B. and C.P. All authors have read and agreed to the published version of the manuscript.

Funding: This research received no external funding.

Institutional Review Board Statement: Not applicable.

Informed Consent Statement: Not applicable.

Data Availability Statement: Not applicable.

Acknowledgments: Qiagen and bioMérieux provided the reagents free of charge for the study. National reference centers for enteroviruses (Lyon) and *Chlamydia trachomatis* (Bordeaux) kindly provided us Enterovirus-A71-C1, Echovirus-30 and Parechovirus-1 strains and *Mycoplasma pneumoniae* M129 strain, respectively.

Conflicts of Interest: The corresponding author states on behalf of all the authors that all potential conflicts of interest have been disclosed.

References

1. Choi, J.J.; Westblade, L.F.; Gottesdiener, L.S.; Liang, K.; Li, H.A.; Wehmeyer, G.T.; Glesby, M.J.; Simon, M.S. Impact of a multiplex polymerase chain reaction panel on duration of empiric antibiotic therapy in suspected bacterial meningitis. *Open Forum Infect. Dis.* **2021**, *8*, ofab467. [CrossRef] [PubMed]
2. Clague, M.; Kim, C.; Zucker, J.; Green, D.A.; Sun, Y.; Whittier, S.; Thakur, K.T. Impact of implementing the cerebrospinal fluid FilmArray Meningitis/Encephalitis panel on duration of intravenous acyclovir treatment. *Open Forum Infect. Dis.* **2022**, *9*, ofac356. [CrossRef]
3. Hoen, B.; Varon, E.; de Debroucker, T.; Fantin, B.; Grimprel, E.; Wolff, M.; Duval, X.; Expert and Reviewing Group. Management of acute community-acquired bacterial meningitis (excluding newborns). Long version with arguments. *Med. Mal. Infect.* **2019**, *49*, 405–441. [CrossRef] [PubMed]
4. Menasalvas-Ruiz, A.I.; Salvador-Garcia, C.; Moreno-Docon, A.; Alfayate-Miguelez, S.; Perez Canovas, C.; Sanchez-Solis, M. Enterovirus reverse transcriptase polymerase chain reaction assay in cerebrospinal fluid: An essential tool in meningitis management in childhood. *Enferm. Infecc. Microbiol. Clin.* **2013**, *31*, 71–75. [CrossRef] [PubMed]
5. Trujillo-Gomez, J.; Tsokani, S.; Arango-Ferreira, C.; Atehortua-Munz, S.; Jimenez-Villegas, M.J.; Serrano-Tabares, C.; Veroniki, A.A.; Florez, I.D. Biofire Filmarray Meningitis/Encephalitis panel for the aetiological diagnosis of central nervous system infections: A systematic review and diagnostic test accuracy meta-analysis. *EClinicalMedicine* **2022**, *44*, 101275. [CrossRef] [PubMed]
6. Aberle, S.W.; Puchhammer-Stöckl, E. Diagnosis of herpesvirus infections of the central nervous system. *J. Clin. Virol.* **2002**, *25* (Suppl. 1), S79–S85. [CrossRef]
7. Binnicker, M.J.; Espy, M.J.; Irish, C.L. Rapid and direct detection of herpes simplex virus in cerebrospinal fluid by use of a commercial real-time PCR assay. *J. Clin. Microbiol.* **2004**, *52*, 4361–4362. [CrossRef]
8. Ziyaeyan, M.; Alborzi, A.; Borhani Haghighi, A.; Jamalidoust, M.; Moeini, M.; Pourabbas, B. Diagnosis and quantitative detection of HSV DNA in samples from patients with suspected herpes simplex encephalitis. *Braz. J. Infect. Dis.* **2011**, *15*, 211–214. [CrossRef]

9. Ramirez, K.A.; Choudhri, A.F.; Patel, A.; Lenny, N.T.; Thompson, R.E.; Berkelhammer Greenberg, L.; Clanton Watson, N.; Kocak, M.; DeVincenzo, J.P. Comparing molecular quantification of herpes simplex virus (HSV) in cerebrospinal fluid (CSF) with quantitative structural and functional disease severity in patients with HSV encephalitis (HSVE): Implications for improved therapeutic approaches. *J. Clin. Virol.* **2018**, *107*, 29–37. [CrossRef]
10. Saraya, A.W.; Wacharapluesadee, S.; Petcharat, S.; Sittidetboripat, N.; Ghai, S.; Wilde, H.; Hemachudha, T. Normocellular CSF in herpes simplex encephalitis. *BMC Res. Notes* **2016**, *9*, 95. [CrossRef]
11. Schloss, L.; van Loon, A.M.; Cinque, P.; Cleator, G.; Echevarria, J.M.; Falk, K.I.; Klapper, P.; Schirm, J.; Vestergaard, B.F.; Niesters, H.; et al. An international external quality assessment of nucleic acid amplification of herpes simplex virus. *J. Clin. Virol.* **2003**, *28*, 175–185. [CrossRef] [PubMed]
12. Schnuriger, A.; Vimont, S.; Godmer, A.; Gozlan, J.; Gallah, S.; Macé, M.; Lalande, V.; Saloum, K.; Perrier, M.; Veziris, N.; et al. Differential performance of the FilmArray Meningitis/Encephalitis assay to detect bacterial and viral pathogens in both pediatric and adult populations. *Microbiol. Spectr.* **2022**, *10*, e0277421. [CrossRef] [PubMed]
13. Kuypers, J.; Jerome, K.R. Applications of digital PCR for clinical microbiology. *J. Clin. Microbiol.* **2017**, *55*, 1621–1628. [CrossRef] [PubMed]
14. Tapparel, C.; Siegrist, F.; Petty, T.J.; Kaiser, L. Picornavirus and enterovirus diversity with associated human diseases. *Infect. Genet. Evol.* **2013**, *14*, 282–293. [CrossRef]
15. Wang, M.; Ren, Q.; Zhang, Z.; Zhang, L.; Carr, M.J.; Li, J.; Zhou, H.; Shi, W. Rapid detection of hand, foot and mouth disease enterovirus genotypes by multiplex PCR. *J. Virol. Methods* **2018**, *258*, 7–12. [CrossRef]
16. Volle, R.; Bailly, J.L.; Mirand, A.; Pereira, B.; Marque-Juillet, S.; Chambon, M.; Regagnon, C.; Brebion, A.; Henquell, C.; Peigue-Lafeuille, H.; et al. Variations in cerebrospinal fluid viral loads among enterovirus genotypes in patients hospitalized with laboratory-confirmed meningitis due to enterovirus. *J. Infect. Dis.* **2014**, *210*, 576–584. [CrossRef]
17. Sooksawasdi Na Ayudhya, S.; Sips, G.J.; Bogers, S.; Leijten, L.M.E.; Laksono, B.M.; Smeets, L.C.; Bruning, A.; Benschop, K.; Wolthers, K.; van Riel, D.; et al. Detection of intrathecal antibodies to diagnose enterovirus infections of the central nervous system. *J. Clin. Virol.* **2022**, *152*, 105190. [CrossRef]
18. Tansarli, G.S.; Chapin, K.C. Diagnostic test accuracy of the BioFire® FilmArray® meningitis/encephalitis panel: A systematic review and meta-analysis. *Clin. Microbiol. Infect.* **2020**, *26*, 281–290. [CrossRef]
19. La Scolea, L.J.; Dryja, D. Cerebrospinal fluid and blood of children with meningitis and its diagnostic significance. *J. Clin. Microbiol.* **1984**, *19*, 187–190. [CrossRef]
20. Boudet, A.; Pantel, A.; Carles, M.J.; Boclé, H.; Charachon, S.; Enault, C.; Stéphan, R.; Cadot, L.; Lavigne, J.P.; Marchandin, H. A review of a 13-month period of FilmArray Meningitis/Encephalitis panel implementation as a first-line diagnosis tool at a university hospital. *PLoS ONE* **2019**, *14*, e0223887. [CrossRef]
21. Bouam, A.; Vincent, J.J.; Drancourt, M.; Raoult, D.; Levy, P.Y. Preventing contamination of PCR-based multiplex assays including the use of a dedicated biosafety cabinet. *Lett. Appl. Microbiol.* **2021**, *72*, 98–103. [CrossRef] [PubMed]
22. Seme, K.; Mocilnik, T.; Fujs Komlos, K.; Doplihar, A.; Persing, D.H.; Poljak, M. GeneXpert enterovirus assay: One-year experience in a routine laboratory setting and evaluation on three proficiency panels. *J. Clin. Microbiol.* **2008**, *46*, 1510–1513. [CrossRef] [PubMed]
23. Baraldés, M.A.; Domingo, P.; Mauri, A.; Monmany, J.; Castellanos, M.; Pericas, R.; Vázquez, G. Group A streptococcal meningitis in the antibiotic era. *Eur. J. Clin. Microbiol. Infect. Dis.* **1999**, *18*, 572–578. [CrossRef] [PubMed]
24. van de Beek, D.; Drake, J.M.; Tunkel, A.R. Nosocomial bacterial meningitis. *N. Engl. J. Med.* **2010**, *362*, 146–154. [CrossRef] [PubMed]

diagnostics

MDPI

Article

Prevalence of *Schistosoma haematobium* and Intestinal Helminth Infections among Nigerian School Children

Tolulope Alade [1], Thuy-Huong Ta-Tang [2,*], Sulaiman Adebayo Nassar [3], Akeem Abiodun Akindele [3,4], Raquel Capote-Morales [2], Tosin Blessing Omobami [3] and Pedro Berzosa [2]

1 Department of Medical Laboratory Science, Niger Delta University, Wilberforce Island 560103, Nigeria
2 Malaria and Neglected Tropical Diseases Laboratory, National Centre of Tropical Medicine, Biomedical Research Networking Center of Infectious Diseases (CIBERINFEC), Instituto de Salud Carlos III, Avenida Monforte de Lemos, 5, Pabellón 13, 28029 Madrid, Spain
3 Medical Laboratory Science Department, Ladoke Akintola University of Technology, Ogbomoso 210101, Nigeria
4 Centre for Emerging and Re-Emerging Infectious Diseases, Ladoke Akintola University of Technology, Ogbomoso 210101, Nigeria
* Correspondence: thuyhuong.tatang@gmail.com

Abstract: Schistosomiasis and soil-transmitted helminthiases (STH) are two parasitic diseases mainly affecting school children. The purpose of this study was to estimate the current prevalence and infection intensity, in addition to the associations of these infections with age and sex, in children aged 4–17 years living in Osun State, Nigeria. From each participant (250 children), one urine and one stool sample were taken for the study, for the microscopic detection of eggs or larvae in faeces by means of the Kato–Katz method and eggs in filtrated urine. The overall prevalence of urinary schistosomiasis was 15.20%, with light infection. The intestinal helminthic species identified (and their prevalence) were *S. stercoralis* (10.80%), *S. mansoni* (8%), *A. lumbricoides* (7.20%), hookworm (1.20%), and *T. trichiura* (0.4%), all of them being classified as light infections. Single infections (67.95%) are more frequent than multiple infections (32.05%). With this study, schistosomiasis and STH are still endemic in Osun State, but with a light to moderate prevalence and light infection intensity. Urinary infection was the most prevalent, with higher prevalence in children over 10 years. The >10 years age group had the highest prevalence for all of the intestinal helminths. There were no statistically significant associations between gender and age and urogenital or intestinal parasites.

Keywords: *Schistosoma mansoni*; *Schistosoma haematobium*; soil-transmitted helminths; neglected tropical diseases; Kato-Katz; Nigeria

Citation: Alade, T.; Ta-Tang, T.-H.; Nassar, S.A.; Akindele, A.A.; Capote-Morales, R.; Omobami, T.B.; Berzosa, P. Prevalence of *Schistosoma haematobium* and Intestinal Helminth Infections among Nigerian School Children. *Diagnostics* **2023**, *13*, 759. https://doi.org/10.3390/diagnostics13040759

Academic Editor: Hsin-Yao Wang

Received: 24 December 2022
Revised: 3 February 2023
Accepted: 14 February 2023
Published: 16 February 2023

1. Introduction

Schistosomiasis is a parasitic disease caused by infection with *Schistosoma* spp. trematodes. The disease affects poor rural communities but has spread to urban areas and to tourists visiting endemic areas [1]. There are two main types of the disease: (i) intestinal schistosomiasis, caused by *S. mansoni*, *S. japonicum*, *S. mekongi*, *S. guineensis*, and *S. intercalatum*; and (ii) urogenital schistosomiasis, caused only by *S. haematobium* [2]. Human transmission occurs through contact with water (e.g., bathing, swimming, washing clothes in water containing the infective cercariae) infested with larval forms (cercariae) that develop in freshwater snails, the intermediate host; inadequate sanitation increases the risk of transmission [1–3].

As of January 2020, schistosomiasis is endemic in 78 tropical and subtropical countries, of which 51 countries have moderate to severe transmission and require preventive chemotherapy with praziquantel. Approximately 236 million are people infected worldwide, with more than 90% living in Africa, causing about 24,000 deaths in 2016 and 2.5 million disability-adjusted life years (DALYs). Deaths and DALYs are likely underestimated due to underreporting, the methods used to assess disability and other factors [4,5].

Soil-transmitted helminthiases (STH) are caused by infection with intestinal parasites (*Ascaris lumbricoides* and *Trichuris trichiura*), hookworms (*Necator americanus* and *Ancylostoma duodenale*) and roundworms (*Strongyloides stercoralis*). Human transmission occurs through eggs or larvae in faeces, which contaminate soil in areas with poor sanitation. *S. stercoralis* is transmitted similarly to other STH, requires a different diagnostic method and can cause hyper-infection syndrome leading to death [4,6,7].

In 2019, 92 countries were endemic for *A. lumbricoides*, *T. trichiura*, and hookworm, and required mass drug administration (MDA) with albendazole or mebendazol. Approximately 1.5 billion people estimated to be infected with STH, about 6300 deaths and 3.5 million DALYs in 2016. The burden of *S. stercoralis* should be quantified precisely [4,5].

In Nigeria, only two *Schistosoma* species cause human schistosomiasis, *S. mansoni*, which causes intestinal schistosomiasis, and *S. haematobium*, which causes urinary schistosomiasis. In Nigeria, schistosomiasis is a disease of considerable and growing importance, mainly affecting rural areas and vulnerable age groups. School children are the major victims of this disease [8].

Nigeria is among the countries with the highest burden of STH disease in Africa. STH mainly affects children, causing anemia, Vitamin A deficiency, malnutrition, loss of appetite, retarded growth, reduced ability to learn, etc., in them. The prevalence of this disease is moderate (<50%)–high (≥50%).

The World Health Organization (WHO) classifies schistosomiasis and STH as neglected tropical diseases (NTDs), but not *S. stercoralis* [5,9]. These NTDs in Nigeria are targeted to for their control, elimination, and eradication by the Federal Ministry of Health and Government of Nigeria, in collaboration with various stakeholders and partners. The National Schistosomiasis Control Programme was initiated in 1988, and the goal of the programme is to control/eliminate schistosomiasis in the region through MDA, delivering regular praziquantel tablets, donated by Merck KGaA Germany since 2009, to at least 75% of school-age children in endemic areas in the country in line with WHO recommendation. The STH control programme was initiated in 2007. In line with WHO recommendations, the programme has set a target of regular administration of mebendazole tablets, donation from Johnson and Johnson, to at least 75% of school-age children in endemic areas in the country at risk of morbidity. Regarding strongyloidiasis, in those areas where MDA with ivermectin has been used to control onchocerciasis or lymphatic filariasis, the prevalence of strongyloidiasis seems to have reduced, but further investigation is needed.

The purpose of this study was to estimate the current prevalence and infection intensity of *Schistosoma* and intestinal parasitic infections in a group of school children (aged 4–17 years) living in a recognized endemic area at Ore community in Odo-Otin Local Government of Osun State, Nigeria. We also evaluated the associations between the acquisition of these infections and age and sex.

2. Materials and Methods

2.1. The Study Area

This study was carried out in the Ore community in Odo-Otin Local Government of Osun State, Nigeria (Figure 1). Osun State has an estimated population of 4,275,526 people (Nigeria Population Census 2006). The community is in stable malaria transmission zone. Malaria is present during all months of the year, with a marked increase in the wet season, which normally runs from April to October. The soil in the communities can be described as well drained, moderately leached, and with moderate humus content. Farming and petty trading are the major occupations. The study was executed from September 2021 to December 2021, which spanned the dry and rainy months.

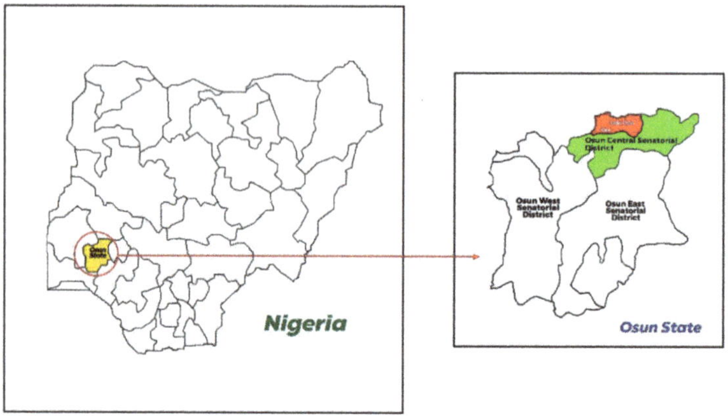

Figure 1. Map of Osun State (yellow in left map), Nigeria showing Ore community in Odo-Otin Local Government (red in right map) where the study was carried out. This community belongs to Osun Central Senatorial District (green in right map).

2.2. Ethical Considerations

Ethical clearance for the study was given by the Research and Ethics Committee of Osun State, Ministry of Health, Osogbo, Nigeria (ref no: OSHREC/PRS/569T/131). Before sample collection, meetings were held with community leaders, teachers, and community members. The aim of the study, the study procedures, types of specimens required, and benefits of the study to individuals and to the community as a whole and risks involved were included in the informed consent letters and fully explained to parents and children. Parents and legal guardians were asked to give their verbal consent for the children who were willing to be sampled after being given proper information about the study. The ethical committee allowed the use of oral consent because majority of the parents were not educated.

2.3. Study Population and Sampling

School children (one primary and one secondary school) were recruited into the study. A total of 250 children aged between 4 and 17 years old were selected and from each participant, one urine sample and one stool sample were taken for *S. haematobium*, *S. mansoni*, *S. stercoralis*, *A. lumbricoides*, *A. duodenale* (hookworm), and *T. trichiura* studies, using microscopic detection of eggs in faeces by means of the Kato–Katz (KK) method and eggs in urine using urine filtration. Both stool and urine samples were collected separately from each pupil using two sterile, leak-proof, and transparent wide-mouthed containers. The sample containers were pre-labelled with the participant's identification number. The collected samples were transported within 2 h of collection to the laboratory for analysis.

Furthermore, a blood sample was also taken to determine the packed cell volume (PCV). Of the three schools in the community, only two participated in the study. The association of parents of the third school refused to participate.

2.4. Study Design and Eligibility Criteria

This cross-sectional study was conducted on school children in the community. All of the school children who were willing to be part of the study and reside in the study area, and who had not taken anti-helminth drugs within six months before the study, were recruited into the study. Children whose parents gave consent to participate in the study and those without a severe medical condition were recruited into the study. The exclusion criteria included anyone who was too sick to participate or who could not provide informed consent or obtain it from a parent or guardian.

2.5. Determination of Packed Cell Volume (PCV)

Anticoagulated blood with heparin was centrifuged in a sealed capillary tube at 10,000× *g* for 5 min. The tubes were placed in the micro-haematocrit reader and children with PCV values < 31% were considered as anaemic, which was further classified as mild (21–30%), moderate (15–20%), or severe (≤15%) [10].

2.6. Microscopic Examination

Microscopy was performed on one KK slide per fecal sample by a skilled, well-trained research microscopist who is an expert in detecting helminth eggs. In total, 20% of prepared (previously examined) Kato–Katz slides were randomly selected for quality control and examined by a second experienced microscopist who was blinded to the previous test results.

2.7. Urine Filtration Analysis

The presence of *S. haematobium* eggs was assessed using the urine filtration technique, the standard for the diagnosis of urogenital schistosomiasis recommended by WHO, as previously described [11]. Briefly, 10 mL of the freshly passed urine sample was filtered through a micro-filter membrane with a pore size of 10–12 µm (MF, Whatman, NJ, USA) using a syringe. The micro-filter membrane was then carefully placed on a glass slide, mounted on a microscope, and examined using a light microscope's low-power objective (10×). *Schistosoma* eggs were counted and recorded as the number of eggs/10 mL of urine. Infection intensity was classified as light (<50 eggs/10 mL of urine) or heavy (≥50 eggs/10 mL of urine), as previously described by Atalabi et al. [12].

2.8. Detection and Quantification of Intestinal Helminths

The KK thick smear technique, the standard method for STH according to the WHO, was used for the quantitative determination of helminth ova on one KK slide per sample. The intensity of infection was expressed as the number of eggs per gram (epg) of faeces. The number of helminth eggs were counted and multiplied by 24 in order to quantify the number of epg of faeces. To ensure consistency of the result and as a form of quality control, 20% of the slides were randomly selected and read again. The epg was classified according to the WHO classification as light infection (epg < 100), moderate infection (epg 100–399), and heavy infection (epg ≥ 400) [13].

2.9. Statistical Analysis

Data obtained from microscopic examinations were entered in Microsoft Excel prior to statistical analyses (mean, range, percentage, and estimated prevalence) for urinary schistosomiasis and intestinal helminths, calculated using the free software WinEpi: Working in Epidemiology [14]. The confidence intervals (CI) were established at 95%. Graphs and tables were created with Microsoft Excel. Results were compared and associations between qualitative variables were determined using a Chi-square test (χ^2), included in the free software WinEpi. *p*-values were also calculated, considering *p*-values < 0.05 to be statistically significant.

3. Results

3.1. Study Population

A total of 250 children aged 4–17 years were screened using microscopy test for schistosomiasis and STH evaluation. The mean age of the 250 recruited children was 9.72 years, 135 out of 250 were boys (54%) and 115 out of 250 were girls (46%). The mean age for the boys was 9.91 and that for the girls was 9.50. Children were distributed in three age groups: <5 years (2/250, 0.8%); 5–10 years (157/250, 62.8%); >10 years (91/250, 36.4%).

3.2. Packed Cell Volume and Anaemia

From the 250 children tested for anaemia, according to PCV values, 99 (39.6%) were found to be anaemic (PCV < 31%), with most of them displaying mild anaemia (95/99, 95.96%). Prevalence of anaemia was higher in males (54, 54.55%) than in females (45, 45.45%), although it was not statistically significant ($\chi^2 = 0.020$, $p = 0.8886$). The age group most affected was 5–10-year-olds (52, 52.53%). Anaemia prevalence was significantly higher in 5–10-year-old children compared with other age groups ($\chi^2 = 9.590$, $p = 0.0083$).

In this study, considering *Schistosoma* and STH as a risk factor for anaemia, there was a significant positive correlation between parasite-infected children and anaemia ($\chi^2 = 38.093$, $p < 0.0001$). The most prevalent parasite in the anaemic children group was *S. haematobium*, and there was a significant association between urinary schistosomiasis and anaemia ($\chi^2 = 40.680$, $p < 0.0001$).

3.3. Microscopic Examination

Overall, 172 (68.8%) participants were found to be negative for *Schistosoma* spp. and intestinal helminths by means of the methods used in the present study, and 78 (31.2%) participants were found to be positive for at least one of the parasites studied. Out of the 78 positive children, 41 (52.56%) were boys and 37 (47.44%) were girls.

Overall, 53 out of 78 (67.95%) of the children had a single infection and 25 out of 78 (32.05%) had more than one parasite (Table 1). The most frequent combinations for multiple parasitism can be visualized in Table 1. The maximum number of parasites found in the same child was three. All of the children with multiple parasites were boys (8–14 years), and the intensity of infection was light.

Table 1. Distribution of urogenital and intestinal schistosomiasis and intestinal helminths in the population studied and the most frequent combination of parasites.

	Parasites	Boys	Girls	Subtotal	Total
Single infection	SH	14	13	27	53
	SM	3	3	6	
	SS	6	5	11	
	AL	3	6	9	
	HOOKWORM	0	0	0	
	TT	0	0	0	
Total		26	27	53	
Multiple parasitism	AL + TT	0	1	1	25
	SM + SS + AL	2	0	2	
	SS + HOOKWORM	1	2	3	
	SM + SS	3	1	4	
	SS + AL	1	0	1	
	SM + AL	0	3	3	
	SH + SS	3	1	4	
	SH + SM	1	2	3	
	SH + SM + SS	2	0	2	
	SH + AL	2	0	2	
Total		15	10	25	78

SH: *Schistosoma haematobium*; SM: *Schistosoma mansoni*; SS: *Strongyloides stercoralis*; AL: *Ascaris lumbricoides*; TT: *Trichuris trichiura*.

3.4. Prevalence and Intensity of Schistosomiasis Infection

The overall prevalence of urinary schistosomiasis among the children tested was 15.20%, 38 out of 250 (95% CI: 10.75%, 19.65%); 57.89% (22 out of 38) were boys and 42.11% (16 out of 38) were girls (Table 2). Most of them had a light infection with <50 eggs/10 mL of urine, and only in four out of 38 (10.53%) participants was the infection heavy (>50 eggs/10 mL of urine). Urogenital schistosomiasis was the most prevalent parasitic infection in the population studied, with a higher prevalence in children over 10 years (19.78%).

Table 2. Total number of positive infections based on the species of parasite according to sex.

	SH		SM		SS		AL		HOOKWORM		TT		TOTAL
	P	N	P	N	P	N	P	N	P	N	P	N	N°
BOYS	22	113	11	124	18	117	8	127	1	134	0	135	**135**
GIRLS	16	99	9	106	9	106	10	105	2	113	1	114	**115**
TOTAL	38	212	20	230	27	223	18	232	3	247	1	249	**250**

P: Positive; N: Negative; SH: *Schistosoma haematobium*; SM: *Schistosoma mansoni*; SS: *Strongyloides stercoralis*; AL: *Ascaris lumbricoides*; TT: *Trichuris trichiura*.

Regarding intestinal schistosomiasis, the overall prevalence was 8.00% (20 out of 250; 95% CI: 4.64%, 11.36%); 55% (11 out of 20) were boys and 45% (nine out of 20) were girls (Table 2). From the 20 KK positive cases, the epg range observed was from 48 to 2256, with a mean of 304.8 epg, giving in all cases moderate infection.

3.5. Prevalence and Intensity of STH Infection

The intestinal helminthic species identified and their prevalence, from highest to lowest, were *S. stercoralis* (10.80%; 27 cases; 95% CI: 6.95%, 14.65%), *A. lumbricoides* (7.20%; 18 cases; 95% CI: 4.00%, 10.40%), hookworm (1.20%, three cases; 95% CI: 0.00%, 2.55%), and *T. trichiura* (0.4%; one case; 95% CI: 0.000%, 1.182%) (Table 3). The gender-related prevalence of the intestinal helminths in the study area is shown in Table 2, and the age-related prevalence is summarized in Table 3. Among boys and girls, *S. stercoralis* revealed the highest difference, with 18 and nine positive cases, respectively, although the bivariate analysis did not confirm a significant association between gender and infection with *S. stercoralis*, ($p = 0.1626$; 95% CI, χ^2: 1.955). Regarding the intensity of infection, *A. lumbricoides* had the statistically highest mean intensity (3958.67 epg), followed by *S. stercoralis* (387.56 larvae/g), *T. trichiura* (192 epg), and hookworm (64 epg).

Table 3. Urogenital and intestinal infections classified by age group.

Age Group	SH			SM			SS			AL			HOOKWORM			TT			TOTAL
	P	N	%	P	N	%	P	N	%	P	N	%	P	N	%	P	N	%	N°
<5 YEARS OLD	0	2	0.00	0	2	0.00	0	2	0.00	0	2	0.00	0	2	0.00	0	2	0	2
5–10 YEARS OLD	20	137	12.74	11	146	7.01	15	142	9.55	10	147	6.37	1	156	0.64	0	157	0.00	157
>10 YEARS OLD	18	73	19.78	9	82	9.89	12	79	13.19	8	83	8.79	2	89	2.20	1	90	1.10	91
TOTAL	38	212	15.20	20	230	8.00	27	223	10.80	18	232	7.20	3	247	1.20	1	249	0.4	250

P: Positive; N: Negative; SH: *Schistosoma haematobium*; SM: *Schistosoma mansoni*; SS: *Strongyloides stercoralis*; AL: *Ascaris lumbricoides*; TT: *Trichuris trichiura*.

The >10 years age group had the highest prevalence in any of the intestinal helminths. However, we cannot affirm that age and intestinal helminth infection are significatively associated.

4. Discussion

This study intended to determine the prevalence and intensity of urinary schistosomiasis and intestinal parasitic infections in school children in Osun State, Nigeria. Prior to this study, three similar reports existed on intestinal parasitic infections in the same State, but not on urinary schistosomiasis involving school children [15–17]. Ten years after Adefioye et al. and Sowemimo and Asaolu's studies [15,17], whose authors reported an overall prevalence of 52.0% and 34.4%, respectively, our study reported an overall decreased prevalence of 27.60%, which is consistent with the rate of intestinal parasitic infection (24%) in a recent study conducted by Olopade et al., 2022 [16]. This indicates that in Osun State, the Federal Ministry of Health and Government of Nigeria's interventions have made great achievements in the control of intestinal parasitic infections, and consequently there has been a prevalence reduction of these intestinal parasites [18]. In the past, the prevalence of STH in Osun State, Nigeria has been reported to be between moderate and high among children, and nowadays the prevalence is moderate [18].

Adefioye et al. and Olopade et al. recorded *A. lumbricoides* as the most prevalent intestinal parasite, at 36.2% and 22.1%, respectively, and the least prevalent parasites were *S. stercoralis* (0.7%) and *Hymenolepis nana* (0.3%), respectively [15,16]. In another study conducted by Aribodor et al. in Enugu State (Nigeria), they also found *A. lumbricoides* as the most prevalent STH, with a prevalence rate of 40.3%, followed by *T. trichiura* (15.3%) and hookworm (8.9%) [19]. Otherwise, in the present study, the most prevalent parasite was *S. stercoralis* (10.80%, 27 out of 250) and the least prevalent was *T. trichiura* (0.4%, one out of 250). Therefore, our study is not in congruence with most of the recent reports regarding intestinal parasites' prevalence [15,16,19–21]. The true reason for these discrepant results in the area studied is not fully clear. It might have been due to the different diagnostic methods used, the amount of faeces utilized, or the number of stool samples used for the KK.

It should be noted that the KK technique presents a great variability in the considerable diagnostic results, due to the irregular distribution of eggs in the faeces depending on the samples. This explains the poorer performance of the KK technique and the low sensitivity of fecal examinations by microscopy [1,13,22,23].

In contrast, this study does agree with some previous reports in that none of the parasitic helminths were statistically gender-dependent or age-dependent, while this study also demonstrates that the parasitic intensity was light–moderate in all cases, except for *A. lumbricoides*, which had a high intensity [15,16,21].

Currently, the anthelminthic drugs recommended by the WHO for use in public health interventions to control STH infections are albendazole, levamisole, mebendazole and pyrantel [24]. The control of schistosomiasis and STH in Nigeria has employed preventive chemotherapy which involves the mass distribution of praziquantel and albendazole to school-aged children across endemic local government areas [18]. However, less than half (50%) of the treated endemic local government areas met the 75% effective coverage target in the last eight years. The unavailability of drugs and the logistics required to drive mass treatment campaigns are amongst the issues limiting coverage. These challenges were particularly worsened during the COVID-19 pandemic. Our study revealed the presence of schistosomiasis infection with a prevalence rate of 15.20% for *S. haematobium* and 8% for *S. mansoni*, indicating a moderate and low prevalence, respectively. Both *Schistosoma* species had, in general, light parasitic intensity, but unexpectedly 10.53% of the urinary schistosomiasis had a high infection rate (>50 eggs/10 mL of urine). These results are similar to others obtained in a study conducted in 2019, in which S. haematobium was detected in 13.6% of the students, while *S. mansoni* infection prevalence was 7.2% [19]. On the other hand, lower prevalence of *S. haematobium* (0.6%) and *S. mansoni* (2.3%) was recorded by Agbolade et al. compared to the present study [21,25]. Differences in geographical location, snail distribution, local endemicity of the parasites, and laboratory techniques used could explain the differing prevalence. The highest schistosomiasis prevalence was recorded among children over 10 years old compared to other age groups, but, as shown by this survey, age was not significantly associated with urinary and/or intestinal schistosomiasis.

The presence of human schistosomiasis is often related to sanitary deficiencies, contaminated water sources for domestic chores, bathing, and insufficient health education in the population or a deficiency in the control of the intermediate snail host. Temperature is also an important determinant of transmission of schistosomiasis, influencing parasite development and the lifecycle of snail intermediate hosts [1,13,23]. When praziquantel became available in the 1980s, given as oral tablets at a dose of 40 mg/kg body weight in Africa, MDA campaigns against schistosomiasis were slowly adopted as the major control strategy [26]. In Nigeria, MDA for schistosomiasis was first carried out in 2009 and aimed at reducing infection and morbidity [4,18]. The results presented here could be important not only to assess the control programs' success and the prevalence reduction, but also to observe any changes in the incidence, distribution, and control of schistosomiasis disease and other factors relating to health resulting from schistosomiasis MDA.

The occurrence of anemia was statistically significantly associated with age. Children between five and 10 years old have a higher risk of developing anemia than other groups, and there is likely a considerable connection between anemia, intestinal helminth infections, and urinary schistosomiasis, with these parasites affecting hemoglobin levels in different ways, and this anemia is exacerbated when there is co-infection with *P. falciparum* [10,27,28]. Unfortunately, data regarding malaria parasites were not obtained in this study. This study shows that there was a significant association between anemia and helminth infection, especially with *S. haematobium*. A prevalence of 39.6% for anemia in our study reveals a worrying public health issue in Osun State. Fortunately, most of these cases were not severe anemia. Anemia is very common in developing countries, and it is generally a serious problem in school children [20].

5. Conclusions

In this study, it is observed that schistosomiasis and STH are still endemic in Osun State, but with a mild to moderate prevalence. Moreover, the intensity of infection has been found to be mild. Urinary infection was the most prevalent among the children recruited, with a higher prevalence in children over 10 years. The >10 years age group had the highest prevalence for all of the intestinal helminths. The association between gender and age and urogenital or intestinal parasites was not statistically significant.

Author Contributions: Conceptualization, T.A., S.A.N., T.B.O. and A.A.A.; methodology, T.A., T.B.O. and A.A.A.; software, T.-H.T.-T. and P.B.; validation, T.A., S.A.N., A.A.A. and T.B.O.; formal analysis, A.A.A. and T.-H.T.-T.; investigation, T.A., T.B.O. and A.A.A.; resources, A.A.A.; data curation, T.A., A.A.A. and T.-H.T.-T.; writing—original draft preparation, T.-H.T.-T. and P.B.; writing—review and editing, T.-H.T.-T., A.A.A. and P.B.; visualization, T.A., S.A.N., R.C.-M. and T.B.O.; supervision, T.-H.T.-T.; project administration, S.A.N. and A.A.A.; funding acquisition, S.A.N. and A.A.A. All authors have read and agreed to the published version of the manuscript.

Funding: This research received no external funding.

Institutional Review Board Statement: The study was conducted in accordance with the Declaration of Helsinki and approved by the Research & Ethic Committee of Osun State, Ministry of Health, Osogbo, Nigeria (ref no: OSHREC/PRS/569T/131).

Informed Consent Statement: Informed consent was obtained from all subjects involved in the study. Written informed consent has been obtained from the patient(s) to publish this paper.

Data Availability Statement: Not applicable.

Acknowledgments: The authors are sincerely grateful to all consented pupils, their parents and the school teachers for their cooperation.

Conflicts of Interest: The authors declare no conflict of interest. The funders had no role in the design of the study; in the collection, analyses, or interpretation of data; in the writing of the manuscript; or in the decision to publish the results.

References

1. Colley, D.G.; Bustinduy, A.L.; Secor, W.E.; King, C.H. Human Schistosomiasis. *Lancet* **2014**, *383*, 2253–2264. [CrossRef]
2. Webster, B.L.; Southgate, V.R.; Littlewood, D.T.J. A Revision of the Interrelationships of Schistosoma Including the Recently Described *Schistosoma guineensis*. *Int. J. Parasitol.* **2006**, *36*, 947–955. [CrossRef]
3. CDC. CDC—Schistosomiasis—FAQs. Available online: https://www.cdc.gov/parasites/schistosomiasis/gen_info/faqs.html (accessed on 21 March 2021).
4. WHO 2020 Ending the Neglect to Attain the Sustainable Development Goals: A Road Map for Neglected Tropical Diseases 2021–2030. Available online: https://www.who.int/publications-detail-redirect/9789240010352 (accessed on 12 November 2021).
5. WHO Neglected Tropical Diseases. Available online: https://www.who.int/neglected_diseases/diseases/en/ (accessed on 26 July 2020).

6. Ekundayo, O.J.; Aliyu, M.H.; Jolly, P.E. A Review of Intestinal Helminthiasis in Nigeria and the Need for School-Based Intervention. *J. Rural. Trop. Public Health* **2007**, *7*, 33–39.
7. Hailu, T.; Amor, A.; Nibret, E.; Munshea, A.; Anegagrie, M.; Flores-Chavez, M.D.; Tang, T.-H.T.; Saugar, J.M.; Benito, A. Evaluation of Five Diagnostic Methods for *Strongyloides stercoralis* Infection in Amhara National Regional State, Northwest Ethiopia. *BMC Infect. Dis.* **2022**, *22*, 297. [CrossRef]
8. ESPEN. ESPEN | Expanded Special Project for Elimination Neglected Tropical Diseases. Available online: https://espen.afro.who.int/ (accessed on 29 March 2021).
9. Taylor, E.M. NTD Diagnostics for Disease Elimination: A Review. *Diagnostics* **2020**, *10*, 375. [CrossRef]
10. Nkuo-Akenji, T.K.; Chi, P.C.; Cho, J.F.; Ndamukong, K.K.J.; Sumbele, I. Malaria and Helminth Co-Infection in Children Living in a Malaria Endemic Setting of Mount Cameroon and Predictors of Anemia. *J. Parasitol.* **2006**, *92*, 1191–1195. [CrossRef] [PubMed]
11. Ojurongbe, O.; Sina-Agbaje, O.R.; Busari, A.; Okorie, P.N.; Ojurongbe, T.A.; Akindele, A.A. Efficacy of Praziquantel in the Treatment of *Schistosoma haematobium* Infection among School-Age Children in Rural Communities of Abeokuta, Nigeria. *Infect. Dis. Poverty* **2014**, *3*, 30. [CrossRef] [PubMed]
12. Atalabi, T.E.; Lawal, U.; Ipinlaye, S.J. Prevalence and Intensity of Genito-Urinary Schistosomiasis and Associated Risk Factors among Junior High School Students in Two Local Government Areas around Zobe Dam in Katsina State, Nigeria. *Parasit Vectors* **2016**, *9*, 388. [CrossRef] [PubMed]
13. Wiegand, R.E.; Secor, W.E.; Fleming, F.M.; French, M.D.; King, C.H.; Deol, A.K.; Montgomery, S.P.; Evans, D.; Utzinger, J.; Vounatsou, P.; et al. Associations between Infection Intensity Categories and Morbidity Prevalence in School-Age Children Are Much Stronger for *Schistosoma haematobium* than for *S. mansoni*. *PLoS Negl. Trop. Dis.* **2021**, *15*, e0009444. [CrossRef]
14. Win Epi Working in Epidemiology. Available online: http://winepi.net/ (accessed on 26 July 2020).
15. Adefioye, O.; Efunshile, A.; Ojurongbe, O.; Akindele, A.; Adewuyi, I.; Bolaji, O.; Adedokun, S.; Adeyeba, A. Intestinal Helminthiasis among School Children in Ilie, Osun State, Southwest, Nigeria. *Sierra Leone J. Biomed. Res.* **2011**, *3*, 43–48. [CrossRef]
16. Olopade, B.O.; Charles-Eromosele, T.O.; Olopade, O.B. Clinical Presentation and Intensity of Infection with Intestinal Helminths among School Children in Ile-Ife, Osun State, Nigeria. *West Afr. J. Med.* **2022**, *39*, 568–572. [PubMed]
17. Sowemimo, O.A.; Asaolu, S.O. Current Status of Soil-Transmitted Helminthiases among Pre-School and School-Aged Children from Ile-Ife, Osun State, Nigeria. *J. Helminthol.* **2011**, *85*, 234–238. [CrossRef]
18. ESPEN-NIGERIA Nigeria | ESPEN. Available online: https://espen.afro.who.int/countries/nigeria (accessed on 10 November 2021).
19. Aribodor, D.N.; Bassey, S.A.; Yoonuan, T.; Sam-Wobo, S.O.; Aribodor, O.B.; Ugwuanyi, I.K. Analysis of Schistosomiasis and Soil-Transmitted Helminths Mixed Infections among Pupils in Enugu State, Nigeria: Implications for Control. *Infect. Dis. Health* **2019**, *24*, 98–106. [CrossRef]
20. Osazuwa, F.; Ayo, O.M.; Imade, P. A Significant Association between Intestinal Helminth Infection and Anaemia Burden in Children in Rural Communities of Edo State, Nigeria. *N. Am. J. Med. Sci.* **2011**, *3*, 30–34. [CrossRef] [PubMed]
21. Agbolade, O.M.; Agu, N.C.; Adesanya, O.O.; Odejayi, A.O.; Adigun, A.A.; Adesanlu, E.B.; Ogunleye, F.G.; Sodimu, A.O.; Adeshina, S.A.; Bisiriyu, G.O.; et al. Intestinal Helminthiases and Schistosomiasis among School Children in an Urban Center and Some Rural Communities in Southwest Nigeria. *Korean J. Parasitol.* **2007**, *45*, 233–238. [CrossRef] [PubMed]
22. Fenta, A.; Hailu, T.; Alemu, M.; Amor, A. Performance Evaluation of Diagnostic Methods for *Schistosoma mansoni* Detection in Amhara Region, Northwest Ethiopia. *Biomed. Res. Int.* **2020**, *2020*, 5312512. [CrossRef] [PubMed]
23. Weerakoon, K.G.A.D.; Gobert, G.N.; Cai, P.; McManus, D.P. Advances in the Diagnosis of Human Schistosomiasis. *Clin. Microbiol. Rev.* **2015**, *28*, 939–967. [CrossRef]
24. WHO Expert Committee on the Selection, Use of Essential Medicines, & World Health Organization. *The Selection and Use of Essential Medicines: Report of the WHO Expert Committee, 2013 (Including the 18th WHO Model List of Essential Medicines and the 4th WHO Model List of Essential Medicines for Children)*; World Health Organization: Geneva, Switzerland, 2006; ISBN 978-92-4-120933-5.
25. Agbolade, O.M.; Akinboye, D.O.; Awolaja, A. Intestinal Helminthiasis and Urinary Schistosomiasis in Some Villages of Ijebu North, Ogun State, Nigeria. *Afr. J. Biotechnol.* **2003**, *3*, 206–209. [CrossRef]
26. Olliaro, P.L.; Vaillant, M.T.; Belizario, V.J.; Lwambo, N.J.S.; Ouldabdallahi, M.; Pieri, O.S.; Amarillo, M.L.; Kaatano, G.M.; Diaw, M.; Domingues, A.C.; et al. A Multicentre Randomized Controlled Trial of the Efficacy and Safety of Single-Dose Praziquantel at 40 Mg/Kg vs. 60 Mg/Kg for Treating Intestinal Schistosomiasis in the Philippines, Mauritania, Tanzania and Brazil. *PLoS Negl. Trop. Dis.* **2011**, *5*, e1165. [CrossRef] [PubMed]
27. Degarege, A.; Veledar, E.; Degarege, D.; Erko, B.; Nacher, M.; Madhivanan, P. Plasmodium Falciparum and Soil-Transmitted Helminth Co-Infections among Children in Sub-Saharan Africa: A Systematic Review and Meta-Analysis. *Parasit Vectors* **2016**, *9*, 344. [CrossRef]
28. M'bondoukwé, N.P.; Kendjo, E.; Mawili-Mboumba, D.P.; Koumba Lengongo, J.V.; Offouga Mbouoronde, C.; Nkoghe, D.; Touré, F.; Bouyou-Akotet, M.K. Prevalence of and Risk Factors for Malaria, Filariasis, and Intestinal Parasites as Single Infections or Co-Infections in Different Settlements of Gabon, Central Africa. *Infect. Dis. Poverty* **2018**, *7*, 6. [CrossRef] [PubMed]

diagnostics

MDPI

Article

Gram Stain and Culture of Sputum Samples Detect Only Few Pathogens in Community-Acquired Lower Respiratory Tract Infections: Secondary Analysis of a Randomized Controlled Trial

Mariana B. Cartuliares [1,2,*], Helene Skjøt-Arkil [1,2], Christian B. Mogensen [1,2], Thor A. Skovsted [3], Steen L. Andersen [4], Andreas K. Pedersen [2,5] and Flemming S. Rosenvinge [6,7]

1 Emergency Department, University Hospital of Southern Denmark, 6200 Aabenraa, Denmark
2 Department of Regional Health Research, University of Southern Denmark, 6200 Aabenraa, Denmark
3 Department of Biochemistry and Immunology, University Hospital of Southern Denmark, 6200 Aabenraa, Denmark
4 Department of Clinical Microbiology, University Hospital of Southern Denmark, 6200 Aabenraa, Denmark
5 Department of Clinical Research, University Hospital of Southern Denmark, 6200 Aabenraa, Denmark
6 Department of Clinical Microbiology, Odense University Hospital, 5000 Odense, Denmark
7 Research Unit of Clinical Microbiology, University of Southern Denmark, 5000 Odense, Denmark
* Correspondence: mbc@rsyd.dk

Abstract: Identification of the bacterial etiology of lower respiratory tract infections (LRTI) is crucial to ensure a narrow-spectrum, targeted antibiotic treatment. However, Gram stain and culture results are often difficult to interpret as they depend strongly on sputum sample quality. We aimed to investigate the diagnostic yield of Gram stain and culture from respiratory samples collected by tracheal suction and expiratory technique from adults admitted with suspected community-acquired LRTI (CA-LRTI). In this secondary analysis of a randomized controlled trial, 177 (62%) samples were collected by tracheal suction, and 108 (38%) by expiratory technique. We detected few pathogenic microorganisms, and regardless of sputum quality, there were no significant differences between the sample types. Common pathogens of CA-LRTI were identified by culture in 19 (7%) samples, with a significant difference between patients with or without prior antibiotic treatment ($p = 0.007$). The clinical value of sputum Gram stain and culture in CA-LRTI is therefore questionable, especially in patients treated with antibiotics.

Keywords: lower respiratory tract infection; emergency department; sputum; Gram stain; culture; microbiology; tracheal suction; expiratory technique; antibiotic treatment

Citation: Cartuliares, M.B.; Skjøt-Arkil, H.; Mogensen, C.B.; Skovsted, T.A.; Andersen, S.L.; Pedersen, A.K.; Rosenvinge, F.S. Gram Stain and Culture of Sputum Samples Detect Only Few Pathogens in Community-Acquired Lower Respiratory Tract Infections: Secondary Analysis of a Randomized Controlled Trial. *Diagnostics* **2023**, *13*, 628. https://doi.org/10.3390/diagnostics13040628

Academic Editor: Hsin-Yao Wang

Received: 9 December 2022
Revised: 5 February 2023
Accepted: 6 February 2023
Published: 8 February 2023

1. Introduction

The diagnostic value of sputum samples in lower respiratory tract infection (LRTI) has been questioned for many years. In clinical practice, microbiological analysis of sputum by Gram stain and culture can determine the etiological agent of LRTI and enable targeted antibiotic treatment [1–3].

Sputum samples can be collected by tracheal suctioning, induction with saline inhalation, self-expectoration using expiratory techniques, or other methods [4–7]. A randomized controlled trial (RCT) identified tracheal suction (TS) as the best method to obtain sputum samples of good quality compared to forced expiratory technique combined with induced sputum (FETIS) [8]. This leaves a question of whether good quality sputum samples obtained by TS are better than FETIS for detecting pathogenic microorganisms by Gram stain and culture.

American clinical guidelines recommend that laboratories only culture samples of acceptable quality [9]. Gram stain is used to assess sputum quality, but there is no gold standard and different criteria and thresholds have been suggested. Commonly, quality is defined by the number of squamous epithelial cells (SEC) indicating contamination by oropharyngeal microbiota and polymorphonuclear leukocytes (PMNL) indicating inflammation. In addition, some studies assess quality by calculating the ratio of PMNL/SEC [10–16].

Community-acquired LRTI (CA-LRTI) is usually caused by common pathogens such as *Streptococcus pneumoniae* and *Haemophilus influenzae*. Enteric and non-fermenting Gram-negative bacilli are notable pathogens in selected patients but are infrequent causes of CA-LRTI, and detection often reflects upper airway colonization [17]. Gram stain is reported to be highly specific for diagnosing *S.pneumoniae*, *H. influenzae*, and other Gram-negative bacilli and can therefore contribute to clinical decisions before pathogens are verified by culture [2,18]. However, the reliability of sputum analysis decreases if the patient has been treated with antibiotics before admission, reducing the clinical usefulness of the results [13,19,20].

It is unknown and therefore important to investigate how sample type (TS and FETIS), different sputum quality criteria, and recent antibiotic treatment affect the detection of pathogenic bacteria in CA-LRTI.

We hypothesized that good quality sputum samples collected by TS would detect more potential pathogens of CA-LRTI than samples collected by FETIS. The objectives were (i) to investigate if there was a difference in microorganisms detected by Gram stain and culture from good quality sputum samples obtained by TS and FETIS and (ii) to investigate the impact of prior antibiotic treatment on sputum culture results.

2. Materials and Methods

This study is a secondary analysis of a RCT, and for detailed information about the primary trial, we refer to the statistical analysis plan [21] and the primary study [8]. The trial was conducted from 9 November 2020 to 5 July 2021 at 2 Danish emergency departments (EDs) at Hospital Sønderjylland, with a catchment area of approximately 225,000 inhabitants. Microbiological analyses were performed at the hospital's Department of Clinical Microbiology.

Processing of personal data was approved by the Region of Southern Denmark (20/41767) in accordance with the EU General Data Protection Regulation. Furthermore, the study was registered by clinicaltrials.org (NCT04595526 20 October 2020 and completed 5 July 2021) and was approved by the Regional Committee for Health Research Ethics in Southern Denmark (S-20200133).

2.1. Participants

Adults (>18 years of age) admitted to the ED with suspected CA-LRTI were invited by ED project assistants and enrolled in the study, if they gave verbal and written consent, and if the attending physician identified at least one of the following pulmonary symptoms: dyspnea, cough, expectoration, chest pain, or fever. Patients were excluded if participation delayed urgent treatment, transfer to an intensive care unit, or if the patient had severe immunodeficiency [21].

2.2. Randomization

Patients were randomly assigned (1:1) to either tracheal suction (TS) (usual care) or forced expiratory technique (FET) combined with sputum induction (FETIS) (intervention). Randomization was computer generated [22] and performed by the project assistants before collecting the sputum sample [21].

2.3. Sampling Methods

Respiratory samples (tracheal secretions and expectorated sputa) were collected after the initial clinical assessment or within 24 h of admission. TS was performed according to local guidelines. The patient was placed in Fowler's position and encouraged to clear the airways with a deep cough. The suction catheter (EXTRUDAN Surgery Aps, Denmark,

CH12, 530 mm) tip was lubricated with Xylocaine (lidocaine HCl) 2% jelly, inserted into the nares during inhalation, and gently advanced about 40 cm without applying suction. Suction was performed at 200–400 mmHg negative pressure before withdrawing the catheter. FETIS was performed according to a standardized protocol [21] and was based on the patients' attempts to deliver a sputum sample. It included ng FET alone and induced sputum (IS) combined with FET [5,23]. The patient was placed in a 90° sitting position, the mouth was cleared with water to minimize oropharyngeal contamination, and the sample was obtained by forced exhalation and coughing [5]. Using the same procedure, a second sputum sample was obtained after inhalation of nebulized isotonic saline (Unomedical Opti-Mist TM, 2.1 m, ref. 93–772 mm) [23]. Hence, each patient in the intervention group (FETIS) could deliver two samples. Participants in the intervention group who could not deliver a sputum sample by FETIS underwent tracheal suction (TS-IG); these samples were also included in the secondary analysis [21].

2.4. Gram Stain and Culture

A part of the sputum specimen was placed on a microscope slide with a cotton swab, and a second slide was used to distribute the material on the surface. The smear was then heat fixed and Gram stained. For each sputum sample, the number of SEC and PMNL per field of view (10× objective) were recorded. Sputum samples were classified as good quality by three different criteria: (i) <10 SEC, (ii) <10 SEC and >25 PMNL, or (iii) PMNL/SEC ratio > 5. Samples with SEC < 10 and PMNL > 25 were defined as purulent.

Microorganisms were classified as Gram-positive or Gram-negative and by morphology (rods, cocci (pairs, chains, clusters), yeast) (×100 objective).

The remaining part of the sputum sample was transferred to a 5% sheep blood agar plate (Beckton Dickinson, BD, Sparks, MD, USA) and a Chrom Orientation agar plate (BD) and streaked over the agar surface with a sterile inoculation loop. Blood agar plates were inoculated with a *Staphylococcus aureus* streak to allow growth of *H. influenzae*. Agar plates were incubated at 35 °C in normal atmospheric conditions (Chrom-agar Orientation) and in a 5% CO_2 atmosphere (5% blood agar).

After 1–2 days of incubation, pathogens were identified by matrix-assisted laser desorption/ionization–time of flight. In addition, "no growth of pathogens" and "upper airway microbiota" were reported. If culture and microscopy were incongruous, microscopy was re-evaluated, and the agar plates were incubated for two more days.

Microscopy and culture results were registered in the microbiological laboratory information system (MADS, Aarhus University Hospital, Aarhus, Denmark) and were accessible from the patient's medical chart.

2.5. Group of Pathogens

Detected microorganisms were classified into four groups:

(1). Common pathogens of CA-LRTI (*S. pneumoniae*, *H. influenzae*, and *Moraxella catarrhalis*);
(2). Possible pathogens of CA-LRTI (*Pseudomonas aeruginosa* and *S. aureus*);
(3). Unlikely pathogens of CA-LRTI (*Enterobacterales*, *Enterococcus* sp., *Neisseria meningitidis*, *S. maltophila*, *Streptococcus agalactiae*, and yeast);
(4). Upper airway microbiota.

Respiratory pathogens classified as 'common pathogens' represent the most predominant etiologies of CA-LRTI [24–28]. 'Possible pathogens' may cause CA-LRTI, especially in patients with underlying respiratory diseases, but more often represent colonization [29]. 'Unlikely pathogens' represents pathogens that rarely cause CA-LRTI and usually originate from upper airway colonization [17,28].

2.6. Statistical Analysis

The secondary analyses included specimens collected from patients randomized to TS and FETIS. Tracheal secretions from patients randomized to the FETIS group who could not deliver a sample by self-expectoration and therefore underwent tracheal suction were also included. Hence, two groups were analyzed: TS (included TS-SG from standard care group and TS-IG from intervention group) and FETIS (FET and IS). Sensitivity analyses were performed for the four sampling methods (TS-SG, TS-IG, FET, and IS).

Fisher's exact test was performed to compare the yield of microorganisms identified by Gram stain and culture from (1) TS and FETIS and (2) TS and FETIS stratified on the different quality criteria (<10 SEC, <10 SEC and ≥25 PML, >5 PMNL/SEC).

The impact of antibiotic treatment on the yield of pathogens from culture was presented descriptively and using the Chi-Square test based on the defined pathogen groups.

The analysis was based on complete cases and no multiple imputation was performed. A *p*-value less than 0.05 was considered statistically significant, and no adjustments for multiple testing were utilized. Statistical analyses were performed using STATA 17.0 (TX, USA).

3. Results

In total, 285 specimens were collected from 280 patients between 10 November 2020 and 5 July 2021. We included 177 (62%) tracheal secretions (120 TS-SG and 57 TS-IG) and 108 (38%) sputum samples (50 FET and 58 IS) (Figure 1).

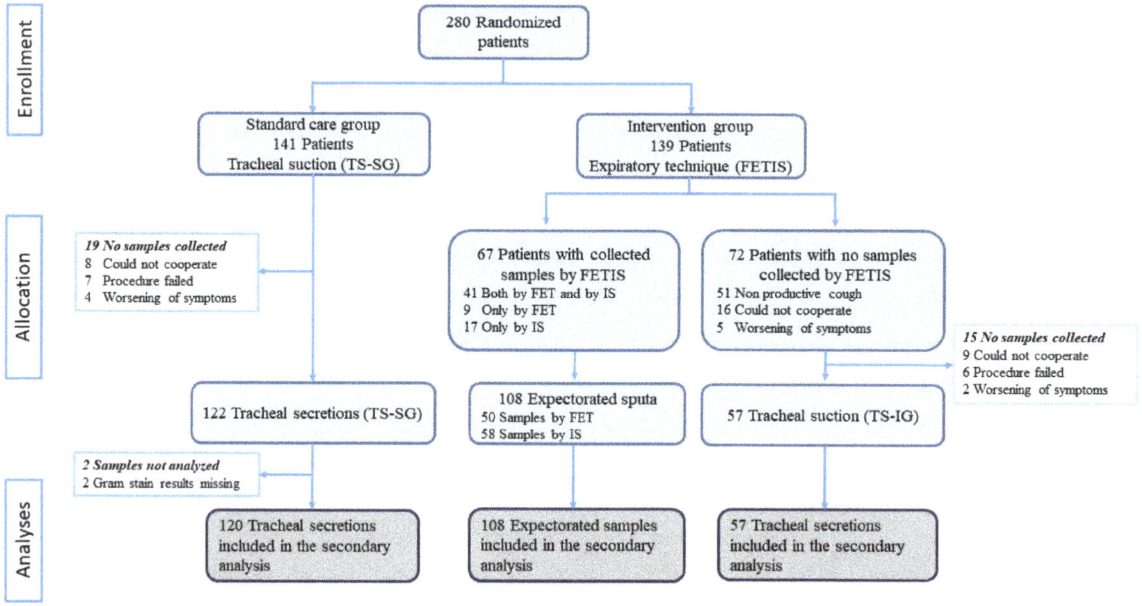

Figure 1. Trial profile and description of the collection of samples. FET: forced expiratory technique; IS: induced sputum; FETIS: forced expiratory technique and induced sputum; TS-SG: tracheal suction standard care group; TS-IG: tracheal suction intervention group.

Gram stains and culture results from samples collected by TS and FETIS are presented in Table 1. Sensitivity analysis from Gram stains and culture results from samples collected by TS and FET and TS and IS are presented in the Supplementary Materials (Tables S1 and S2).

Gram stain detected possible pathogens in 59 samples (21%). A total of 2 or more different possible pathogens were detected by Gram stain in 16 (6%) samples: 8 (6%) from TS and 8 (7%) from FETIS. There was no significant difference between detected pathogens from TS and FETIS (p = 0.384). TS samples were less contaminated with upper airway microbiota 57 (32%) compared to FETIS 60 (55%) (p = 0.001).

Table 1. Findings from Gram stain and culture from tracheal secretions (TS) and sputum samples collected by FET and IS (FETIS).

		Sampling Method		Total	*p*-Value
Total *n* (%)		TS 177 (62%)	FETIS 108 (38%)	*n* = 285	
Gram stain					
	Number of positive samples	31 (18%)	28 (26%)	59 (21%) *	
	All potential pathogens	39 (22%)	36 (33%)	75 (26%) *	0.384
	Gram-positive cocci chains/pairs	15 (38%)	10 (28%)	25 (33%) #	
	Gram-positive cocci clusters	3 (8%)	3 (8%)	6 (8%) #	
	Gram-negative rods	5 (13%)	12 (33%)	17 (23%) #	
	Gram-positive rods	2 (5%)	1 (3%)	3 (4%) #	
	Gram-positive single	5 (13%)	4 (11%)	9 (12%) #	
	Gram-negative diplococci	3 (8%)	4 (11%)	7 (9%) #	
	Yeast	6 (15%)	2 (6%)	8 (11%) #	
	Upper airway microbiota	57 (32%)	60 (56%)	117 (41%) *	0.001
Culture					
	Number of positive samples *	63 (36%)	42 (39%)	105 (37%) *	
	All potential pathogens *	72 (41%)	48 (44%)	120 (42%) *	0.325
	Streptococcus pneumoniae	4 (6%)	2 (4%)	6 (5%) #	
	Enterococcus sp.	2 (3%)	0 (0%)	2 (1%) #	
	Staphylococcus aureus	19 (26%)	4 (8%)	23 (19%) #	
	Haemophilus influenzae	3 (4%)	4 (8%)	7 (6%) #	
	Enterobacterales	25 (35%)	20 (42%)	45 (38%) #	
	Moraxella catarrhalis	3 (4%)	3 (6%)	6 (5%) #	
	Pseudomonas aeruginosa	1 (1%)	1 (2%)	2 (1%) #	
	Other	1 (1%)	2 (4%)	3 (3%) #	
	Yeast	14 (19%)	12 (25%)	26 (22%) #	
	Upper airway microbiota *	27 (15%)	15 (14%)	42 (15%) *	0.765
	No growth of pathogens	67 (38%)	31 (29%)	98 (34%) *	0.174

* percentage of total; # percentage of all potential pathogens.

We identified microorganisms by culture in 105 samples (37%). In 15 (6%) samples, more than 1 microorganism was identified. Overall, there was no significant difference between culture results when comparing TS and FETIS in relation to identified microorganisms ($p = 0.325$), "upper airway microbiota" ($p = 0.765$), and "no growth of pathogens" ($p = 0.174$).

Culture results for TS and FETIS stratified on the three different quality criteria are presented in Table 2.

In good quality sputa (<10 SEC), we identified more microorganisms in TS samples (49 (28%)) than in FETIS samples (23 (21%)); however, the difference between the groups was not statistically significant ($p = 0.096$). In purulent samples and in samples with a PMNL/SEC ratio ≥ 5, culture results from TS and FETIS were similar ($p = 0.955$ and $p = 0.457$, respectively). Results stratified in the three quality criteria showed no statistical difference between TS and FETIS in relation to "upper airway microbiota" ($p = 0.561$, $p = 0.500$, $p = 0.195$) and "no growth of pathogens" ($p = 0.053$, $p = 0.306$, $p = 0.124$).

The 260 culture results were categorized as 'Common pathogens of CA-LRTI' [19 (7.3%): *H. influenzae* (7 (2.7%)), *S. pneumoniae* (6 (2. 3%)), *M. catarrhalis* (6 (2.3%))], 'Possible pathogens of CA-LRTI' [25 (9.6%): *S. aureus* (23 (8.8%)), *P. aeruginosa* (2 (0.8%))], 'Unlikely pathogens of CA-LRTI' [76 (29.2%): *Enterobacterales* (45 (17.3%)), yeast (26 (10%)), other (5 (2%))], 'Upper airway microbiota' (42 (16%)), and 'No growth of pathogens' (98 (37.7%)). The associations between the pathogen group, sampling method, Gram stain quality criteria, and prior antibiotic treatment are shown in Figure 2. Most samples of good quality (<10 SEC) were obtained by TS and 'Common pathogens of CA-LRT' were most often identified in good quality samples (14 (5.4%)), where 8 (3%) were from purulent samples (<10 SEC and >25 PMNL). Most purulent samples (2/3) were obtained by FETIS.

Table 2. Culture results for TS and FETIS stratified on different quality criteria.

Quality Criteria		Sampling Method		Total	*p*-Value
Total *n* (%)		TS 177 (62%)	FETIS 108 (38%)	*n* = 285	
<10 SEC †					
	Number of positive samples	45 (25%)	21 (19%)	66 (23%) *	
	All potential pathogens	49 (28%)	23 (21%)	72 (25%) *	0.096
	Streptococcus pneumoniae	3 (6%)	2 (9%)	5 (7%) #	
	Haemophilus influenzae	1 (2%)	2 (9%)	3 (4%) #	
	Pseudomonas aeruginosa	1 (2%)	0 (0%)	1 (1%) #	
	Moraxella catarrhalis	3 (6%)	3 (13%)	6 (8%) #	
	Staphylococcus aureus	13 (27%)	1 (4%)	14 (19%) #	
	Enterobacterales	17 (35%)	8 (34%)	25 (35%) #	
	Enterococcus sp.	1 (2%)	0 (0%)	1 (1%) #	
	Yeast	10 (20%)	5 (22%)	15 (21%) #	
	Other *	0 (0%)	2 (9%)	2 (3%) #	
	Upper airway microbiota	11 (6%)	3 (3%)	14 (5%) *	0.561
	No growth of pathogens	43 (24%)	7 (6%)	50 (17%) *	0.053
<10 SEC and >25 PMNL ††					
	Number of positive samples	5 (3%)	8 (7%)	13 (5%) *	
	All potential pathogens	6 (3%)	10 (9%)	16 (6%) *	0.955
	Streptococcus pneumoniae	1 (17%)	1 (10%)	2 (12%) #	
	Haemophilus influenzae	1 (17%)	2 (20%)	3 (19%) #	
	Moraxella catarrhalis	1 (17%)	2 (20%)	3 (19%) #	
	Staphylococcus aureus	1 (17%)	0 (0%)	1 (6%) #	
	Enterobacteriaceae	2 (33%)	4 (40%)	6 (38%) #	
	Other **	0 (0%)	1 (10%)	1 (6%) #	
	Upper airway microbiota	2 (1%)	1 (1%)	3 (1%) *	0.500
	No growth of pathogens	3 (2%)	1 (1%)	4 (1%) *	0.306
≥5 PMNL/SEC					
	Number ofpositive samples	9 (5%)	9 (8%)	18 (6%) *	
	All potential pathogens	11 (6%)	11 (10%)	22 (8%) *	0.457
	Streptococcus pneumoniae	1 (9%)	1 (9%)	2 (9%) #	
	Haemophilus influenzae	1 (9%)	2 (18%)	3 (14%) #	
	Moraxella catarrhalis	1 (9%)	2 (18%)	3 (14%) #	
	Staphylococcus aureus	3 (27%)	0 (0%)	3 (14%) #	
	Enterobacterales	4 (36%)	4 (36%)	8 (36%) #	
	Yeast	1 (9%)	0 (0%)	1 (4%) #	
	Other ***	0 (0%)	2 (18%)	2 (9%) #	
	Upper airway microbiota	1 (<1%)	3 (3%)	4 (1%) *	0.195
	No growth of pathogens	10 (6%)	3 (3%)	13 (5%) *	0.124

* percentage of total; # percentage of all potential pathogens; † SEC: squamous epithelial cells; †† PMNL: polymorph nuclear leucocytes; * Other: *N. meningitidis* and *S. maltophila*; ** Other: *S. maltophila*; *** Other: *N. meningitidis* and *S. maltophila*. A total of 43 and 44 samples were missing from the <10 SEC and >25 PMNL and ≥PMNL/SEC group, respectively.

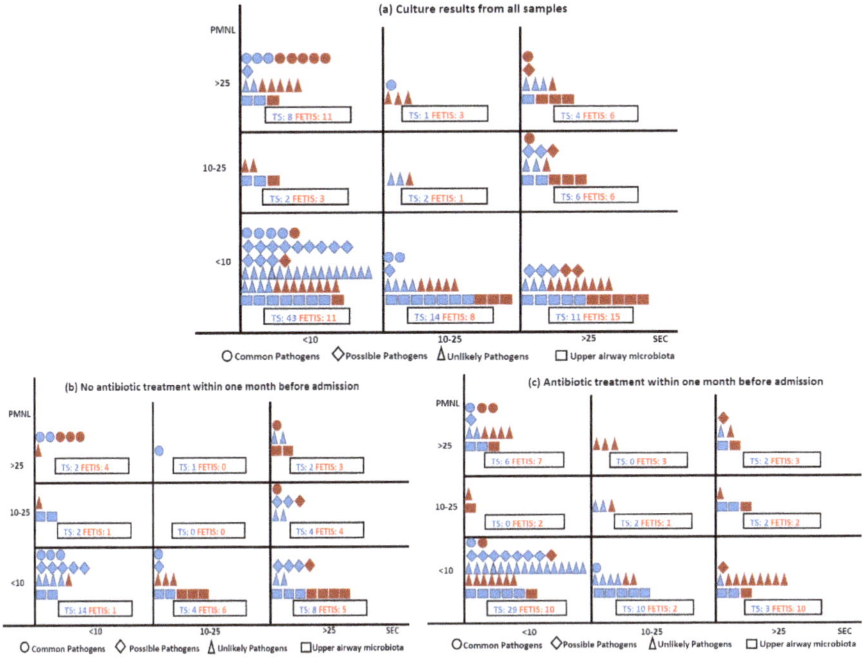

Figure 2. Samples collected by TS and FETIS distributed according to Gram stain quality criteria, culture results (**a**), and samples without and with prior antibiotic treatment (**b**,**c**). Sampling methods: TS blue, FETIS red. Culture results are presented in four groups: ○: common pathogens of CA-LRTI (*S. pneumoniae*, *H. influenzae*, and *M. catarrhalis*), ◊: possible pathogens of CA-LRTI (*P. aeruginosa* and *S. aureus*), Δ: unlikely pathogens of CA-LRTI (*Enterobacterales*, *Enterococcus* sp., *N. meningitidis*, *S. maltophila*, *S. agalactiae*, and yeast), and □: upper airway microbiota. A total of 9 culture results were missing: ○ 1 FETIS (<10 SEC), ◊ 1 TS (<10 SEC), Δ 6 TS (<10 SEC), □ 1 TS (<10 SEC).

Compared to patients without prior antibiotic treatment, samples from patients treated with antibiotics within one month before admission yielded significantly fewer common pathogens ($p = 0.007$), possible pathogens ($p = 0.018$), and significantly more unlikely pathogens ($p < 0.001$) of CA-LRTI (Table 3). Sensitivity analysis of detected pathogens (common, possible, and unlikely) stratified by sampling methods (TS and FET, TS and IS) did not change the overall results and are presented in the Supplementary Materials (Table S3). Identified microorganisms from patients untreated and treated with antibiotics are presented in the Supplementary Materials (Table S4).

Table 3. Detected pathogens: relation to antibiotic treatment within one month before admission.

	Antibiotics (NO)	**Antibiotic (YES)**	**Total**	***p*-Value**
	***n* = 128 (45%)**	***n* = 157 (55%)**	***n* = 285**	
Number of positive samples	40 (31%)	65 (41%)	105 (37%) *	
Common pathogens of CA-LRTI	12 (9%)	7 (4%)	19 (7%) *	0.007
Possible pathogens of CA-LRTI	14 (11%)	11 (7%)	25 (9%) *	0.018
Unlikely pathogens of CA-LRTI	17 (13%)	59 (38%)	76 (27%) *	<0.001
Upper airway microbiota	18 (14%)	24 (15%)	42 (15%) *	0.784

* percentage of total. Culture results of four groups of pathogens: (1) common pathogens of CA-LRT (*S. pneumoniae*, *H. influenzae*, and *M. catarrhalis*), (2) possible pathogens of CA-LRTI (*P. aeruginosa* and *S. aureus*), (3) unlikely pathogens of CA-LRT (*Enterobacterales*, *Enterococcus* sp. *N. meningitidis*, *S. maltophila*, *S. agalactiae*, and yeast).

4. Discussion

In this study, we described the Gram stain and culture findings in 285 sputum samples collected by TS and FETIS from CA-LRTI patients. Regardless of different quality criteria, there was no statistically significant difference in culture results between TS and FETIS. Samples obtained by TS were assessed to be less contaminated with upper airway microbiota by Gram stain. This result indicates that TS is better than FETIS for obtaining samples from the lower airways. Few common pathogens of CA-LRTI (*H. influenzae*, *S. pneumoniae*, and *M. catarrhalis*) were identified by culture. Not surprisingly, samples from patients not treated with antibiotics before admission yielded almost twice as many common pathogens of CA-LRTI compared to samples from patients treated with antibiotics.

A retrospective multicenter study from 2022 reported a different result, concluding that the diagnostic yield was higher for expectorated and induced sputum compared to tracheal secretions [24]. However, the study included very few patients in the TS group (21 (1.6%)), indicating sample bias.

We identified common pathogens of CA-LRTI in 19 (7.3%) of the 260 culture results—almost all 14 (5.4%) from good quality samples with <10 SEC and over half were from purulent samples (<10 SEC and >25 PMNL). These findings, in accordance with earlier observations, showed that good quality sputum with <10 SEC and >25 PMNL was 3.8 times more likely to grow pathogenic bacteria compared to poor quality sputum [30]. A recent systematic review found an increased diagnostic yield of the Gram stain in identifying bacterial etiologies of CAP when samples of good quality were obtained [2]. It indicates that quality classification by Gram stain is important and contributes to accurate diagnostics of CAP pathogens.

No pathogen was detected by culture in 140 (49%) samples. There are several possible explanations for the low yield of the Gram stain and culture. An explanation could be that the pathogens of LRTI generally are difficult to detect. A study with a high level of patient participation (95%) failed to determine the etiology for 47% of the patients [26]. Meanwhile, another study comparing paired sputa and transtracheal aspirated samples revealed that if a specimen of good quality (<10 SEC and >25 PMNL) did not identify a pathogen, there was still a 45% chance that a pathogen was detected in the paired transtracheal aspirate [10]. These findings suggest that bacterial culture has a low sensitivity in detecting causative pathogens of CA-LRTI.

Patients were enrolled in this study based on clinical symptoms (dyspnea, cough, expectoration, chest pain, or fever), and before results from chest X-rays, blood tests, and urine tests were available. These symptoms are common in patients with bacterial CA-LRTI but also in patients with viral infections [31]. Therefore, another explanation for the low number of culture-positive sputa could be that a high number of patients in our study was admitted with viral infections. Unfortunately, the only registered viral agent was SARS-CoV-2 as data were prospectively collected with pre-specified variables. Forty (14%) patients were infected with SARS-CoV-2 [8]. On the other hand, surveillance data show that there was a very low transmission in Denmark of other common respiratory viruses during the SARS-CoV-2 pandemic [29]. This might have reduced the number of admissions caused by viral infections and may also have reduced the risk of secondary bacterial pneumonia—possibly in part explaining the low detection of bacterial pathogens in our study.

Finally, another probable explanation is that patients with chronic obstructive pulmonary disease (COPD) might have been included in the study with acute exacerbation rather than CA-LRTI as they are often admitted with similar clinical symptoms, e.g., increased sputum production, sputum purulence, and dyspnea. There is an etiological overlap, but acute exacerbations in COPD are often caused by non-bacterial etiologies (e.g., viral infections and environmental factors) [27,28,32].

In line with the literature, many samples in our study, 157 (55%), were analyzed from patients receiving antibiotics within one month before admission [26]. It is well recognized that consumption of antibiotics decreases the diagnostic yield of Gram stain and culture [13,19,33]. A previous study reported an association between prior antibiotic treatment and a four-fold reduction in diagnostic yield [33]. Furthermore, the detection of causative pathogens of LRTI is significantly reduced if antibiotics are consumed within 24 h before collecting a sputum sample [13,19]. Our study correlates well with these studies, with a statistically significant difference in culture results from patients with or without previous antibiotic treatment. Our study also supports the observation from other studies that more unlikely pathogens of CA-LRTI, such as *Enterobacterales*, are detected in patients previously treated with antibiotics [13,19]. *Enterobacterales* rarely cause pneumonia in a community setting and the detection is probably a result of antibiotic selective pressure and oropharyngeal overgrowth [25]. Albeit an infrequent cause, the bacteria may cause severe LRTI, highlighting the importance of separating etiology and colonization [17]. Antibiotic therapy may also explain the observation that in this study almost half of TS samples, despite good quality, had no growth of pathogens. The question remaining is: "Do samples from patients previously treated with antibiotics add value to clinical practice?"

The major strengths of this study are the high rate of obtained specimens (88%) from patients with suspected CA-LRTI and the randomized prospective design of the primary study minimizing sampling bias. In addition, samples were collected, Gram stained, and cultured by standardized and closely monitored procedures. A major limitation is, similar to other studies, the low number of microorganisms identified, especially common pathogens of CA-LRTI. If significantly more samples had been included, we may have detected a difference in diagnostic yield, but the study size was fixed by the primary study [8]. Another limitation was not including patient discharge diagnosis, viral test results, and blood culture results, which may have confirmed or supplemented our results. Many samples were from patients who received antibiotics before admission (55%). However, this is not regarded as a limitation as this prospective study gives insights into real-world practice and challenges in managing acutely admitted patients with suspected CA-LRTI.

5. Conclusions

We detected very few relevant pathogens of CA-LRTI regardless of sample type (TS/FETIS), sample quality, and microbiological test (Gram stain/culture), especially in patients treated with antibiotics. Future research should focus on methods to mitigate this problem. It is possible that molecular methods, e.g., syndromic test panels, will have a higher diagnostic sensitivity, will be less sensitive to prior antibiotic treatment, and in addition, allow the detection of both viral and bacterial pathogens. Regardless of the method, it will still be essential to ensure specimens of optimal quality as most bacterial pathogens also are commensals of the upper airways.

Supplementary Materials: The following supporting information can be downloaded at: https://www.mdpi.com/article/10.3390/diagnostics13040628/s1, Table S1: Sensitivity analysis of Gram stain and culture from samples obtained by TS (TS-SG, TS-IG) and FET. Table S2: Sensitivity analysis of Gram stain and culture from samples obtained by TS (TS-SG, TS-IG) and IS. Table S3: Sensitivity analysis of the detected pathogens in relation to antibiotic treatment stratified by the collected methods TS (TS-SG, TS-IG) and FET, TS (TS-SG, TS-IG) and IS. Table S4: Identified microorganisms in samples from patients untreated and treated with antibiotics.

Author Contributions: M.B.C., H.S.-A., C.B.M., T.A.S., S.L.A., A.K.P., and F.S.R. were involved in the study's design. M.B.C. performed the literature search and drafted the original work in collaboration with F.S.R., M.B.C. was the study investigator and coordinated the project with participant recruitment and data collection. A.K.P. supervised the statistical analyses. H.S.-A. was the chief research officer responsible for supervising the overall study. S.L.A. contributed substantially to the data quality and monitoring of sputum samples. All authors have read and agreed to the published version of the manuscript.

Funding: The study was funded by the University of Southern Denmark (17/10636), University Hospital of Southern Denmark (20/20505), Knud and Edith Eriksens Mindefond (62786–2020), and Fabrikant Mads Clausens Fond (SHS.59.1-11.13582). The funders of this study had no role in the study design, data collection, data analysis, data interpretation, or writing of the report.

Institutional Review Board Statement: The study was conducted according to the guidelines of the Declaration of Helsinki and approved by the Regional Committee on Health Research Ethics for Southern Denmark (S-20200133) 22 September 2020.

Informed Consent Statement: Informed consent was obtained both in writing and orally from all participants included in the study.

Data Availability Statement: Due to Danish laws on personal data, data cannot be shared publicly. To request data, please contact the corresponding author for more information. The person responsible for the research was the principal investigator and corresponding author (MBC) in collaboration with the Department of Health Research and the University Hospital of Southern Denmark. These organizations own the data and can provide access to the final data set.

Acknowledgments: The authors appreciate text editing from Caroline Moos, research consultant, University Hospital of Southern Denmark.

Conflicts of Interest: The authors declare no conflict of interest.

References

1. Bartlett, J.G. Diagnostic tests for agents of community-acquired pneumonia. *Clin. Infect. Dis.* **2011**, *52*, S296–S304. [CrossRef]
2. Ogawa, H.; Kitsios, G.D.; Iwata, M.; Terasawa, T. Sputum Gram Stain for Bacterial Pathogen Diagnosis in Community-acquired Pneumonia: A Systematic Review and Bayesian Meta-analysis of Diagnostic Accuracy and Yield. *Clin. Infect. Dis.* **2020**, *71*, 499–513. [CrossRef]
3. Metlay, J.P.; Waterer, G.W.; Long, A.C.; Anzueto, A.; Brozek, J.; Crothers, K.; Cooley, L.A.; Dean, N.C.; Fine, M.J.; Flanders, S.A. Diagnosis and treatment of adults with community-acquired pneumonia. An official clinical practice guideline of the American Thoracic Society and Infectious Diseases Society of America. *Am. J. Respir. Crit. Care Med.* **2019**, *200*, e45–e67. [CrossRef]
4. Bartlett, J.G.; Finegold, S.M. Bacteriology of expectorated sputum with quantitative culture and wash technique compared to transtracheal aspirates. *Am. Rev. Respir. Dis.* **1978**, *117*, 1019–1027. [CrossRef]
5. Lewis, L.K.; Williams, M.T.; Olds, T.S. The active cycle of breathing technique: A systematic review and meta-analysis. *Respir. Med.* **2012**, *106*, 155–172. [CrossRef]
6. Bandyopadhyay, T.; Gerardi, D.A.; Metersky, M.L. A comparison of induced and expectorated sputum for the microbiological diagnosis of community acquired pneumonia. *Respiration* **2000**, *67*, 173–176. [CrossRef]
7. Gunasekaran, J.; Saksena, R.; Jain, M.; Gaind, R. Can sputum gram stain be used to predict lower respiratory tract infection and guide empiric antimicrobial treatment: Experience from a tertiary care hospital. *J. Microbiol. Methods* **2019**, *166*, 105731. [CrossRef]
8. Cartuliares, M.B.; Rosenvinge, F.S.; Mogensen, C.B.; Skovsted, T.A.; Andersen, S.L.; Pedersen, A.K.; Skjøt-Arkil, H. Expiratory Technique versus Tracheal Suction to Obtain Good-Quality Sputum from Patients with Suspected Lower Respiratory Tract Infection: A Randomized Controlled Trial. *Diagnostics* **2022**, *12*, 2504. [CrossRef]
9. Miller, J.M.; Binnicker, M.J.; Campbell, S.; Carroll, K.C.; Chapin, K.C.; Gilligan, P.H.; Gonzalez, M.D.; Jerris, R.C.; Kehl, S.C.; Patel, R. A guide to utilization of the microbiology laboratory for diagnosis of infectious diseases: 2018 update by the Infectious Diseases Society of America and the American Society for Microbiology. *Clin. Infect. Dis.* **2018**, *67*, e1–e94.
10. Geckler, R.W.; Gremillion, D.H.; McAllister, C.K.; Ellenbogen, C. Microscopic and bacteriological comparison of paired sputa and transtracheal aspirates. *J. Clin. Microbiol.* **1977**, *6*, 396–399. [CrossRef]
11. Murray, P.R.; Washington, J.A. Microscopic and baceriologic analysis of expectorated sputum. *Mayo Clin. Proc.* **1975**, *50*, 339–344.
12. Joyce, S.M. Sputum analysis and culture. *Ann. Emerg. Med.* **1986**, *15*, 325–328. [CrossRef]
13. Miyashita, N.; Shimizu, H.; Ouchi, K.; Kawasaki, K.; Kawai, Y.; Obase, Y.; Kobashi, Y.; Oka, M. Assessment of the usefulness of sputum Gram stain and culture for diagnosis of community-acquired pneumonia requiring hospitalization. *Med. Sci. Monit.* **2008**, *14*, CR171–CR176.
14. Fukuyama, H.; Yamashiro, S.; Kinjo, K.; Tamaki, H.; Kishaba, T. Validation of sputum Gram stain for treatment of community-acquired pneumonia and healthcare-associated pneumonia: A prospective observational study. *BMC Infect. Dis.* **2014**, *14*, 534. [CrossRef]
15. Mizrachi, H.H.; Valenstein, P.N. Randomized trial interpreting sputum quality in a clinical laboratory. *J. Clin. Microbiol.* **1987**, *25*, 2327–2329. [CrossRef]
16. Lee, D.-H.; Kim, S. Clinical Analysis of Sputum Gram Stains and Cultures to Improve the Quality of Sputum Cultures. *J. Lab. Med. Qual. Assur.* **2020**, *42*, 33–39. [CrossRef]

17. Villafuerte, D.; Aliberti, S.; Soni, N.J.; Faverio, P.; Marcos, P.J.; Wunderink, R.G.; Rodriguez, A.; Sibila, O.; Sanz, F.; Martin-Loeches, I.; et al. Prevalence and risk factors for Enterobacteriaceae in patients hospitalized with community-acquired pneumonia. *Respirology* **2020**, *25*, 543–551. [CrossRef]
18. Del Rio-Pertuz, G.; Gutiérrez, J.F.; Triana, A.J.; Molinares, J.L.; Robledo-Solano, A.B.; Meza, J.L.; Ariza-Bolívar, O.M.; Acosta-Reyes, J.; Garavito, A.; Viasus, D.; et al. Usefulness of sputum gram stain for etiologic diagnosis in community-acquired pneumonia: A systematic review and meta-analysis. *BMC Infect. Dis.* **2019**, *19*, 403. [CrossRef]
19. Musher, D.M.; Montoya, R.; Wanahita, A. Diagnostic value of microscopic examination of Gram-stained sputum and sputum cultures in patients with bacteremic pneumococcal pneumonia. *Clin. Infect. Dis.* **2004**, *39*, 165–169. [CrossRef]
20. Lidman, C.; Burman, L.G.; Lagergren, A.; Ortqvist, A. Limited value of routine microbiological diagnostics in patients hospitalized for community-acquired pneumonia. *Scand. J. Infect. Dis.* **2002**, *34*, 873–879. [CrossRef]
21. Cartuliares, M.B.; Skjøt-Arkil, H.; Rosenvinge, F.S.; Mogensen, C.B.; Skovsted, T.A.; Pedersen, A.K. Effectiveness of expiratory technique and induced sputum in obtaining good quality sputum from patients acutely hospitalized with suspected lower respiratory tract infection: A statistical analysis plan for a randomized controlled trial. *Trials* **2021**, *22*, 675. [CrossRef]
22. Harris, P.A.; Taylor, R.; Minor, B.L.; Elliott, V.; Fernandez, M.; O'Neal, L.; McLeod, L.; Delacqua, G.; Delacqua, F.; Kirby, J.; et al. The REDCap consortium: Building an international community of software platform partners. *J. Biomed. Inform.* **2019**, *95*, 103208. [CrossRef]
23. Chanez, P.; Holz, O.; Ind, P.; Djukanović, R.; Maestrelli, P.; Sterk, P. Sputum induction. *Eur. Respir. J.* **2002**, *20*, 3s–8s.
24. Waagsbø, B.; Buset, E.M.; Longva, J.; Bjerke, M.; Bakkene, B.; Ertesvåg, A.S.; Holmen, H.; Nikodojevic, M.; Tran, T.T.; Christensen, A.; et al. Diagnostic stewardship aiming at expectorated or induced sputum promotes microbial diagnosis in community-acquired pneumonia. *BMC Infect. Dis.* **2022**, *22*, 203. [CrossRef]
25. Finegold, S.M.; Johnson, C.C. Lower respiratory tract infection. *Am. J. Med.* **1985**, *79*, 73–77. [CrossRef]
26. Bjarnason, A.; Westin, J.; Lindh, M.; Andersson, L.M.; Kristinsson, K.G.; Löve, A.; Baldursson, O.; Gottfredsson, M. Incidence, Etiology, and Outcomes of Community-Acquired Pneumonia: A Population-Based Study. *Open Forum Infect. Dis.* **2018**, *5*, ofy010. [CrossRef]
27. Murphy, T.F.; Parameswaran, G.I. Moraxella catarrhalis, a human respiratory tract pathogen. *Clin. Infect. Dis.* **2009**, *49*, 124–131. [CrossRef]
28. Torres, A.; Blasi, F.; Peetermans, W.; Viegi, G.; Welte, T. The aetiology and antibiotic management of community-acquired pneumonia in adults in Europe: A literature review. *Eur. J. Clin. Microbiol. Infect. Dis.* **2014**, *33*, 1065–1079. [CrossRef]
29. Institut, S.S. Influenza Season 2020–2021—Report on Disease Occurrence. Available online: https://en.ssi.dk/surveillance-and-preparedness/surveillance-in-denmark/annual-reports-on-disease-incidence/influenza-season-2020-2021---report-on-disease-occurrence (accessed on 29 August 2022).
30. Budayanti, N.S.; Suryawan, K.; Iswari, I.S.; Sukrama, D.M. The Quality of Sputum Specimens as a Predictor of Isolated Bacteria From Patients with Lower Respiratory Tract Infections at a Tertiary Referral Hospital, Denpasar, Bali-Indonesia. *Front. Med.* **2019**, *6*, 64. [CrossRef]
31. Vos, L.M.; Bruyndonckx, R.; Zuithoff, N.P.A.; Little, P.; Oosterheert, J.J.; Broekhuizen, B.D.L.; Lammens, C.; Loens, K.; Viveen, M.; Butler, C.C.; et al. Lower respiratory tract infection in the community: Associations between viral aetiology and illness course. *Clin. Microbiol. Infect.* **2021**, *27*, 96–104. [CrossRef]
32. Li, X.J.; Li, Q.; Si, L.Y.; Yuan, Q.Y. Bacteriological differences between COPD exacerbation and community-acquired pneumonia. *Respir. Care* **2011**, *56*, 1818–1824. [CrossRef] [PubMed]
33. Ewig, S.; Schlochtermeier, M.; Goke, N.; Niederman, M.S. Applying sputum as a diagnostic tool in pneumonia: Limited yield, minimal impact on treatment decisions. *Chest* **2002**, *121*, 1486–1492. [PubMed]

diagnostics

MDPI

Article

Effect of the Hematocrit and Storage Temperature of Dried Blood Samples in the Serological Study of Mumps, Measles and Rubella

Mariano Rodríguez-Mateos [1], Javier Jaso [1], Paula Martínez de Aguirre [1,2], Silvia Carlos [2,3,4,*], Leire Fernández-Ciriza [1], África Holguín [5] and Gabriel Reina [1,2,4]

1 Microbiology Department, Clínica Universidad de Navarra, 31008 Pamplona, Spain
2 ISTUN, Institute of Tropical Health, Universidad de Navarra, 31008 Pamplona, Spain
3 Department of Preventive Medicine and Public Health, Universidad de Navarra, 31008 Pamplona, Spain
4 IdiSNA, Navarra Institute for Health Research, 31008 Pamplona, Spain
5 HIV-1 Molecular Epidemiology Laboratory, Microbiology and Parasitology Department, University Hospital Ramón y Cajal-IRYCIS and CIBEREsp-RITIP, 28034 Madrid, Spain
* Correspondence: scarlos@unav.es; Tel.: +34-948-425-600 (ext. 826636)

Abstract: Dried blood spots (DBSs) are an economical and convenient alternative to serum/plasma, which allow for the serological and molecular study of different pathogens. Sixty-four blood samples were collected by venipuncture and spotted onto Whatman™ 903 cards to evaluate the utility of DBSs and the effect of the storage temperature for 120 days after sample collection to carry out serological diagnosis. Mumps, measles and rubella IgG were investigated from DBSs and plasma using an automated chemiluminescent immunoassay. Using a calculated optimal cut-off value, the serological evaluation of mumps, measles and rubella using DBSs achieved high sensitivity (100%, 100% and 82.5%, respectively) and specificity (100%, 87.5% and 100%, respectively). The correlation observed between the plasma and the DBSs processed after sample collection was high (0.914–0.953) for all antibodies studied, both considering hematocrit before sample elution or not. For the different storage conditions, the correlation with plasma was high at 4 °C (0.889–0.925) and at −20 °C (0.878–0.951) but lower at room temperature (0.762–0.872). Measles IgG results were more affected than other markers when DBSs were stored at any temperature for 120 days. To summarize, hematocrit does not affect the processing of DBSs in the study of serological markers of mumps, measles and rubella. DBS stability for serological diagnosis of mumps and rubella is adequate when samples are stored at −20 °C or 4 °C, but not at room temperature, for a period of 4 months.

Keywords: dried blood spots (DBSs); serology; chemiluminescence; immunoassay; measles; rubella; mumps

Citation: Rodríguez-Mateos, M.; Jaso, J.; Martínez de Aguirre, P.; Carlos, S.; Fernández-Ciriza, L.; Holguín, Á.; Reina, G. Effect of the Hematocrit and Storage Temperature of Dried Blood Samples in the Serological Study of Mumps, Measles and Rubella. *Diagnostics* **2023**, *13*, 349. https://doi.org/10.3390/diagnostics13030349

Academic Editor: Hsin-Yao Wang

Received: 15 December 2022
Revised: 10 January 2023
Accepted: 14 January 2023
Published: 18 January 2023

1. Introduction

Dried blood spots (DBSs) are a form of sampling in which a few drops of blood are placed on filter paper, which are then allowed to dry at room temperature for several hours and can be easily stored. Ivar Christian Bang is credited for the development of the idea of using blood collected on a paper for analysis when he determined glucose levels from DBSs eluates in 1913 [1]. In 1963, Robert Guthrie began to use DBSs to detect phenylketonuria in newborns using the heel prick test [2]. Since then, several investigators have reported the use of DBSs for serological testing, and it has been used in the surveillance of numerous diseases such as HIV, hepatitis, syphilis and measles [3]. Several studies have demonstrated that antibodies can be detected using DBSs and that the diagnostic accuracy of DBSs is high compared to serum/plasma, indicating that DBSs are a useful alternative to serum [4,5]. In addition, DBSs can also be a reliable sample for molecular testing, as previously reported [3–8].

DBSs are an inexpensive, non-invasive and convenient alternative to serum/plasma, easily obtained without the necessary equipment for venipuncture or the qualified healthcare personnel. Furthermore, a low blood volume is required, which can be important in pediatric diagnosis. Its use can be beneficial in low- and middle-income countries where it is difficult to obtain and test serum/plasma samples due to a lack of laboratory resources [9,10]; and also in high-income countries to reach patients not linked to the healthcare system, as those attending Substance Abuse and Mental Health Services, where fingerstick whole-blood samples for DBSs allow the carrying out of serological and molecular diagnosis [7,11,12]. Consequently, this type of sample is well accepted by patients and study participants and may improve the linkage to care [11].

Moreover, the storage and shipment of DBSs are easier than serum/plasma as these cards require less space than a blood tube, are lighter in weight and are not considered infectious material [13]. Due to these advantages, the World Health Organization (WHO) supports the use of DBSs as an alternative to venipuncture [14].

Regardless of the broad use of DBSs for a wide range of serologic studies, there is still not enough evidence for the reliability of DBSs for the analysis of additional biomarkers, such as vaccine-preventable diseases, such as measles, mumps and rubella. This tool, if valid, may facilitate the diagnosis and surveillance of these infectious diseases. Furthermore, differences in the correlation between the serum/plasma and DBSs results have been reported for different pathogens, suggesting that antibodies against certain microorganisms in DBSs may be less stable than others [15]. In addition, there are still no guidelines on how DBSs should be stored to preserve the stability of the different antibodies to be investigated. Therefore, there is a need to guarantee the conditions of DBSs processing and storage to carry out these analyses.

The aim of our study was to evaluate the ability of DBSs to detect serological indicators of three infectious diseases (measles, mumps and rubella) using an indirect chemiluminescent immunoassay (CLIA) and to test the effects of different storage temperatures of DBSs on the stability of these serological markers. In addition, we evaluated the effect of hematocrit on the serological diagnosis of these infections.

2. Materials and Methods

2.1. Study Design and Participants

A cross-sectional study of 64 adult patients who attended Clínica Universidad de Navarra (Pamplona, Spain) between October and December 2019 was carried out. All of the patients were >18 years old and were selected while taking into account that there was a proportional distribution of men and women, as well as the different age groups and hematocrit levels of the participants. Pregnant women and patients with autoimmune diseases or infectious mononucleosis were excluded due to the higher probability of false positives in the serological analysis. Patients' names were codified at sampling to maintain confidentiality.

2.2. Sample Collection and Storage

For each patient, a blood sample anticoagulated with EDTA was obtained by venipuncture to carry out a complete blood count analysis, including hematocrit value. These samples were collected for routine analysis, and once it was finished, they were selected and used for the research. From this specimen, five DBSs were prepared by spotting 70 μL of whole blood per DBSs on a Whatman™ 903 card (GE Healthcare) that was allowed to dry for 24 h at room temperature. The remaining volume of blood was centrifuged for ten minutes at 2000× g to obtain the plasma. After drying, all five DBSs were cut with sterile scissors and inserted into individual Eppendorf microtubes. Of the five spots collected, two dots were processed following sample collection (DBS-A and DBS-B), and the remaining three dots were stored at different temperatures to evaluate stability (at −20 °C (DBS-C), at 4 °C (DBS-D) and at room temperature (DBS-E)) for 4 months before carrying out the analysis.

2.3. DBS Elution

Immediately after sample collection (time 0), one dot (DBS-A) was eluted with an adjusted volume of phosphate-buffered saline (PBS), taking into account the hematocrit, to achieve an exact equivalence with the plasma volume used in standard tests (5 μL/assay). The remaining dots were universally eluted (DBS-B, DBS-C, DBS-D and DBS-E) with 1 mL of PBS without considering the hematocrit (Figure 1); all of the dots were incubated at 37 °C for 1 h. To improve elution, the tubes were shaken in a vortex every 15 min. When the elution was finished, the remaining paper was removed from the tube to avoid obstructions in the instrument.

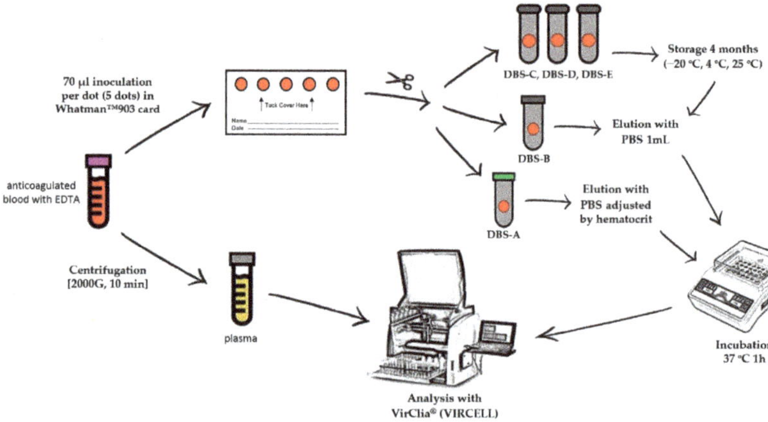

Figure 1. DBS/plasma storage conditions and processing for serological diagnosis. PBS: phosphate-buffered saline; DBS-A: DBSs processed without delay and eluted with an adjusted volume of PBS considering the hematocrit value; DBS-B: DBSs without delay and eluted universally with 1 mL of PBS; DBS-C: DBSs stored at −20 °C for 4 months; DBS-D: DBSs stored at 4 °C for 4 months; DBS-E: DBSs stored at room temperature for 4 months.

2.4. Serological Testing

The detection of IgG against measles, mumps and rubella was performed by indirect chemiluminescent immunoassay (CLIA) using the VirClia® automated system (Vircell), both in DBSs and plasma. Two VirClia® protocols developed by the manufacturer were used, one for plasma with a sample volume of 5 μL and another for eluted DBSs with a volume of 105 μL. The interpretation of the results was carried out following the manufacturer's instructions considering as gold standard the cut-off values provided for the three pathogens in the plasma/serum, which provides a sensitivity of 96–100% and specificity of 100% according to the manufacturer.

2.5. Statistical Analysis

Descriptive statistics were calculated using Excel for Microsoft 365, version 2208. The differences between subpopulations were calculated using a Chi-square test. The assay results for the plasma and DBSs were compared, and correlation was evaluated using Spearman's test due to the lack of a normal distribution in the samples. To assess the degree of agreement between the two DBS elution methods, the kappa coefficient was calculated. To optimize the use of DBSs for IgG measurements, sensitivity, specificity, positive (PPV) and negative (NPV) predictive values of the tests were calculated for each of the three parameters, considering as gold standard, the results obtained with the plasma. An optimal cut-off index for the interpretation of the DBS results for each parameter was obtained by calculating the area under the curve (AUC) of the receiver operating characteristics (ROC) curves.

3. Results

The median age of the 64 participants in the study was 42.6 years, 52% were female, and 90.6% were born in Spain. The general characteristics of the study population can be seen in Table 1.

Table 1. Characteristics of the study population according to age groups.

	Male	**Female**	**Total**
n (%)	31 (48%)	33 (52%)	64
Median age at sampling [IQR]	42.8 [37.6–58.3]	41.8 [31.6–56.7]	42.6 [36.5–58.1]
Age Groups, n (%)			
<30	5 (16%)	7 (21%)	12 (18.8%)
30–45	12 (39%)	12 (36%)	24 (37.5%)
45–60	7 (23%)	8 (24%)	15 (23.4%)
>60	7 (23%)	6 (18%)	13 (20.3%)
Hematocrit, median [IQR]	**42.7 [38.9–45.7]**	**39.8 [37.2–41.7]**	**41.0 [37.8–43.6]**
Age groups			
<30	42.7%	40.5%	41.9%
30–45	44.8%	41.0%	42.1%
45–60	43.2%	38.6%	41.0%
>60	38.2%	38.1%	38.2%
Pathogen immunity (plasma)			
Measles IgG (%)	**71.0%**	**87.9%**	**79.7%**
Age groups			
<30	40.0%	85.7%	66.7%
30–45	58.3%	91.7%	75.0%
45–60	100%	87.5%	93.3%
>60	85.7%	83.3%	84.6%
Mumps IgG (%)	**80.6%**	**87.9%**	**84.4%**
Age groups			
<30	100%	85.7%	91.7%
30–45	75.0%	91.7%	83.3%
45–60	71.4%	87.5%	80.0%
>60	85.7%	83.3%	84.6%
Rubella IgG (%)	**87.1%**	**90.9%**	**89.1%**
Age groups			
<30	80.0%	85.7%	83.3%
30–45	91.7%	91.7%	91.7%
45–60	71.4%	100%	86.7%
>60	100%	83.3%	92.3%

IQR: interquartile range; Age in years; Hematocrit in %.

3.1. Immunization Levels in Plasma

Protective IgG levels varied for each disease in the study cohort. We found that protection against measles, mumps and rubella was high, being >75% in all cases (Table 1). The protection coverage rate was higher in women than in men, but the differences were not statistically significant ($p > 0.05$). The percentage of patients with indeterminate plasma results was low (7.8% measles, 1.6% mumps, and 3.1% rubella).

3.2. Correlation between DBS and Plasma

The results obtained with the DBS samples showed a strong correlation with those from the plasma samples (Figure 2, Table 2). However, the quantitative results in the immunoassay using DBS samples were slightly higher than those of plasma samples, leading to decreased specificity if the interpretation of the DBS results was performed using the manufacturer's cut-off values for plasma (1.1). When this cut-off was applied to the interpretation of the DBS results, the percentage of immunized patients for all pathogens was higher than when the plasma results were analyzed, and the specificity was reduced to 60% for measles, 88.5% for mumps and 60% for rubella. Therefore, a new optimized DBS cut-off was calculated for each target using ROC curves to achieve optimal sensitivity and/or specificity in the detection of IgG using DBSs. These values were 1.569, 2.791 and 1.450 for the detection of IgG against mumps, measles and rubella, respectively (Table 3, Figure 3). When the optimized DBS cut-off was applied, the percentage of immunized patients was lower than using plasma for measles (−6.9%), mumps (−1.8%) and rubella (−23%). The use of this new DBS cut-off increased the specificity, PPV and NPV of the tests (Table 3).

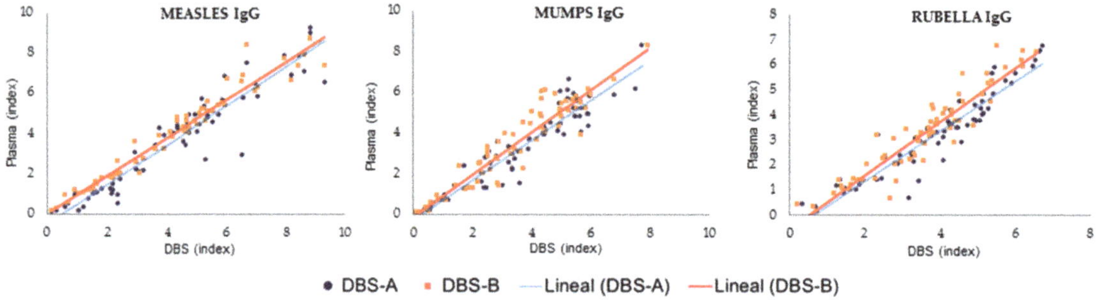

Figure 2. Comparison of DBSs and plasma results for measles, mumps and rubella processed after sample collection. DBS-A: DBSs eluted with a volume of PBS adjusted by hematocrit; DBS-B: DBSs eluted with 1 mL of PBS.

Table 2. Spearman's correlation coefficient between plasma and DBSs results.

	Plasma/DBS-A	Plasma/DBS-B	Plasma/DBS-C	Plasma/DBS-D	Plasma/DBS-E
MEASLES	0.939	0.948	0.878	0.889	0.762
MUMPS	0.914	0.928	0.905	0.917	0.882
RUBELLA	0.953	0.940	0.951	0.925	0.872

DBS-A: DBSs processed without delay and eluted with an adjusted volume of PBS, taking into account the hematocrit; DBS-B: DBSs without delay and eluted with 1 mL of PBS; DBS-C: DBSs stored at −20 °C for 4 months; DBS-D: DBSs stored at 4 °C for 4 months; DBS-E: DBSs stored at room temperature for 4 months.

Table 3. Results of VirClia®-IgG test for the detection of protective IgG against measles, mumps and rubella.

		MEASLES *				MUMPS **				RUBELLA ***			
		Sen	**Spe**	**PPV**	**NPV**	**Sen**	**Spe**	**PPV**	**NPV**	**Sen**	**Spe**	**PPV**	**NPV**
DBS-A	Plasma cut-off	100%	57.1%	94.4%	100%	100%	87.5%	98.2%	100%	100%	60%	96.6%	100%
	DBS cut-off **	100%	87.5%	98.1%	100%	98.1%	100%	100%	90%	84.2%	80%	98%	30.8%
DBS-B	Plasma cut-off	100%	60%	96.2%	100%	100%	88.9%	98.2%	100%	100%	60%	96.6%	100
	DBS cut-off	100%	87.5%	98.1%	100%	100%	100%	100%	100%	82.5%	100%	100%	33.3%

Table 3. *Cont.*

		MEASLES *				MUMPS **				RUBELLA ***			
		Sen	Spe	PPV	NPV	Sen	Spe	PPV	NPV	Sen	Spe	PPV	NPV
DBS-C	Plasma cut-off	96.1%	50%	94.2%	60%	100%	87.5%	98.2%	100%	98.2%	60%	96.6%	75%
	DBS cut-off	92.2%	87.5%	97.9%	63.3%	98.1%	100%	100%	90%	80.7%	100%	100%	31.3%
DBS-D	Plasma cut-off	98%	42.9%	92.6%	75%	100%	62.5%	94.7%	100%	100%	60%	96.6%	100%
	DBS cut-off	94.1%	62.5%	94.1%	62.5%	98.1%	88.9%	98.1%	88.9%	84.2%	100%	100%	35.7%
DBS-E	Plasma cut-off	96%	0%	88.9%	0%	100%	28.6%	91.5%	100%	100%	40%	95%	100%
	DBS cut-off	94.1%	50%	92.3%	57.1%	98.1%	55.6%	93%	83.3%	80.7%	80%	97.9%	26.7%

* Measles cut-off, plasma: 1.1; DBS: 1.569; ** Mumps cut-off, plasma: 1.1; DBS: 2.791; *** Rubella cut-off, plasma: 1.1; DBS: 1.450. Sen: Sensitivity; Spe: Specificity; PPV: Positive predictive value; NPV: Negative predictive value. DBS-A: DBSs processed without delay and eluted with an adjusted volume of PBS, taking into account the hematocrit; DBS-B: DBSs without delay and eluted with 1 mL of PBS; DBS-C: DBSs stored at −20 °C for 4 months; DBS-D: DBSs stored at 4 °C for 4 months; DBS-E: DBSs stored at room temperature for 4 months.

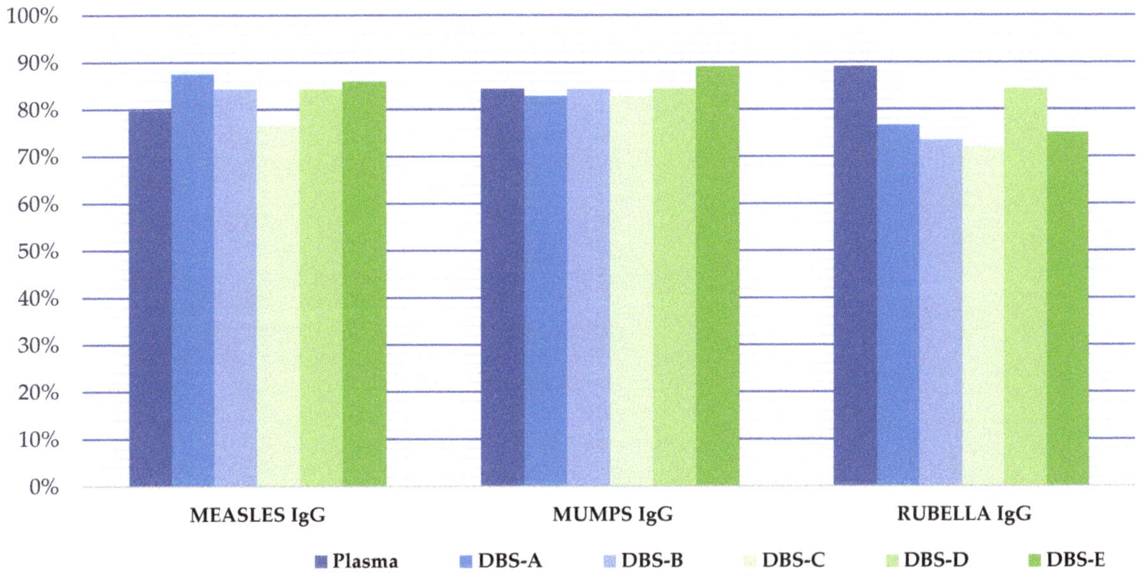

Figure 3. Pathogen immunity against measles, mumps and rubella in our study population considering the manufacturer cut-off for plasma and the optimized DBSs cut-off for all DBSs analysis. DBS-A: DBSs processed without delay and eluted with an adjusted volume of PBS, taking into account the hematocrit; DBS-B: DBSs without delay and eluted with 1 mL of PBS; DBS-C: DBSs stored at −20 °C for 4 months; DBS-D: DBSs stored at 4 °C for 4 months; DBS-E: DBSs stored at room temperature for 4 months.

3.2.1. Effect of the Hematocrit

When the DBSs were eluted with an adjusted volume of PBS, considering the hematocrit value to analyze exactly the equivalent volume of plasma in standard tests (DBS-A), the results were similar to those obtained when the DBSs were universally eluted with 1 mL of PBS for the three serological markers evaluated (DBS-B) (Figure 2). Both methods obtained excellent concordance between them, with kappa values of 1.0, 0.924 and 1.0 for measles, mumps and rubella, respectively.

3.2.2. DBS Stability

The serological values obtained from the DBSs stored at room temperature for 4 months (DBS-E) differed from those obtained with the DBSs stored at −20 °C (DBS-C) or 4 °C (DBS-

D), compared to the results obtained from plasma processed immediately after sample collection (reference result). In addition, DBS-C and DBS-D yielded results comparable to those obtained with DBSs processed without delay (DBS-A and DBS-B), except for the investigation of IgG against measles, where the storage caused a negative effect at any temperature (Table 2). The 4-month processing delay of DBSs reduced the correlation with plasma in 2.43–7.46% when the DBSs were stored at −20 °C, 1.20–6.28% when the DBSs were stored at 4 °C and 4.91–19.61% when the DBSs were stored at room temperature. This drop in the correlation of the DBS samples processed after storage caused a marked reduction in the specificity of the three serological markers. However, since the serological values obtained from DBSs tend to be higher than those from the plasma, the sensitivity of the assays was not affected, except for the evaluation of measles (Table 3). As mentioned above, measles serology results were more affected than mumps or rubella values when the DBSs were preserved for 4 months, with drops in the correlation with the plasma of 7.46%, 6.28% and 19.61% after storage at −20 °C, 4 °C and room temperature, respectively.

4. Discussion

The use of DBSs is becoming more and more popular as it is a convenient and suitable sample to carry out different laboratory tests. This study demonstrated equivalent detection of antibodies against measles, mumps and rubella using DBSs compared to plasma. In addition, a universal procedure of DBSs elution independent of hematocrit data has been able to obtain excellent results for antibody detection. Moreover, we observed that the storage of DBSs up to 4 months at low temperatures was adequate to preserve these samples.

Our results demonstrate that DBS samples are valid to verify prior exposure or immunization against some infections, such as measles, mumps and rubella, using an automated chemiluminescent immunoassay. This procedure may also allow the study of the seroprevalence against these vaccinable-preventable diseases and provide useful information to check whether herd immunity has been achieved within a community or target vaccination campaigns. We also report the optimal cut-off values when DBSs specimens are used in the VirClia® automated platform (Vircell) to obtain high sensitivity and specificity when these IgG antibodies are investigated.

The correlation of the quantitative index results obtained from the plasma and DBSs processed immediately after sample collection was excellent, reaching coefficients of 0.914–0.953. Both DBS-A and DBS-B, blood spot specimens processed considering hematocrit level (DBS-A) or not (DBS-B), showed results comparable to those obtained from the plasma. Therefore, it is demonstrated that DBSs elution for serological diagnosis can be performed with a universal elution volume, not exactly adjusted to the hematocrit, thus facilitating the lab work when the patient's hematocrit data are unknown. This good linearity of the DBSs matrix and plasma with no effect of physiological hematocrit levels on assay performance has been reported previously to measure antibodies against Epstein–Barr or hepatitis E [16,17]; however, the hematocrit may adversely affect the accuracy of therapeutic drug monitoring results where DBSs are a popular sample [18]. Nevertheless, new devices for DBSs collection have recently been proposed to overcome the heterogeneity and hematocrit issues and allow more efficient quantitation [19].

The procedure used with DBSs to carry out the chemiluminescence tests was slightly different to that used with the plasma, as a different sample volume was used to improve the sensitivity and specificity of the analysis. Then, for DBS testing, 105 microlitres of the eluted DBSs were inoculated in the sample well, while the diagnosis from the plasma sample was conducted using 5 microlitres of a sample with 100 microlitres of diluent (1/21 dilution). The optimal cut-off values for the evaluation of the chemiluminescence results of each parameter were calculated by constructing ROC curves. These values were higher than the cut-off index applied to plasma samples (1.1) and allowed for the improvement of the interpretation of the results obtained from the DBSs when compared to those from the plasma. In this way, the procedure for the serological evaluation of measles, mumps and rubella using DBSs achieved high sensitivity (100%, 81% and 100%) and specificity (88%, 100% and 100%), respectively, as previously reported to study infants samples from resource-limited settings [20].

To assess the stability of the DBS samples for serological analysis after a long storage (120 days), three different conditions were evaluated (−20 °C, 4 °C and room temperature). For the different storage conditions, the correlation with the plasma results was high at 4 °C (0.888–0.925) and at −20 °C (0.878–0.951) but lower at room temperature (0.762–0.882). Hence, the storage of DBS samples at room temperature may be suboptimal to carry out serological analysis four months after sample collection, but a shorter period (15–20 days) has not been evaluated and should be validated in the future. Therefore, the long-term storage of DBSs intended for subsequent testing should be undertaken at low temperatures, as previously reported for anti-HIV, HBsAg, anti-HBc, anti-HCV or anti-HEV [21–23], as a marked loss of Western blot positivity and low titer antibody signals have been observed if cold storage is not carried out [24].

The negative effect on DBS preservation of storage above 4 °C was observed for the three different antibodies investigated, but, in particular, the values of measles serology were more affected than the other markers. Then, for measles investigation, the diagnosis can be made using DBS since the correlation obtained immediately after collection was high (0.948), but it should be made without delay. The effect of storage may be variable for different biomarkers, as has been observed with different types of antibodies or drug monitoring [25–27].

The validation of a commercially available chemiluminescence assay using DBSs for the detection of mumps, measles, and rubella IgG may facilitate the investigation of these markers in low- and middle-income countries where nursing facilities or equipment are not available for sample collection. In addition, the availability of DBSs in high-income countries may be very convenient as a minimally invasive sample, allowing for self-sampling and direct shipment to a clinical laboratory using regular mail. This procedure allows for the investigation of these antibodies, either to study the population that does not regularly attend healthcare services or those in which sample collection may be challenging. Surveillance studies to verify protection against these pathogens are regularly conducted in different situations, especially in occupational safety and health services, and also during pregnancy, after exposure, or previous to international travelling.

Multiple determinants have been identified for lower vaccination uptake among migrants for routine and COVID-19 targets. A tailored, culture-sensitive and evidence-informed strategy has been suggested to strengthen vaccination programmes in high-income countries [28]. The collection of DBSs may enable testing vulnerable people to propose catch-up vaccination campaigns, particularly among populations at greater risk, such as migrants or those born years before universal vaccination against these three pathogens was implemented, mainly between 1960 and 1980 in most high-income countries [29]. However, several authors have highlighted the need for additional validation studies of these techniques to carry out serological surveillance from DBSs as a lack of standardization has been observed in the collection, storage and testing methods [30].

Our study is subject to a number of potential limitations. The first is that the vaccination history of participants was unknown, so no information on the expected biomarkers could be obtained. Second, the pre-infection rate was also not available; however, the high vaccination coverage within our population could reassure the possibility of assessing these antibodies. The results are given by subgrouping the data according to age group and hematocrit, although the study was performed after making a homogeneous selection of the participants in terms of age, sex and hematocrit. The study has several notable strengths, including the use of standardized, commercial and validated robust serological platforms to measure values of interest for the study.

In conclusion, this study confirms the validity of DBS samples for the study of serological markers of mumps, measles and rubella. Moreover, the hematocrit does not affect the processing of DBSs to carry out chemiluminescent immunoassays. DBS stability for use in antibody detection against mumps and rubella is adequate when the samples are stored at −20 °C or 4 °C, but not at room temperature, for a period of 4 months.

Author Contributions: Conceptualization, G.R., Á.H. and S.C.; methodology, M.R.-M., J.J., P.M.d.A. and G.R.; validation, M.R.-M., J.J. and G.R.; formal analysis, M.R.-M., L.F.-C. and S.C.; investigation, M.R.-M., J.J. and S.C.; resources, Á.H. and G.R.; writing—original draft preparation, M.R.-M., J.J., S.C. and G.R.; writing—review and editing, P.M.d.A., L.F.-C. and Á.H. All authors have read and agreed to the published version of the manuscript.

Funding: This research received no external funding. The APC was funded by *Diagnostics*.

Institutional Review Board Statement: The planning, conduct and reporting of the studies were in line with the Declaration of Helsinki. The project was approved by the Human Subjects Review at the University of Navarra (Pamplona, Spain) (Reference: 2019.152. Code: Virclia-DBS).

Informed Consent Statement: Written informed consent was obtained from enrolled participants. All methods were carried out in accordance with relevant guidelines and regulations (CPMP/ICH/135/95). All data and samples were coded and confidentially managed.

Data Availability Statement: The data presented in this study are openly available in the Harvard Dataverse https://dataverse.harvard.edu/dataset.xhtml?persistentId=doi:10.7910/DVN/PGJKA9 (accessed on 15 December 2022).

Acknowledgments: We thank all the people who participated in the study, as well as professionals responsible for the appointments, and sample/data collection. We thank VIRCELL S.L. for providing the serological tests.

Conflicts of Interest: The authors declare no conflict of interest.

References

1. Schmidt, V. Ivar Christian Bang (1869–1918), founder of modern clinical microchemistry. *Clin. Chem.* **1986**, *32*, 213–215. [CrossRef] [PubMed]
2. Guthrie, R. Blood Screening for Phenylketonuria. *JAMA* **1961**, *178*, 863. [CrossRef]
3. Grüner, N.; Stambouli, O.; Ross, R.S. Dried blood spots–preparing and processing for use in immunoassays and in molecular techniques. *J. Vis. Exp.* **2015**, *13*, 52619. [CrossRef] [PubMed]
4. Hannon, W.H.; Therell, B.L. Overview of the history and applications of dried blood spot samples. In *Dried Blood Spots: Applications and Techniques*; Li, W., Lee, M.S., Eds.; Wiley Hoboken: East Hanover, NJ, USA, 2014; Volume 3, pp. 3–15.
5. Su, X.; Carlson, B.F.; Wang, X.; Li, X.; Zhang, Y.; Montgomery, J.P.; Ding, Y.; Wagner, A.L.; Gillespie, B.; Boulton, M.L. Dried blood spots: An evaluation of utility in the field. *J. Infect. Public Health* **2018**, *11*, 373–376. [CrossRef]
6. Carrasco, T.; Barquín, D.; Ndarabu, A.; Fernández-Alonso, M.; Rubio-Garrido, M.; Carlos, S.; Makonda, B.; Holguín, Á.; Reina, G. HCV Diagnosis and Sequencing Using Dried Blood Spots from Patients in Kinshasa (DRC): A Tool to Achieve WHO 2030 Targets. *Diagnostics* **2021**, *11*, 522. [CrossRef] [PubMed]
7. Catlett, B.; Hajarizadeh, B.; Cunningham, E.; Wolfson-Stofko, B.; Wheeler, A.; Khandaker-Hussain, B.; Feld, J.J.; Martró, E.; Chevaliez, S.; Pawlotsky, J.M.; et al. Diagnostic Accuracy of Assays Using Point-of-Care Testing or Dried Blood Spot Samples for the Determination of Hepatitis C Virus RNA: A Systematic Review. *J. Infect. Dis.* **2022**, *226*, 1005–1021. [CrossRef] [PubMed]
8. Rubio-Garrido, M.; Ndarabu, A.; Reina, G.; Barquín, D.; Fernández-Alonso, M.; Carlos, S.; Holguín, Á. Utility Of POC Xpert HIV-1 Tests For Detection-Quantification Of Complex HIV Recombinants Using Dried Blood Spots From Kinshasa, D. R. *Congo. Sci. Rep.* **2019**, *9*, 5679. [CrossRef] [PubMed]
9. Barquín, D.; Ndarabu, A.; Carlos, S.; Fernández-Alonso, M.; Rubio-Garrido, M.; Makonda, B.; Holguín, Á.; Reina, G. HIV-1 diagnosis using dried blood spots from patients in Kinshasa, DRC: A tool to detect misdiagnosis and achieve World Health Organization 2030 targets. *Int. J. Infect. Dis.* **2021**, *111*, 253–260. [CrossRef] [PubMed]
10. Øverbø, J.; Aziz, A.; Zaman, K.; Julin, C.H.; Qadri, F.; Stene-Johansen, K.; Biswas, R.; Islam, S.; Bhuiyan, T.R.; Haque, W.; et al. Stability and Feasibility of Dried Blood Spots for Hepatitis E Virus Serology in a Rural Setting. *Viruses* **2022**, *14*, 2525. [CrossRef]
11. Ryan, P.; Valencia, J.; Cuevas, G.; Troya, J.; Torres-Macho, J.; Muñoz-Gómez, M.J.; Muñoz-Rivas, N.; Canorea, I.; Vázquez-Morón, S.; Resino, S. HIV screening and retention in care in people who use drugs in Madrid, Spain: A prospective study. *Infect. Dis. Poverty* **2021**, *10*, 111. [CrossRef]
12. Bajis, S.; Grebely, J.; Hajarizadeh, B.; Applegate, T.; Marshall, A.D.; Harrod, M.E.; Byrne, J.; Bath, N.; Read, P.; Edwards, M.; et al. Hepatitis C virus testing, liver disease assessment and treatment uptake among people who inject drugs pre- and post-universal access to direct-acting antiviral treatment in Australia: The LiveRLife study. *J. Viral Hepat.* **2020**, *27*, 281–293. [CrossRef] [PubMed]
13. International Air Transport Association Dangerous (IATA) Goods Regulations (62nd Edition). Available online: https://www.iata.org/contentassets/b08040a138dc4442a4f066e6fb99fe2a/dgr-62-en-3.6.2.pdf (accessed on 21 November 2022).

14. WHO Manual for HIV Drug Resistance Testing Using Dried Blood Spot Specimens. Available online: https://www.who.int/publications/i/item/9789240009424 (accessed on 24 November 2022).
15. Amini, F.; Auma, E.; Hsia, Y.; Bilton, S.; Hall, T.; Ramkhelawon, L.; Heath, P.T.; Le Doare, K. Reliability of dried blood spot (DBS) cards in antibody measurement: A systematic review. *PLoS ONE* **2021**, *16*, e0248218. [CrossRef] [PubMed]
16. Eick, G.; Urlacher, S.S.; McDade, T.W.; Kowal, P.; Snodgrass, J.J. Validation of an Optimized ELISA for Quantitative Assessment of Epstein-Barr Virus Antibodies from Dried Blood Spots. *Biodemography Soc. Biol.* **2016**, *62*, 222–233. [CrossRef]
17. Sultana, R.; Bhuiyan, T.R.; Sathi, A.S.; Sharmin, S.; Yeasmin, S.; Uddin, M.I.; Bhuiyan, S.; Mannoor, K.; Karim, M.M.; Zaman, K.; et al. Developing and validating a modified enzyme linked immunosorbent assay method for detecting HEV IgG antibody from dried blood spot (DBS) samples in endemic settings. *Microbes Infect.* **2022**, *24*, 104890. [CrossRef] [PubMed]
18. Palmer, O.M.P.; Dasgupta, A. Review of the Preanalytical Errors That Impact Therapeutic Drug Monitoring. *Ther. Drug Monit.* **2021**, *43*, 595–608. [CrossRef]
19. Whittaker, K.; Mao, Y.-Q.; Lin, Y.; Zhang, H.; Zhu, S.; Peck, H.; Huang, R.-P. Dried blood sample analysis by antibody array across the total testing process. *Sci. Rep.* **2021**, *11*, 20549. [CrossRef]
20. Rodríguez-Galet, A.; Rubio-Garrido, M.; Valadés-Alcaraz, A.; Rodríguez-Domínguez, M.; Galán, J.C.; Ndarabu, A.; Reina, G.; Holguín, A. Immune surveillance for six vaccinable pathogens using paired plasma and dried blood spots in HIV infected and uninfected children in Kinshasa. *Sci. Rep.* **2022**, *12*, 7920. [CrossRef]
21. Eisenberg, A.L.; Patel, E.U.; Packman, Z.; Fernandez, R.; Piwowar-Manning, E.; Hamilton, E.L.; MacPhail, C.; Hughes, J.P.; Pettifor, A.; Kallas, E.; et al. Short Communication: Dried Blood Spots Stored at Room Temperature Should Not Be Used for HIV Incidence Testing. *AIDS Res. Hum. Retroviruses* **2018**, *34*, 1013–1016. [CrossRef]
22. McAllister, G.; Shepherd, S.; Templeton, K.; Aitken, C.; Gunson, R. Long term stability of HBsAg, anti-HBc and anti-HCV in dried blood spot samples and eluates. *J. Clin. Virol.* **2015**, *71*, 10–17. [CrossRef]
23. Singh, M.P.; Majumdar, M.; Budhathoki, B.; Goyal, K.; Chawla, Y.; Ratho, R.K. Assessment of dried blood samples as an alternative less invasive method for detection of Hepatitis E virus marker in an outbreak setting. *J. Med. Virol.* **2013**, *86*, 713–719. [CrossRef]
24. Manak, M.M.; Hack, H.R.; Shutt, A.L.; Danboise, B.A.; Jagodzinski, L.L.; Peel, S.A. Stability of Human Immunodeficiency Virus Serological Markers in Samples Collected as HemaSpot and Whatman 903 Dried Blood Spots. *J. Clin. Microbiol.* **2018**, *56*, e00933-18. [CrossRef] [PubMed]
25. Moat, S.J.; Zelek, W.M.; Carne, E.; Ponsford, M.J.; Bramhall, K.; Jones, S.; El-Shanawany, T.; Wise, M.J.; Thomas, A.; George, C.; et al. Development of a high-throughput SARS-CoV-2 antibody testing pathway using dried blood spot specimens. *Ann. Clin. Biochem. Int. J. Biochem. Lab. Med.* **2021**, *58*, 123–131. [CrossRef] [PubMed]
26. Jacobs, C.M.; Wagmann, L.; Meyer, M.R. Development, validation, and application of a quantitative volumetric absorptive microsampling–based method in finger prick blood by means of LC-HRMS/MS applicable for adherence monitoring of antipsychotics. *Anal. Bioanal. Chem.* **2021**, *413*, 1729–1737. [CrossRef] [PubMed]
27. Martens-Lobenhoffer, J.; Hinderhofer, M.; Tröger, U.; Bode-Böger, S.M. Stability of ceftolozane in human plasma and dried blood spots: Implications for transport and storage. *J. Pharmacol. Toxicol. Methods* **2020**, *103*, 106692. [CrossRef]
28. Crawshaw, A.F.; Farah, Y.; Deal, A.; Rustage, K.; E Hayward, S.; Carter, J.; Knights, F.; Goldsmith, L.P.; Campos-Matos, I.; Wurie, F.; et al. Defining the determinants of vaccine uptake and undervaccination in migrant populations in Europe to improve routine and COVID-19 vaccine uptake: A systematic review. *Lancet Infect. Dis.* **2022**, *22*, e254–e266. [CrossRef]
29. Hinman, A.; Orenstein, W. Immunisation practice in developed countries. *Lancet* **1990**, *335*, 707–710. [CrossRef]
30. Holroyd, T.A.; Schiaffino, F.; Chang, R.H.; Wanyiri, J.W.; Saldanha, I.J.; Gross, M.; Moss, W.J.; Hayford, K. Diagnostic accuracy of dried blood spots for serology of vaccine-preventable diseases: A systematic review. *Expert Rev. Vaccines* **2022**, *21*, 185–200. [CrossRef]

diagnostics

MDPI

Article

A Comparative Study on Visual Detection of *Mycobacterium tuberculosis* by Closed Tube Loop-Mediated Isothermal Amplification: Shedding Light on the Use of Eriochrome Black T

Alireza Neshani [1], Hosna Zare [1], Hamid Sadeghian [1,2], Hadi Safdari [1,2], Bamdad Riahi-Zanjani [3] and Ehsan Aryan [1,4,*]

1 Antimicrobial Resistance Research Center, Mashhad University of Medical Sciences, Mashhad 91967-73113, Iran
2 Department of Laboratory Sciences, School of Paramedical Sciences, Mashhad University of Medical Sciences, Mashhad 91779-48964, Iran
3 Medical Toxicology Research Center, Mashhad University of Medical Sciences, Mashhad 91779-48564, Iran
4 Department of Medical Microbiology, Ghaem University Hospital, Mashhad University of Medical Sciences, Mashhad 91766-99199, Iran
* Correspondence: ehsanaryan@hotmail.com; Tel.: +98-511-3845-3019; Fax: +98-511-3711-2596

Abstract: Loop-mediated isothermal amplification is a promising candidate for the rapid detection of *Mycobacterium tuberculosis*. However, the high potential for carry-over contamination is the main obstacle to its routine use. Here, a closed tube LAMP was intended for the visual detection of Mtb to compare turbidimetric and two more favorable colorimetric methods using calcein and hydroxy naphthol blue (HNB). Additionally, a less studied dye (i.e., eriochrome black T (EBT)) was optimized in detail in the reaction for the first time. Mtb purified DNA and 30 clinical specimens were used to respectively determine the analytical and diagnostic sensitivities of each method. The turbidimetric method resulted in the best analytical sensitivity (100 fg DNA/reaction), diagnostic sensitivity and specificity (100%), and time-to-positivity of the test (15 min). However, this method is highly prone to subjective error in reading the results. Moreover, HNB-, calcein-, and EBT-LAMP could respectively detect 100 fg, 1 pg, and 1 pg DNA/reaction (the analytical sensitivities) in 30, 15, and 30 min, while the diagnostic sensitivity and specificity were respectively 93.3% and 100% for them all. Interestingly, EBT-LAMP showed the lowest potential for subjective error in reading the results. This report helps judiciously choose the most appropriate visual method, taking a step forward toward the field applicability of LAMP for the detection of Mtb, particularly in resource-limited settings.

Keywords: LAMP; *Mycobacterium tuberculosis*; visual detection; EBT; calcein; HNB

Citation: Neshani, A.; Zare, H.; Sadeghian, H.; Safdari, H.; Riahi-Zanjani, B.; Aryan, E. A Comparative Study on Visual Detection of *Mycobacterium tuberculosis* by Closed Tube Loop-Mediated Isothermal Amplification: Shedding Light on the Use of Eriochrome Black T. *Diagnostics* **2023**, *13*, 155. https://doi.org/10.3390/diagnostics13010155

Academic Editor: Hsin-Yao Wang

Received: 29 November 2022
Revised: 29 December 2022
Accepted: 29 December 2022
Published: 2 January 2023

1. Introduction

Tuberculosis (TB) has been a human disease since the beginning of the Neolithic period, as studies on bones dating back over 6000 years suggest that some prehistoric people also had TB [1–3]. TB is caused by the acid-fast bacillus *Mycobacterium tuberculosis*, spreading via respiratory aerosols during the active pulmonary form of the disease [4]. According to the World Health Organization's (WHO) latest annual TB report, there has been an increase in the global TB deaths between 2019 and 2021. In 2021, nearly 10.6 million new cases of TB and 1.6 million TB-related deaths were reported worldwide [5]. Treatment of TB requires a prolonged course of multiple drugs. The prompt and effective treatment of TB is crucial for controlling and preventing the emergence of potentially lethal resistant strains of *Mycobacterium tuberculosis*. To avoid delayed appropriate treatment of TB, which may facilitate disease transmission, it is crucial to diagnose infectious TB cases promptly and effectively [6]. Despite modern medical advances, the diagnosis and treatment of TB remain a formidable challenge, rendering an ancient disease a contemporary problem [7,8].

Although conventional methods such as smear microscopy and mycobacterial culture remain the major diagnostic tests for TB in resource-limited settings and most developing countries, these tests suffer from certain limitations [9,10]. As an example, smear microscopy has low sensitivity for the detection of acid-fast bacilli (AFB) in clinical specimens (5–10 $\times$ 10^4 AFB/mL), and mycobacterial culture is a time-consuming method, taking 3–8 weeks to conclude [11].

On the other hand, a pathogen's genome is a diagnostic biomarker for accurately identifying the causative agent of an infectious disease, and polymerase chain reaction (PCR) is the gold standard for identifying nucleic acids. To this end, PCR-based molecular methods have been widely studied to detect *Mycobacterium tuberculosis* (Mtb) with promising results [6,12–14]. Despite being highly sensitive and specific, these diagnostic methods have failed to replace smear and culture methods according to a report by the U.S. Centers for Disease Control and Prevention (CDC) [15].

Loop-mediated isothermal amplification (LAMP) is an attractive alternative technique for nucleic acid amplification [16] that has a promising prospect for the diagnosis of TB and has been recommended by the WHO for this purpose [17]. LAMP has several advantages over the conventional PCR-based assays: (i) it does not require DNA denaturation to amplify the target gene; (ii) the reaction is performed at a constant temperature obviating the need for expensive equipment; (iii) it is a highly specific reaction due to the use of six primers including two chimeric ones, recognizing eight distinct regions on the target sequence; (iv) the reaction is very efficient and rapid so it can generate more than 10^9 copies of the target gene within 15–60 min of incubation at 60–65 °C; and (v) it is less affected by the presence of inhibitor substances in clinical specimens [16,18].

Consequently, LAMP can be considered as an invaluable diagnostic method for various infectious diseases [18–20], demonstrating a high potential for being a point-of-care test [21,22]. However, LAMP is highly prone to carry-over contamination and the amplicons of the reaction can frequently lead to false-positive results, an issue of immense practical importance [23,24]. To this end, a closed tube LAMP assay has been proposed to address this concern via different approaches [25–28]. In fact, false-positive LAMP results can be avoided by visually reading the results with the naked eye, which is considered as a primary benefit of LAMP, which eliminates the requirement to open the reaction tube. Among the various methods for detecting LAMP products, visual endpoint evaluation of the reaction based on a color change or the presence of turbidity is preferred [22].

Fluorescence or metal ion indicator dyes such as calcein or hydroxy naphthol blue (HNB) are added to the LAMP reaction mixture in colorimetric approaches, and the test result is determined by changing the color of the reaction. Among all of the colorimetric methods studied to date, calcein and HNB are the most frequently used indicator dyes in LAMP assays [20,22,26,28]. Calcein is a fluorescence dye added along with $MnCl_2$ to the LAMP pre-reaction mixture. The primary color of the reaction is orange, since the combination of calcein with Mn^{2+} ions quenches calcein fluorescence. Manganese ions are replaced by Mg^{2+} ions as the LAMP products are produced due to an increased concentration of pyrophosphate ions in the reaction, which deprives the calcein of Mn^{2+} ions. The reaction turns yellow under visible light at this point [29]. Alternatively, HNB is a metal indicator whose color is determined by the concentration of Mg^{2+}. When magnesium ions are present, it turns violet; however, as the LAMP reaction proceeds, pyrophosphate ions are produced and combined with magnesium to form a magnesium pyrophosphate precipitate. The color of the reaction changes from violet to sky blue as the Mg^{2+} level decreases [26].

In the turbidimetric method, the white turbidity or precipitate of magnesium pyrophosphate as a LAMP by-product of the LAMP reaction indicates the reaction's positivity, which can be determined visually or with an optical instrument [27]. Both colorimetric and turbidimetric methods are observable with the naked eye [26–28,30].

Occasionally, DNA amplification may occur due to the formation of primer dimers, producing turbidity as a non-specific positive signal. Therefore, designing valid LAMP primers is critical when the turbidity method is used [22].

Obviously, the colorimetric detection of amplification products through the naked eye could increase the popularity of a molecular diagnostic tool, making it suitable for field application. Among all colorimetric detection methods, using a metal ion indicator dye is highly sensitive, straightforward, economical, and efficient. This kind of indicator is readily available and can be incorporated into the pre-reaction mixture [22,25]. However, the transition from violet to sky blue is too subtle in the HNB-mediated LAMP reaction, allowing for a subjective error in result interpretation [31]. This is also a problem with calcein as a fluorescence dye, whose color changes from orange to yellow under visible light. Therefore, as a major disadvantage, an "experienced eye" is needed to read the LAMP results while using these two colorimetric methods.

As a result, we screened other compounds to identify an alternative indicator for possible improvements in the detection of the LAMP reaction for TB diagnosis through the naked eye. In this regard, an alternative metal indicator with the same mechanism of action as HNB was identified and evaluated to detect Mtb. Eriochrome black T (EBT) is a newer and less studied magnesium ion indicator dye that can be directly added to the LAMP mixture to interpret the reaction result visually. Only one brief report on using EBT for the visual detection of Mtb by LAMP assay exists [32]. In this prototype study, however, the practical conditions of the optimal reaction and its performance on clinical specimens compared to the most frequently employed LAMP monitoring methods were not clarified.

Considering these facts, the present study aims to determine the optimal conditions of the EBT-mediated LAMP reaction and its diagnostic performance for visually detecting Mtb through naked eye observations. This study was conducted to determine whether EBT is an appropriate alternative to HNB/calcein to be applied in LAMP. In addition, we designed a closed tube LAMP assay to eliminate carry-over contamination from previous LAMP assays. This is the first report to our knowledge that compares the diagnostic performance of EBT-, HNB-, calcein-, and turbidity-based LAMP assays for the diagnosis of TB. The results may pave the way for the field application of LAMP technology for the rapid, dependable, and cost-effective detection of Mtb, particularly in settings with limited resources.

2. Materials and Methods

A flow chart representing the experimental approach of this study is shown in Figure 1. In detail, a primary step for LAMP reaction optimization is to prepare a template DNA after choosing the appropriate primer sets. Purified and crude DNA were obtained from Mtb cells and clinical specimens, respectively. LAMP primers can be newly designed using PrimerExplorer V4 software (Eiken Chemical Co. LTD, Tokyo, Japan) freely available from the Eiken Chemical Co. (https://primerexplorer.jp/e/, accessed on 21 December 2022), or obtained from previous studies, as conducted in this study [33]. Six primers were used in the LAMP reaction including two inner (FIP and BIP), two outer (F3 and B3), and two loop primers (FLP and BLP). Other necessary components of the pre-reaction mixture, in addition to the primer sets, are deoxyribonucleotides (dNTPs), Bst DNA polymerase, and a reaction buffer containing $MgSO_4$, used for the turbidimetric method. Additionally, HNB, calcein, and EBT were each individually added to the pre-reaction solution of the relevant LAMP assays to be monitored via colorimetric methods. In particular, EBT was optimized in the relevant reaction by utilizing different concentrations. Furthermore, various amounts of dNTPs and magnesium were individually added to the reaction of each method to determine their optimal levels. The optimal reaction time and limit of detection were identified for each detection method, respectively, by applying different duration times and Mtb DNA concentrations to each reaction. All reactions were performed at a constant temperature of 64 °C without requiring denaturation and annealing temperatures. Finally, each monitoring method was independently applied to the clinical specimens to evaluate their clinical performance and analyzed by StatsDirect version 3 (StatsDirect Ltd., Wirral, UK) and the McNemar's chi-square test.

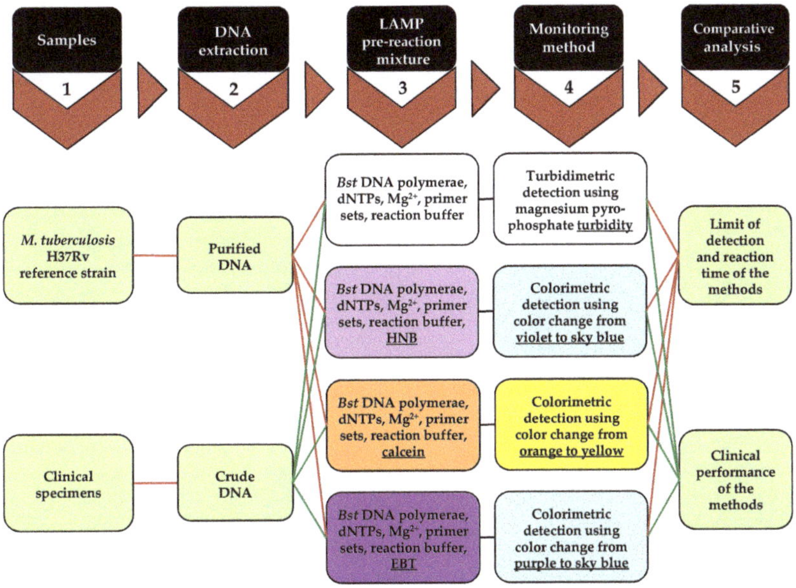

Figure 1. Flowchart representing the experimental approach including stages and methods utilized for comparative closed tube TB-LAMP using the four naked eye methodology for amplification detection. LAMP: loop-mediated isothermal amplification; HNB: hydroxy naphthol blue; EBT: eriochrome black T.

2.1. DNA Extraction

Genomic DNA used in the present study was extracted and purified from the *M. tuberculosis* H37Rv reference strain to optimize the LAMP reactions and determine the limit of detection (LOD) of each method. For this purpose, mycobacterial colonies were suspended in TE buffer (10 mM Tris-HCl, pH 8.0, and 1 mM EDTA) and heat killed at 80 °C for one hour. The mixture was incubated overnight at 37 °C in the presence of 1 mg/mL lysozyme (Sigma-Aldrich, St. Louis, MO, USA) while shaking. Bacterial lysis was performed by the addition of 1.5% SDS and 100 µg/mL proteinase K (Fermentas Life Sciences, Vilnius, Lithuania), followed by incubation at 65 °C for 10 min. Then, the suspension was treated by 5 M NaCl and CTAB-NaCl solution (10% CTAB plus 0.7 M NaCl) at 65 °C for another 10 min. Genomic DNA was purified and precipitated, respectively, using chloroform–isoamyl alcohol (24:1) and isopropanol. Finally, the pellet was washed with 70% ethanol and dissolved in 50 µL of TE buffer for use in the subsequent experiments [34].

To determine the clinical performance of each assay, clinical specimens were initially processed by Petroff's method [35]. Then, DNA was extracted from the clinical specimens by a simple boiling method described by Afghani and Stutman [36]. Briefly, after washing each specimen with TE buffer twice, the pellet was boiled for 5–10 min followed by a quick spin down of the tube. The supernatant was kept at −20 °C before use as the template DNA in the subsequent experiments.

2.2. LAMP Primers and Assays

The LAMP reactions were carried out using six primers targeting the *M. tuberculosis* 16S rRNA gene as previously described by Pandey et al. [33]. The primer sequences were as follows: F3, 5′-CTGGCTCAGGACGAACG-3′; B3, 5′-GCTCATCCCACACCGC-3′; FIP, 5′-CACCCACGTGTTACTCATGCCAGTCGAACGGAAAGGTCT-3′; BIP, 5′-TCGGGA-

TAAGCCTGGACCACCAGACATGCATCCCGT-3′; FLP, 5′- GTTCGCCACTCGAGTAT-CTCCG-3′; and BLP, 5′-GAAACTGGGTCTAAATACCGG-3′.

LAMP assays were performed in a total volume of 25 μL containing 1.6 μM each of the inner primers (FIP and BIP), 0.2 μM each of the outer primers (F3 and B3), 0.8 μM each of the loop primers (FLP and BLP), 0.8 M betaine (Sigma-Aldrich, St. Louis, MO, USA), 1X ThermoPol reaction buffer (New England Biolabs, Ipswich, MA, USA), 8 U *Bst* DNA polymerase (New England Biolabs), and 1 ng purified DNA from *M. tuberculosis* H37Rv. To determine the optimal condition leading to the most distinct visual result, various concentrations of $MgSO_4$ (Figure 2) and dNTPs (Figure 3) were also applied to the LAMP reactions of each monitoring method.

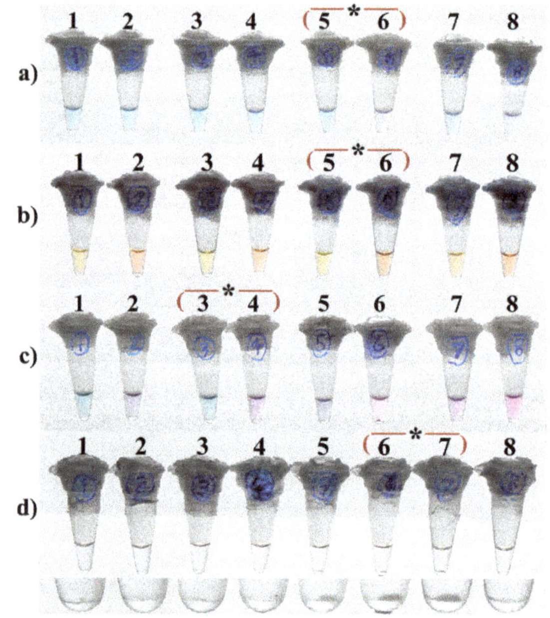

Figure 2. Optimization of Mg^{2+} concentration in HNB-LAMP (**a**), Calcein-LAMP (**b**), EBT-LAMP (**c**), and turbidity-LAMP (**d**) for the detection of *M. tuberculosis*. (**a**,**c**) 2.5 mM (tubes 1 and 2), 3.5 mM (tubes 3 and 4), 4.5 mM (tubes 5 and 6), and 5.5 mM (tubes 7 and 8) $MgSO_4$. (**b**) 4 mM (tubes 1 and 2), 6 mM (tubes 3 and 4), 8 mM (tubes 5 and 6), and 10 mM (tubes 7 and 8) $MgSO_4$. Tubes with even and odd numbers, respectively, represent negative and positive reactions. In (**d**), tubes 1 to 7 are positive reactions, respectively, containing 2, 3, 4, 5, 6, 8, and 10 mM $MgSO_4$, and tube 8 is the negative control. The image on the bottom shows the close-up view of (**d**) focused on the pellets of pyrophosphate magnesium. The asterisks indicate the optimal concentration of Mg^{2+}.

For colorimetric LAMP reactions, 25 μM calcein (Sigma-Aldrich) plus 0.5 mM $MnCl_2$ (Sigma-Aldrich), and 9 mM HNB (Sigma-Aldrich) were also added to calcein- and HNB-LAMP assays, respectively.

Due to the limited studies, the EBT concentration was additionally optimized in the relevant reaction (Table 1). For this purpose, 40, 60, 80, 100, and 120 mM EBT (Sigma-Aldrich) were individually applied to the LAMP reaction along with a negative control for each concentration. The negative controls contained all components of the reaction except the template DNA, which was replaced by sterile distilled water. The optimal concentration of EBT was determined by visually inspecting the reaction tubes every 15 min up to 180 min to obtain the most distinct color change between the test tube and its relevant negative control.

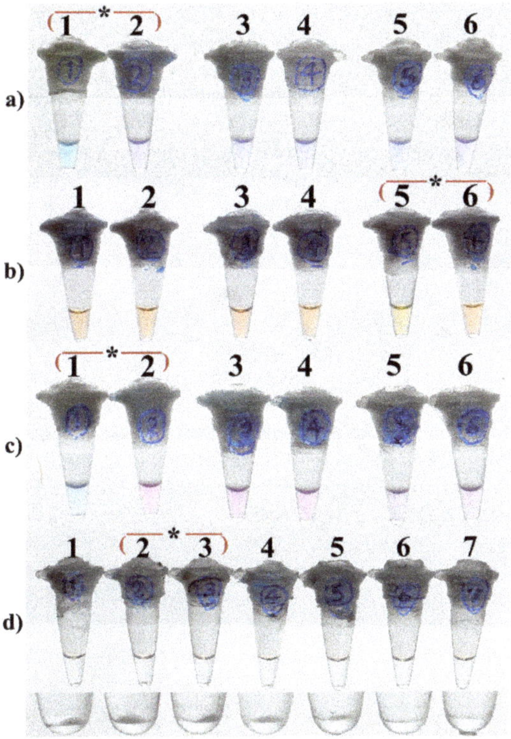

Figure 3. Optimization of the dNTP concentration in HNB-LAMP (**a**), Calcein-LAMP (**b**), EBT-LAMP (**c**), and turbidity-LAMP (**d**) for the detection of *M. tuberculosis*. (**a–c**) 0.5 mM (tubes 1 and 2), 1 mM (tubes 3 and 4), and 1.4 mM (tubes 5 and 6) dNTPs. Tubes with even and odd numbers, respectively, represent negative and positive reactions. In (**d**), tubes 1 to 6 are positive reactions, respectively, containing 0.5, 1, 1.4, 2, 2.5, and 3 mM dNTPs, and tube 7 is the negative control. The image on the bottom shows the close-up view of (**d**) focused on the pellets of pyrophosphate magnesium. The asterisks indicate the optimal concentration of Mg^{2+}.

Table 1. Determination of the optimal concentration of EBT in the LAMP assay by applying different duration times to the reactions.

LAMP Reaction Time (min)	EBT Concentrations (μM)				
	40	60	80	100	120
15	−	−	−	−	−
30	+	+	−	−	−
45	+	+	−	−	−
60	+	+	−	−	−
75	+	+	−	−	−
90	+	+	−	−	−
105	+	+	−	−	−
120	+	+	−	−	−
135	+	+	−	−	−
150	+	+	+	−	−
180	+	+	+	−	−

Note. The most distinct color change was observed at 60 μM EBT between the positive and negative reactions after 30 min (pink-colored column). Although the reactions were positive at 40 and 80 μM EBT, respectively, after 30 and 150 min, the color change between the positive and negative reactions were less distinctive at these concentrations (grey-colored column). +, positive LAMP reaction; −, negative LAMP reaction; EBT, eriochrome black T.

The color changes in the reactions from orange to yellow in calcein-LAMP, violet to sky blue in HNB-LAMP, and purple to sky blue in EBT-LAMP were considered as a positive result.

For turbidity-LAMP, the presence and the size of a white pellet at the bottom of the reaction tube following a quick spin-down were respectively considered as a positive and an optimal result (Figures 2d and 3d).

All the reactions were incubated at 64 °C and the results were monitored by the naked eye. To prevent accidental opening of the reaction tubes, the tubes' caps were kept in a sealed position by the use of Parafilm® (Bemis Inc., Neenah, WI, USA). To evaluate reproducibility of the results, each assay was performed three times.

2.3. Limit of Detection and Optimal Reaction Time

First, the concentration of a solution containing purified DNA from *M. tuberculosis* H37Rv was measured three times at 260 nm by a NanoDrop ND-1000 Spectrophotometer (NanoDrop Technologies Inc., Rockland, DE, USA). Afterward, the average of these values was considered as the true concentration to prepare a 10-fold serial dilution of Mtb DNA in 10 mM Tris-HCl (pH 8.8), ranging from 100 ng/µL to 1 fg/µL. To determine the limit of detection (LOD) of the LAMP assays, 1 µL of each dilution was applied to the optimal reactions of each monitoring method as the template DNA. For all of the monitoring methods, the LOD was determined in a single day using the same serial dilution to ensure comparability of the results. To precisely determine the LOD of the LAMP monitoring methods, 20 replicates of the minimum detectable concentration of Mtb DNA were tested by each method, and this concentration was confirmed as the LOD for the respective method, if positive results were obtained in ≥95% of all 20 replicates.

To determine the optimal reaction time, the results were visually inspected and recorded every 15 min for each method. The experiment was performed on two different days using two distinct set of serial dilutions to assess the intra-day reproducibility of the results.

2.4. Clinical Evaluation of LAMP Assays

To evaluate the clinical performance for each monitoring method of LAMP, 30 clinical specimens including 17 sputum and 13 bronchoalveolar lavage (BAL) samples were collected from TB-confirmed patients referred to the Laboratory of Tuberculosis, Ghaem University Hospital, Mashhad, Iran. All of the specimens were smear- and culture-positive for AFB and Mtb, respectively. Mycobacterial culture was used as the gold standard for laboratory confirmation of TB cases. Clinical specimens were included in our study after completion of their routine requested tests and subjected to discard.

Five microliters of crude DNA from each clinical specimen was individually applied to the optimal reaction of each monitoring method of LAMP. Then, the results of the four monitoring methods were compared. Negative and positive controls were always included in each run of the experiment. The negative control contained all reactants minus the target DNA and the positive control contained *M. tuberculosis* H37Rv purified DNA in place of the clinical specimens' DNA.

3. Results

3.1. Optimal Concentration

As can be deduced from Table 1, both LAMP reactions containing 40 and 60 µM EBT were positive after 30 min and remained unchanged by extending the reaction time. In the presence of higher concentrations of EBT, however, LAMP was either positive after 150 min (80 µM EBT) or totally negative (100 and 120 µM EBT), probably due to the inhibitory effect of the indicator dye (Table 1). Because the presence of 60 µM EBT in the LAMP reaction yielded the most distinct color change from purple to sky blue between the negative and positive assays, it was considered as the optimal concentration of EBT in subsequent LAMP assays.

3.2. Optimal Concentrations of Mg^{2+}

As demonstrated in Figure 2a,c, 4.5 and 3.5 mM $MgSO_4$ yielded the most distinctive visual results, respectively, for the HNB-, and EBT-LAMP assays. In the same way, the optimal concentration of $MgSO_4$ for the calcein-LAMP assay was determined as 8 mM (Figure 2b), while both 6 mM and 8 mM $MgSO_4$ resulted in the same pellet size of magnesium pyrophosphate at the bottom of the reaction tubes for the turbidity-LAMP assay (Figure 2d, tubes 6 and 7).

3.3. Optimal Concentrations of dNTPs

As shown in Figure 3a–c, 0.5 and 1.4 mM dNTPs were yielded the most distinct color change between positive and negative reactions respectively for HNB-/EBT- and calcein-LAMP assays. Additionally, the optimal concentration of dNTPs for turbidity-LAMP was 1 or 1.4 mM, as both concentrations resulted in the largest size of magnesium pyrophosphate pellet at the bottom of the reaction tubes (Figure 3d, tubes 2 & 3).

3.4. LOD and Optimal Time of the Reactions

HNB- and turbidity-LAMP assays were able to detect up to 100 fg purified DNA of *M. tuberculosis* H37Rv per reaction (Figure 4a,d). This was achieved through an optimal reaction time of 15 and 30 min, respectively, for the turbidity and HNB-LAMP assays and remained unchanged by extending the duration time of the reactions (Table 2). Moreover, the LOD was 1 pg DNA/reaction for the calcein- and EBT-LAMP assays (Figure 4b,c). The optimal time to positivity of the reactions for the detection of this amount of DNA was 15 and 30 min, respectively, for the calcein- and EBT-LAMP assays. Additionally, no change was observed with extra reaction time (Table 2). In fact, calcein and EBT led to a one-log reduction in the LOD of the relevant LAMP assays compared to the turbidity- and HNB-LAMP assays.

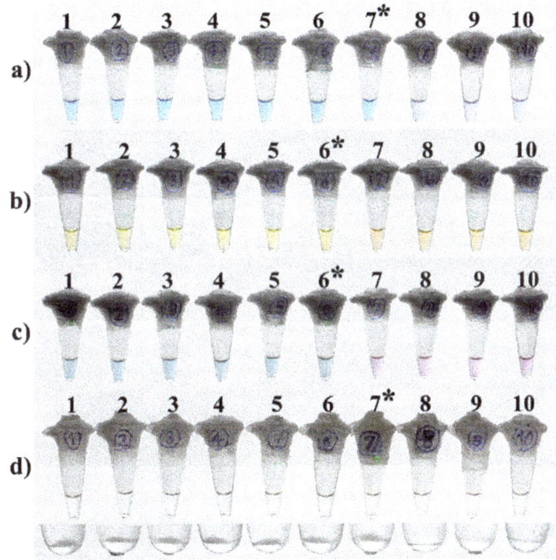

Figure 4. Comparison of the LOD of HNB-LAMP (**a**), Calcein-LAMP (**b**), EBT-LAMP (**c**), and turbidity-LAMP (**d**) for the diagnosis of TB. Tubes 1 to 10, respectively, contain 100 ng, 10 ng, 1 ng, 100 pg, 10 pg, 1 pg, 100 fg, 10 fg, 1 fg, and zero amount of Mtb DNA/reaction. The lower part of the figure shows the close-up view of (**d**) focused on the bottom of the tubes. The asterisks indicate the LOD of each method.

Table 2. LAMP monitoring methods performed on various DNA concentrations/reaction with different duration times of reaction for the determination of the optimal reaction time capable of detecting the lowest amount of the Mtb DNA/reaction.

Reaction Time [a]	Method	Mtb Purified DNA/Reaction (25 μL)									
		100 ng	10 ng	1 ng	100 pg	10 pg	1 pg	100 fg	10 fg	1 fg	0
15 min	HNB-LAMP	−	−	−	−	−	−	−	−	−	−
	Calcein-LAMP	+	+	+	+	+	+	−	−	−	−
	EBT-LAMP	−	−	−	−	−	−	−	−	−	−
	Turbidity-LAMP	+	+	+	+	+	+	+	−	−	−
30 min	HNB-LAMP	+	+	+	+	+	+	+	−	−	−
	Calcein-LAMP	+	+	+	+	+	+	−	−	−	−
	EBT-LAMP	+	+	+	+	+	+	−	−	−	−
	Turbidity-LAMP	+	+	+	+	+	+	+	−	−	−
45 min	HNB-LAMP	+	+	+	+	+	+	+	−	−	−
	Calcein-LAMP	+	+	+	+	+	+	−	−	−	−
	EBT-LAMP	+	+	+	+	+	+	−	−	−	−
	Turbidity-LAMP	+	+	+	+	+	+	+	−	−	−

+, positive LAMP reaction; −, negative LAMP reaction; Mtb, *Mycobacterium tuberculosis*. [a] By extending the reaction time to 120 min, no change was achieved in the results of any monitoring methods of LAMP compared to those obtained in the thirtieth minute of the reactions.

In contrast to the calcein- and turbidity LAMP assays, no positive signal was achieved for HNB- and EBT-LAMP within the first 15 min of the amplification process, even at the higher concentrations of DNA (Table 2). By performing the experiment on two different days and on separate sets of serial dilutions of Mtb DNA, the results were shown to be reproducible. Moreover, all 20 replicates containing 100 fg/μL and 1 pg/μL Mtb DNA (the lowest detectable concentrations) were individually positive with turbidity-/HNB-LAMP and calcein-/EBT-LAMP, respectively.

3.5. Clinical Evaluation

In the present study, all the clinical specimens from TB-confirmed patients were positive by the turbidity-LAMP assay, with a diagnostic sensitivity of 100% (95% CI, 78.2–100%) for this method and perfect agreement between the turbidity-LAMP and mycobacterial culture as the gold standard for TB diagnosis. Only two out of thirty TB-confirmed sputum specimens were negative by the HNB-, calcein-, and EBT-LAMP. Interestingly, these two negative samples belonged to two particular TB patients whose disease could not be detected by all these colorimetric methods. Therefore, diagnostic sensitivity for the HNB-, calcein-, and EBT-LAMP assays was 93.3% (95% CI, 77.9–99.2%). Moreover, all negative controls applied to each run of the experiments were negative, indicating no false-positive result for all the LAMP detection methods evaluated in this study (specificity 100%). Finally, positive and negative predictive values were 100% and 88.2%, respectively, for the colorimetric LAMP methods.

According to the comparative analysis, the HNB-, calcein-, and EBT-LAMP assays each showed an agreement of 95.6% with a Cohen's kappa of 0.91 with turbidity-LAMP, indicating almost complete similarity of the four monitoring methods. However, more distinct color change was observed between the positive and negative EBT-LAMP reactions, proving the lowest error due to subjectivity for this method.

4. Discussion

Although LAMP is superior to conventional nucleic acid amplification techniques in terms of speed and cost, it is more susceptible to carry-over contamination with secondary LAMP products, preventing widespread application [23–25]. This is due to the high efficiency of the reaction, which produces about 100–1000 times more amplicons than other methods such as PCR [37].

Observing the ladder-like pattern of the amplicons during agarose gel electrophoresis of LAMP products stained with a DNA intercalating dye can be used as a reference method for evaluating the assay result [16]. However, it cannot be used as the monitoring method of choice for LAMP because of the need to open the reaction tube cap and subsequent laboratory contamination with LAMP products. Frequently, the contamination problem is so severe that replacing micropipettes, pipette tips, reagents, and tubes and even relocating the testing area is essential [24]. Obviously, this will add some costs to an intrinsically inexpensive technique.

Therefore, improving LAMP monitoring methods is a research priority to facilitate the field application of this invaluable technology. However, care must be taken not to sacrifice LAMP's advantageous characteristics such as its simplicity and cost-effectiveness.

In order to introduce a reliable monitoring method for LAMP, we employed a closed tube system to prevent the contamination of subsequent experiments with amplicons. Consequently, gel electrophoresis analysis was not the method of choice to monitor LAMP products in the current study.

To date, several strategies have been proposed to address the contamination problem utilizing a closed tube system such as the LAMP monitoring method [25,26,28,38]. This system does not allow for the opening of the reaction tube cap for the reasons above-mentioned. Instead, the result of the LAMP assay was determined through the inspection of turbidity or the color change of the reaction. This approach will certainly prevent obtaining false-positive results in downstream LAMP assays [25,38].

Mori et al. introduced this method to improve LAMP-based assays practically for the first time. They interpreted the LAMP results using the turbidity caused by the formation of magnesium pyrophosphate in the reaction. According to reports, this turbidimetric method can be used with the naked eye or, for greater accuracy, a real-time turbidimeter device. Additionally, Mori et al. suggested centrifuging the LAMP tubes at 6000 rpm for several seconds at the end of the reaction [27]. This would aid in a more straightforward visual judgment of the LAMP results by inspecting the white pellet of the magnesium pyrophosphate precipitate at the bottom of the reaction tube. In the current study, this method was also used for the turbidimetric LAMP method. As reported by others [19,39], we concluded that the interpretation of LAMP results based solely on the visual monitoring of the reaction turbidity is a subjective and error-prone judgment, especially while dealing with weak-positive results. We examined the white pellet at the bottom of an illuminated reaction tube with a loupe magnifier to improve this monitoring method. Our findings revealed that the visual monitoring of the reaction turbidity by this modified approach was one of the most sensitive monitoring methods of LAMP evaluated in the present study. Accordingly, this approach found the LOD of the LAMP assay to be 100 fg of the purified Mtb DNA/reaction.

Global efforts to develop a reliable method for monitoring the production of LAMP amplicons in a closed system resulted in an innovation in LAMP technology by employing calcein (plus $MnCl_2$) in the reaction mixture. This metal ion indicator was initially reported in the LAMP reaction by Boehme et al. [29], and Tomita et al. [28] who published a detailed protocol. In this method, calcein is deprived of Mn^{2+} by pyrophosphate ions accumulated in the reaction during the amplification of target DNA, and instead, it binds to magnesium ions. This will result in a more intense bright green fluorescent emission of the reaction under UV light or a visible color change from orange to yellow of the reaction under visible light [28].

Further studies have shown that adding calcein and $MnCl_2$ in the LAMP reaction would reduce the test's sensitivity [40,41]. Yang et al. determined the sensitivity of the LAMP assay targeting IS*1081* for the diagnosis of tuberculous pleurisy [41]. The sensitivity was determined to be 100 fg and 1 pg of purified Mtb DNA using gel electrophoresis and the calcein visual inspection method, respectively. They achieved these results by applying both 60 and 90 min incubation times to the reactions [41]. In our study where the visual turbidimetric method was used instead of gel electrophoresis analysis, calcein-LAMP showed a 10-fold reduction in sensitivity for the detection of Mtb compared to the turbidimetric method (Figure 4b,d). This result is consistent with the findings of Yang et al. and other researchers [40,41], as we previously reported equal detection sensitivity for the turbidimetric and gel electrophoresis methods [18,24]. Two reasons have been proposed for the reduced sensitivity of the calcein-LAMP reaction: (i) the inhibition of LAMP reaction by Mn^{2+} [26,40]; and (ii) the direct interaction between calcein and dsDNA [42]. Nevertheless, calcein is widely used in various LAMP assays [37,41,43], even in the only WHO-recommended LAMP for TB (Loopamp™ MTBC Detection Kit, Eiken Chemical Co., Ltd., Tokyo, Japan) [17].

HNB is an additional metal ion indicator dye initially described by Goto et al. for visually detecting lambda phage DNA using the LAMP technique [26]. This indicator turns violet in the presence of Mg^{2+} when added to the LAMP reaction. During the amplification process, a significant amount of magnesium is used to produce insoluble magnesium pyrophosphate as the main by-product of the reaction. As a result of the decrease in magnesium concentration, the reaction color transforms from violet to sky blue, signifying a positive test result.

Our findings demonstrated that HNB-LAMP was ten times more sensitive than calcein-LAMP for Mtb detection (Figure 4a,b). This is consistent with the lambda phage DNA results reported by Goto et al. [26].

In recent years, EBT's usefulness in the LAMP process for visualizing the reaction's result has garnered increased attention [32,44,45]. The mechanism of action for this metal ion indicator dye is comparable to that of HNB; however, EBT produces distinctive color changes between negative and positive reactions. Briefly, the addition of EBT causes the reaction solution to turn purple because it binds to magnesium ions. As the target DNA is amplified by LAMP, magnesium ions are depleted from EBT due to the production of magnesium pyrophosphate and a decrease in the level of magnesium ions. This leads to the color change of the reaction from purple to sky blue, indicating a positive LAMP assay.

Wang utilized the same set of LAMP primers as Yang et al. in the sole brief report on the use of EBT for the visual detection of Mtb via the LAMP assay [32,41]. Surprisingly, Wang reported a sensitivity of 8 fg Mtb genomic DNA for the EBT-LAMP assay using a 45-min reaction [32]. However, the study lacked an explanation for why a LAMP reaction containing the same set of primers achieved 100-fold higher sensitivity than that reported by Yang et al. More interestingly, this result was obtained with a shorter EBT-LAMP reaction time [32,41]. This is inconsistent with our findings, in which EBT-LAMP showed a 10-fold reduction in sensitivity compared to the turbidimetric LAMP assay. Additionally, we demonstrated that the shorter the reaction time, the lower the test sensitivity (Table 2). In addition, we utilized the identical set of LAMP primers as Pandey et al. In contrast to Wang's findings, the sensitivity of turbidimetric- and HNB-LAMP in our study was comparable to that of real-time turbidimetric-LAMP (100 fg purified Mtb DNA/reaction), as determined by Pandey et al. [33].

Although EBT-LAMP was 10-fold less sensitive than turbidimetric- and HNB-LAMP in the present study, its analytical sensitivity was equivalent to that of the widely used calcein-LAMP method. In addition, reading the results of the EBT-LAMP assay was less susceptible to subjective error than the calcein- and HNB-LAMP assays (Table 3) due to the more distinct color change between its negative and positive reactions (Figure 4). This is of the utmost importance when LAMP is performed by an inexperienced individual, given that one of the primary goals of health organizations is to simplify diagnostic tests, so that they can be utilized in remote and resource-poor settings [46]. Although color change between negative and positive reactions of calcein-LAMP is more distinctive under UV light than visible light, it should be noted that the need for a UV transilluminator device would add an extra cost to the test.

Table 3. A brief comparison among the four monitoring methods of LAMP used in this study for Mtb detection.

	LAMP Monitoring Methods [a]			
	T-LAMP	**C-LAMP**	**H-LAMP**	**E-LAMP**
Principle	Turbidimetry	Colorimetry	Colorimetry	Colorimetry
Mechanism	Mg_2PPi precipitation results in the formation of white turbidity in the reaction	Sequestering of Mn^{2+} from calcein results in the color change of this metal ion indicator dye	Sequestering of Mg^{2+} from hydroxynaphtol Blue leads to a color change of the indicator	Sequestering of Mg^{2+} from eriochrome black T leads to a color change of the indicator
LAMP results (negative/positive)	Clear/Turbid	Orange/Yellow	Violet/Sky blue	Purple/Sky blue
Visual inspection of results	Yes	Yes	Yes	Yes
Performing in closed system	Yes	Yes	Yes	Yes
Potential for subjective error in reading the result	High	High	High	Low
LOD [b]	100 fg	1 pg	100 fg	1 pg
Diagnostic sensitivity (%)	100	93.3	93.3	93.3
Additional cost [c]	None	++	++++	+
O.C. of each indicator/reaction [d]	-	25 μM	4.5 mM	60 μM
Time-to-positivity of LAMP (min.)	15	15	30	30
Inhibitory effect on LAMP reaction	None	Yes, a 10-fold reduction in LOD at optimal concentration	No inhibitory effect at optimal concentration	Yes, a 10-fold reduction in LOD at optimal concentration

[a] T; turbidity, C; calcein, H; HNB (hydroxynaphtol blue), E; EBT (eriochrome black T). [b] LOD; limit of detection. [c] The colorimetric LAMP reactions are slightly more costly to perform compared to the T-LAMP assay because of the additional usage of a metal ion indicator dye in each reaction. Although the extra cost was much less than a dollar, the amount varied among different colorimetric methods. [d] O.C., optimal concentration.

Moreover, our results showed that calcein-LAMP could provide a positive result 15 min earlier than the HNB- and EBT-LAMP assays at the lowest detectable concentration of Mtb DNA (Table 2). We hypothesized that any delay in the positivity of the colorimetric LAMP assays could be attributed to the concentration of each indicator dye in the related reaction. Since the lowest concentration of indicator dye (25 μM) was applied to the calcein-LAMP assay with a time-to-positivity similar to turbidity-LAMP where no indicator dye was used (Table 3), we believe that the 10-fold lower sensitivity of the calcein- and EBT-LAMP assays in comparison to the HNB-LAMP assay may have distinct causes.

First, as previously stated, the functional calcein-LAMP assay depends on the reaction's simultaneous use of $MnCl_2$ and calcein. Thus, based on our findings, the 10-fold less sensitivity of calcein-LAMP appears more likely to be due to the inhibition of the reaction by Mn^{2+} ions than to the calcein itself since (in contrast to HNB and EBT) calcein did not cause any delay in the time-to-positivity of the LAMP reaction at the optimal concentration used in this study (Table 2). This is consistent with the explanations provided by Goto et al. [26] and Wastling et al. [40], in contrast to the earlier-mentioned study by Zhang et al. [42].

Second, EBT and HNB have similar chemical structures except that they contain one and three sulfur trioxide groups (SO_3), respectively. In other words, the negative charge of HNB is twice that of EBT. This means that the possible interaction between EBT and the negatively charged backbone of DNA is more likely to occur in the LAMP reaction than between HNB and DNA. This appears to be the possible reason for our research's 10-fold less sensitivity of EBT-LAMP compared to HNB-LAMP.

Superior to Wang's study, a comparative evaluation of four monitoring methods of LAMP on the clinical specimens was also performed in the current research [32]. We showed that the clinical performance of turbidity-LAMP, lacking any indicator dye in the reaction, was perfect in the TB-confirmed cases (100% positivity rate). However, the LAMP positivity rate was slightly lower (93.3%, 28/30) for all of the colorimetric methods. In fact, two clinical specimens produced false-negative results for all of the colorimetric methods in contrast to the turbidimetric LAMP. We hypothesized that these two samples contained inhibitory substances that interacted synergistically with the indicator dyes or Mn^{2+} ions, in the case of calcein-LAMP, to inhibit the colorimetric reactions. Since these two false-negative results were associated with two specific clinical specimens, our opinion is more probable. Practically, the sensitivity of colorimetric LAMP could be enhanced by adding substances such as guanidine chloride to the reaction, as reported elsewhere [31]. Finally, it should be noted that the clinical performance of a diagnostic tool might be lower for extrapulmonary TB specimens than the pulmonary specimens used in our study. This is due to the paucibacillary nature of the extrapulmonary TB specimens [13]. Therefore, future study needs to be performed to reveal the diagnostic performance of the mentioned LAMP monitoring methods for the extrapulmonary TB specimens.

5. Conclusions

Overall, among the four LAMP monitoring methods evaluated in this study, the following conclusions can be drawn. (1) The visual turbidimetric method provided the best analytical (100 fg) and diagnostic (100%) sensitivities as well as the quickest time-to-positivity (15 min). However, it is highly prone to subjective error while interpreting the results. (2) The HNB method resulted in the highest analytical sensitivity (100 fg) among the visual colorimetric methods, although its diagnostic sensitivity (93.3%) was identical to those of calcein- and EBT-LAMP. (3) Similar to the turbidimetric method, calcein-LAMP demonstrated the shortest time-to-positivity (15 min) compared to the other two colorimetric methods (30 min). (4) The EBT method showed the lowest potential for subjective error while interpreting the results by generating the most distinct color change between negative and positive reactions under visible light. (5) EBT and HNB colorimetric methods for LAMP were performed at the lowest and highest costs, respectively (Table 3). Finally, the findings of this study may contribute to the field applicability of LAMP technology. Nonetheless, it is possible to find other chemical compounds with comparable properties such as murexide, which will need to be investigated in future studies.

Author Contributions: Conceptualization, A.N. and E.A.; Methodology, A.N., H.S. (Hamid Sadeghian), H.S. (Hadi Safdari) and E.A.; Validation, H.S. (Hamid Sadeghian), H.S. (Hadi Safdari) and B.R.-Z.; Formal analysis, A.N., H.S. (Hamid Sadeghian) and H.S. (Hadi Safdari).; Investigation, A.N. and E.A.; Data curation, A.N. and E.A.; Writing—original draft preparation, A.N. and H.Z.; Writing—review and editing, E.A. and B.R.-Z.; Visualization, A.N. and E.A.; Supervision, project administration and funding acquisition, E.A. All authors have read and agreed to the published version of the manuscript.

Funding: This research was funded by the Vice Chancellorship for Research at Mashhad University of Medical Sciences, Mashhad, Iran; grant number 921957.

Institutional Review Board Statement: Not applicable.

Informed Consent Statement: Not applicable.

Data Availability Statement: Not applicable.

Acknowledgments: The authors gratefully thank Samad Aryan, the professional photographer, for taking the high-quality photographs of the LAMP reaction tubes.

Conflicts of Interest: The authors declare no conflict of interest.

References

1. Nicklisch, N.; Maixner, F.; Ganslmeier, R.; Friederich, S.; Dresely, V.; Meller, H.; Zink, A.; Alt, K.W. Rib lesions in skeletons from early neolithic sites in Central Germany: On the trail of tuberculosis at the onset of agriculture. *Am. J. Phys. Anthropol.* **2012**, *149*, 391–404. [CrossRef]
2. Barberis, I.; Bragazzi, N.L.; Galluzzo, L.; Martini, M. The history of tuberculosis: From the first historical records to the isolation of Koch's bacillus. *J. Prev. Med. Hyg.* **2017**, *58*, E9–E12. [PubMed]
3. Cardona, P.J.; Català, M.; Prats, C. Origin of tuberculosis in the Paleolithic predicts unprecedented population growth and female resistance. *Sci. Rep.* **2020**, *10*, 42. [CrossRef] [PubMed]
4. Coleman, M.; Martinez, L.; Theron, G.; Wood, R.; Marais, B. *Mycobacterium tuberculosis* transmission in high-incidence settings-new paradigms and insights. *Pathogens* **2022**, *11*, 1228. [CrossRef] [PubMed]
5. World Health Organization. *Global Tuberculosis Report 2022*; WHO: Geneva, Switzerland, 2022.
6. MacGregor-Fairlie, M.; Wilkinson, S.; Besra, G.S.; Goldberg Oppenheimer, P. Tuberculosis diagnostics: Overcoming ancient challenges with modern solutions. *Emerg. Top. Life Sci.* **2020**, *4*, 435–448.
7. Harries, A.D.; Kumar, A.M.V. Challenges and progress with diagnosing pulmonary tuberculosis in low- and middle-income countries. *Diagnostics* **2018**, *8*, 78. [CrossRef]
8. Böncüoğlu, E.; Akaslan Kara, A.; Bayram, N.; Devrim, İ.; Kiymet, E.; Çağlar, İ.; Demirağ, B.; Eraslan, C.; Bolat, E.; Ertan, Y.; et al. A diagnostic challenge is it tuberculosis? *Pediatr. Infect. Dis. J.* **2022**, *41*, e254. [CrossRef]
9. Parsons, L.M.; Somoskövi, Á.; Gutierrez, C.; Lee, E.; Paramasivan, C.; Abimiku, A.l.; Spector, S.; Roscigno, G.; Nkengasong, J. Laboratory diagnosis of tuberculosis in resource-poor countries: Challenges and opportunities. *Clin. Microbiol. Rev.* **2011**, *24*, 314–350. [CrossRef]
10. Kivihya-Ndugga, L.; van Cleeff, M.; Juma, E.; Kimwomi, J.; Githui, W.; Oskam, L.; Schuitema, A.; van Soolingen, D.; Nganga, L.; Kibuga, D. Comparison of PCR with the routine procedure for diagnosis of tuberculosis in a population with high prevalences of tuberculosis and human immunodeficiency virus. *J. Clin. Microbiol.* **2004**, *42*, 1012–1015. [CrossRef]
11. Gillespie, S.H. Mycobacterium tuberculosis. In *Principles and Practice of Clinical Bacteriology*, 2nd ed.; Gillespie, S.H., Hawkey, P.M., Eds.; John Wiley & Sons Ltd.: Chichester, UK, 2006; pp. 159–169.
12. Sankar, S.; Ramamurthy, M.; Nandagopal, B.; Sridharan, G. An appraisal of PCR-based technology in the detection of *Mycobacterium tuberculosis*. *Mol. Diagn. Ther.* **2011**, *15*, 1–11. [CrossRef]
13. Wang, H.-Y.; Lu, J.-J.; Chang, C.-Y.; Chou, W.-P.; Hsieh, J.C.-H.; Lin, C.-R.; Wu, M.-H. Development of a high sensitivity TaqMan-based PCR assay for the specific detection of *Mycobacterium tuberculosis* complex in both pulmonary and extrapulmonary specimens. *Sci. Rep.* **2019**, *9*, 113. [CrossRef] [PubMed]
14. Mor, P.; Dahiya, B.; Sharma, S.; Sheoran, A.; Parshad, S.; Malhotra, P.; Gulati, P.; Mehta, P.K. Diagnosis of peritoneal tuberculosis by real-time immuno-PCR assay based on detection of a cocktail of *Mycobacterium tuberculosis* CFP-10 and HspX proteins. *Expert Rev. Gastroenterol. Hepatol.* **2022**, *16*, 577–586. [CrossRef] [PubMed]
15. Center for Disease Control and Prevention (CDC). Updated guidelines for the use of nucleic acid amplification tests in the diagnosis of tuberculosis. *Morb. Mortal. Wkly. Rep.* **2009**, *58*, 7–10.
16. Notomi, T.; Okayama, H.; Masubuchi, H.; Yonekawa, T.; Watanabe, K.; Amino, N.; Hase, T. Loop-mediated isothermal amplification of DNA. *Nucleic Acids Res.* **2000**, *28*, e63. [CrossRef] [PubMed]
17. World Health Organization (WHO). *The Use of Loop-Mediated Isothermal Amplification (TB-LAMP) for the Diagnosis of Pulmonary Tuberculosis: Policy Guidance*; World Health Organization: Geneva, Switzerland, 2016.
18. Aryan, E.; Makvandi, M.; Farajzadeh, A.; Huygen, K.; Alvandi, A.-H.; Gouya, M.-M.; Sadrizadeh, A.; Romano, M. Clinical value of IS*6110*-based loop-mediated isothermal amplification for detection of *Mycobacterium tuberculosis* complex in respiratory specimens. *J. Infect.* **2013**, *66*, 487–493. [CrossRef] [PubMed]
19. Wong, Y.P.; Othman, S.; Lau, Y.L.; Radu, S.; Chee, H.Y. Loop-mediated isothermal amplification (LAMP): A versatile technique for detection of micro-organisms. *J. Appl. Microbiol.* **2018**, *124*, 626–643. [CrossRef] [PubMed]
20. Soroka, M.; Wasowicz, B.; Rymaszewska, A. Loop-mediated isothermal amplification (LAMP): The better sibling of PCR? *Cells* **2021**, *10*, 1931. [CrossRef] [PubMed]
21. Njiru, Z.K. Loop-mediated isothermal amplification technology: Towards point of care diagnostics. *PLoS Negl. Trop. Dis.* **2012**, *6*, e1572. [CrossRef]
22. Park, J.W. Principles and applications of loop-mediated isothermal amplification to point-of-care tests. *Biosensors* **2022**, *12*, 857. [CrossRef] [PubMed]
23. Hsieh, K.; Mage, P.L.; Csordas, A.T.; Eisenstein, M.; Soh, H.T. Simultaneous elimination of carryover contamination and detection of DNA with uracil-DNA-glycosylase-supplemented loop-mediated isothermal amplification (UDG-LAMP). *Chem. Commun.* **2014**, *50*, 3747–3749. [CrossRef] [PubMed]
24. Aryan, E.; Makvandi, M.; Farajzadeh, A.; Huygen, K.; Bifani, P.; Mousavi, S.L.; Fateh, A.; Jelodar, A.; Gouya, M.M.; Romano, M. A novel and more sensitive loop-mediated isothermal amplification assay targeting IS*6110* for detection of *Mycobacterium tuberculosis* complex. *Microbiol. Res.* **2010**, *165*, 211–220. [CrossRef] [PubMed]
25. Quoc, N.B.; Phuong, N.D.N.; Chau, N.N.B.; Linh, D.T.P. Closed tube loop-mediated isothermal amplification assay for rapid detection of hepatitis B virus in human blood. *Heliyon* **2018**, *4*, e00561. [CrossRef] [PubMed]

26. Goto, M.; Honda, E.; Ogura, A.; Nomoto, A.; Hanaki, K.-I. Colorimetric detection of loop-mediated isothermal amplification reaction by using hydroxy naphthol blue. *Biotechniques* **2009**, *46*, 167–172. [CrossRef] [PubMed]
27. Mori, Y.; Nagamine, K.; Tomita, N.; Notomi, T. Detection of loop-mediated isothermal amplification reaction by turbidity derived from magnesium pyrophosphate formation. *Bioch. Biophys. Res. Commun.* **2001**, *289*, 150–154. [CrossRef]
28. Tomita, N.; Mori, Y.; Kanda, H.; Notomi, T. Loop-mediated isothermal amplification (LAMP) of gene sequences and simple visual detection of products. *Nat. Protoc.* **2008**, *3*, 877–882. [CrossRef]
29. Boehme, C.C.; Nabeta, P.; Henostroza, G.; Raqib, R.; Rahim, Z.; Gerhardt, M.; Sanga, E.; Hoelscher, M.; Notomi, T.; Hase, T. Operational feasibility of using loop-mediated isothermal amplification for diagnosis of pulmonary tuberculosis in microscopy centers of developing countries. *J. Clin. Microbiol.* **2007**, *45*, 1936–1940. [CrossRef]
30. Aryan, E.; Neshani, A.; Sadeghian, H.; Safdari, H. Visual detection of *Mycobacterium tuberculosis* by loop-mediated isothermal amplification. *Eur. Respir. J.* **2016**, *48*, OA1509.
31. Zhang, Y.; Ren, G.; Buss, J.; Barry, A.J.; Patton, G.C.; Tanner, N.A. Enhancing colorimetric loop-mediated isothermal amplification speed and sensitivity with guanidine chloride. *Biotechniques* **2020**, *69*, 178–185. [CrossRef]
32. Wang, D.G. Visual detection of *Mycobacterium tuberculosis* complex with loop-mediated isothermal amplification and Eriochrome Black T. In *Applied Mechanics and Materials*; Trans Tech Publications Ltd.: Wollerau, Switzerland, 2014; Volume 618, pp. 264–267.
33. Pandey, B.D.; Poudel, A.; Yoda, T.; Tamaru, A.; Oda, N.; Fukushima, Y.; Lekhak, B.; Risal, B.; Acharya, B.; Sapkota, B. Development of an in-house loop-mediated isothermal amplification (LAMP) assay for detection of *Mycobacterium tuberculosis* and evaluation in sputum samples of Nepalese patients. *J. Med. Microbiol.* **2008**, *57*, 439–443. [CrossRef]
34. van Soolingen, D.; Haas, P.E.W.; Kremer, K. Restriction fragment length polymorphism typing of mycobacteria. In *Mycobacterium Tuberculosis Protocols*; Parish, T., Stoker, N.G., Eds.; Humana Press: Totowa, NJ, USA, 2001; pp. 179–180.
35. Petroff, S. A new and rapid method for the isolation and cultivation of tubercle bacilli directly from the sputum and feces. *J. Experiment. Med.* **1915**, *21*, 38–42. [CrossRef]
36. Afghani, B.; Stutman, H.R. Polymerase chain reaction for diagnosis of *M. tuberculosis*: Comparison of simple boiling and a conventional method for DNA extraction. *Biochem. Mol. Med.* **1996**, *57*, 14–18. [CrossRef] [PubMed]
37. Yang, Q.; Domesle, K.J.; Ge, B. Loop-mediated isothermal amplification for Salmonella detection in food and feed: Current applications and future directions. *Foodborne Pathog. Dis.* **2018**, *15*, 309–331. [CrossRef] [PubMed]
38. Liang, C.; Cheng, S.; Chu, Y.; Wu, H.; Zou, B.; Huang, H.; Xi, T.; Zhou, G. A closed-tube detection of loop-mediated isothermal amplification (LAMP) products using a wax-sealed fluorescent intercalator. *J. Nanosci. Nanotechnol.* **2013**, *13*, 3999–4005. [CrossRef] [PubMed]
39. Diribe, O.; North, S.; Sawyer, J.; Roberts, L.; Fitzpatrick, N.; La Ragione, R. Design and application of a loop-mediated isothermal amplification assay for the rapid detection of *Staphylococcus pseudintermedius*. *J. Vet. Diagn. Invest.* **2014**, *26*, 42–48. [CrossRef]
40. Wastling, S.L.; Picozzi, K.; Kakembo, A.S.; Welburn, S.C. LAMP for human African trypanosomiasis: A comparative study of detection formats. *PLoS Negl. Trop. Dis.* **2010**, *4*, e865. [CrossRef]
41. Yang, B.; Wang, X.; Li, H.; Li, G.; Cao, Z.; Cheng, X. Comparison of loop-mediated isothermal amplification and real-time PCR for the diagnosis of tuberculous pleurisy. *Lett. Appl. Microbiol.* **2011**, *53*, 525–531. [CrossRef]
42. Zhang, X.; Li, M.; Cui, Y.; Zhao, J.; Cui, Z.; Li, Q.; Qu, K. Electrochemical behavior of calcein and the interaction between calcein and DNA. *Electroanalysis* **2012**, *24*, 1878–1886. [CrossRef]
43. Wu, D.; Kang, J.; Li, B.; Sun, D. Evaluation of the RT-LAMP and LAMP methods for detection of *Mycobacterium tuberculosis*. *J. Clin. Lab. Anal.* **2018**, *32*, e22326. [CrossRef]
44. Kim, J.-H.; Yoo, I.S.; An, J.H.; Kim, S. A novel paper-plastic hybrid device for the simultaneous loop-mediated isothermal amplification and detection of DNA. *Mater. Lett.* **2018**, *214*, 243–246. [CrossRef]
45. Oh, S.J.; Seo, T.S. Combination of a centrifugal microfluidic device with a solution-loading cartridge for fully automatic molecular diagnostics. *Analyst* **2019**, *144*, 5766–5774. [CrossRef]
46. Caliendo, A.M.; Gilbert, D.N.; Ginocchio, C.C.; Hanson, K.E.; May, L.; Quinn, T.C.; Tenover, F.C.; Alland, D.; Blaschke, A.J.; Bonomo, R.A.; et al. Better tests, better care: Improved diagnostics for infectious diseases. *Clin. Infect. Dis.* **2013**, *57*, S139–S170. [CrossRef] [PubMed]

diagnostics

MDPI

Article

Performance Evaluation of Developed Bangasure™ Multiplex rRT-PCR Assay for SARS-CoV-2 Detection in Bangladesh: A Blinded Observational Study at Two Different Sites

Mamudul Hasan Razu [1], Zabed Bin Ahmed [1], Md. Iqbal Hossain [1], Mohammad Fazle Alam Rabbi [2,3], Maksudur Rahman Nayem [2], Md. Akibul Hassan [2], Gobindo Kumar Paul [1], Md. Robin Khan [1], Md. Moniruzzaman [1], Pranab Karmaker [1] and Mala Khan [1,*]

1 Bangladesh Reference Institute for Chemical Measurements, Dhaka 1205, Bangladesh
2 DNA Solutions Ltd., Dhaka 1207, Bangladesh
3 Department of Soil, Water and Environment, University of Dhaka, Dhaka 1000, Bangladesh
* Correspondence: bricmdg@yahoo.com

Abstract: In this study, we evaluated the performance of the in-house developed rRT-PCR assay for SARS-CoV-2 RNA targeting the envelope (*E*) and nucleocapsid (*N*) genes with internal control as human *RNase P*. A total of 50 positive samples and 50 negative samples of SARS-CoV-2 were tested by a reference kit at site 1 and a subset (30 positives and 16 negatives) of these samples are tested blindly at site 2. The limit of detection (LoD) was calculated by using a replication-deficient complete SARS-CoV-2 genome and known copy numbers, where Pseudo-virus samples were used to evaluate accuracy. On site 1, among the 50 SARS-CoV-2 positive samples 24, 18, and eight samples showed high (Ct < 26), moderate (26 < Ct ≤ 32), and low (32 < Ct ≤ 38) viral load, respectively, whereas in site 2, out of 30 SARS-CoV-2 positive samples, high, moderate, and low viral loads were found in each of the 10 samples. However, SARS-CoV-2 was not detected in the negative sample. So, in-house assays at both sites showed 100% sensitivity and specificity with no difference observed between RT PCR machines. The Ct values of the in-house kit had a very good correlation with the reference kits. LoD was determined as 100 copies/mL. It also displayed 100% accuracy in mutant and wild-type SARS-CoV-2 virus. This Bangasure™ RT-PCR kit shows excellent performance in detecting SARS-CoV-2 viral RNA compared to commercially imported CE-IVD marked FDA authorized kits.

Keywords: Bangasure™; rRT-PCR; SARS-CoV-2; Nucleocapsid; LoD

Citation: Razu, M.H.; Ahmed, Z.B.; Hossain, M.I.; Rabbi, M.F.A.; Nayem, M.R.; Hassan, M.A.; Paul, G.K.; Khan, M.R.; Moniruzzaman, M.; Karmaker, P.; et al. Performance Evaluation of Developed Bangasure™ Multiplex rRT-PCR Assay for SARS-CoV-2 Detection in Bangladesh: A Blinded Observational Study at Two Different Sites. *Diagnostics* **2022**, *12*, 2617. https://doi.org/10.3390/diagnostics12112617

Academic Editor: Hsin-Yao Wang

Received: 24 August 2022
Accepted: 29 September 2022
Published: 28 October 2022

1. Introduction

The coronavirus pandemic caused by severe acute respiratory syndrome coronavirus 2 (SARS-CoV-2) is redefining global public health. The disease was first reported in Wuhan, China in December 2019 [1] and since then it has spread throughout the globe. Till now, the world has lost almost 6.2 million lives to this virus. Bangladesh has reported its first COVID-19 case in March 2020. Since then, the number of positive cases has increased at an exponential rate. As of 13 April 2022, the country observed nearly 1.9 million positive cases of COVID-19 with a cumulative death toll of nearly 30,000 [2,3]. Although vaccination started throughout the country, the pandemic might be far away from over. Moreover, the rise of new variants of concerns of SARS-CoV-2 with a higher transmissibility rate is developing a critical challenge to the response strategy. With the continuous threat of contagion, response measures need to evolve. Diagnostic testing is an important pillar of the response measures in this fight against the COVID- 19 pandemic. Clinical symptoms cannot exclusively define COVID-19 diagnosis. Moreover, 40–50% of the confirmed population with COVID-19 are asymptomatic but can easily infect others [4]. Thus, testing will continue to be important for identifying infected individuals and implementing quarantine and treatment measures. It will also become increasingly more important for surveillance and screening efforts to monitor the effectiveness of control measures and carry out informed public health and economic decisions.

Reverse transcriptase-polymerase chain reaction (rRT-PCR) is the gold standard in the detection of SARS-CoV-2. Distinct rRT-PCR testing protocols were swiftly established and made publicly available by the WHO [5] and by the Centre for Disease Control (CDC), USA [6]. To date, Food and Drug Administration (FDA), USA issued over 200 Emergency Use Authorization (EUA) COVID-19 molecular diagnostic kits. However, many of these rRT-PCR kits have a varying range of lower limit of detection (LoD). Therefore, it is necessary to lower the detection limit to ensure the accuracy and reliability of the test results. Many factors might lead to false-negative results, especially low viral loads [7–9]. Further, the specificity of the confirmatory test relies on the probe-target sequence. The commercially available rRT-PCR kits generally target nucleocapsid (*N*), envelope (*E*) or RNA- dependent RNA polymerase (*RdRp*) gene of SARS-CoV-2 already published by WHO. However, various mutations have been observed within these regions which might hamper sensitivity [10,11]. Dorp et al. found that about 80% of SARS-CoV-2 genome mutations occur in the spike (S) protein, and a large number of mutations are expressed in the *Orf1ab* [12]. Besides that, Neha Kaushal et. al., studied that no mutational frequency was found at *E*-gene of SARS-CoV-2 genome during the beginning months of the outbreak in the USA [13]. An in-silico study was conducted by Changtai Wang, available from the NCBI and GISAID database, and found that SARS-CoV-2 is relatively conserved, especially in the E, 6, 7b regions where no mutation was found. Hotspot mutations in *ORFs* 1a, S, 8, and the *N* region will cause changes in the amino acid sequences of these proteins, and the effects of these mutations on viral replication, transmission, and the induced immune responses need to be further investigated [14]. Moreover, several types of commercial kits have been developed such as singleplex, duplex, or multiplex. The limitation of the singleplex PCR protocol is the requirement to run three or more PCR reactions per sample because all of the probes are labeled with the same dye. Besides that, singleplex uses large amounts of reagents and reduces the laboratory testing capacity, especially in small-scale facilities, which are crucial during the ongoing COVID-19 pandemic, particularly in developing countries. To improve sensitivity, generally, in commercial kits, multiple probes and primers are used in a multi-step PCR workflow.

Bangladesh, a country in Southeast Asia is a densely populated country with a developing economy. The public health of this country is severely challenged due to the limited number of testing facilities and limited access to locally manufactured rapid diagnostic tests [15]. The country is currently highly dependent on imported test kits which are a major concern for the sustainability of response measures. Globally, there is a scarcity of the resources required for the accurate diagnosis of SARS-CoV-2 and dependence on imported kits develops a critical limiting factor for public health measures mainly due to limited assurance for a continued supply. Further, it is difficult to ensure the high quality and quantity of imported kits. Thus, local manufacturing of high-quality test kits might create assurance of supply with self-reliance for diagnostic testing and offer the potential for price rationalization and expanded access to diagnostics.

In this study, we have developed an in-house multiplex assay against SARS-CoV-2 by targeting two viral gene targets from *E* and *N2* genes named Bangasure™. The primer and probe sequence for SARS-CoV-2 *E* and *N2* gene was previously described by Charité—Universitätsmedizin Berlin Institute of Virology, Berlin, Germany [16] and CDC, USA [17] respectively. The Human *RNase P* gene was included as the internal control [18]. This study determines the performance efficiency of this in-house assay at two sites against two commercially imported CE-FDA approved rRT-PCR kits in determining the SARS-CoV-2 among clinical specimens.

2. Methods

2.1. Ethical Approval

Bangladesh Reference Institute for Chemical Measurements (BRiCM) in collaboration with DNA Solution Ltd. (DNAS) carried out a subsequent comparative study of Bangasure™ rRT-PCR assay at two sites, DNAS as site-1 and BRiCM as site-2. All procedures in the study were according to ethical standards of the Helsinki Declaration of 1975, as revised in 2010 [19]. Clinical specimens were collected along with case record forms (CRF) of participants were constructed as per Institute of Epidemiology, Diseases Control and Research (IEDCR) from site 1 by DNAS as they have authorization for COVID-19 test by the Government of Bangladesh. This is only a performance evaluation study of Bangasure™ RT-PCR kit in comparison with a CE-FDA marked reference kit by using secondary data and without disclosing or using demographical data of a participant anywhere, so there was no direct subject enrollment, but written consent was obtained from participants during completion of the CRF. Moreover, the study protocol was approved by the institutional ethics review committee (Ref No#BRiCM2206). The Bangasure™ multiplex rRT-PCR efficacy protocol was also accepted and published on the Clinicaltrials.gov site as an NCT05190016 identification number.

2.2. Primer and Probes

Primer and probe sequences for SARS-CoV-2 viral target genes previously published by CDC, USA (*N1* and *N2*) [17] and Charité—Universitätsmedizin Berlin Institute of Virology, Berlin, Germany (*E* and *RdRP*) [16] were considered for this study. Through literature review, a multiplex combination of *E*, *N2* along with internal control gene *RNase P* was considered for the study [18]. The primer and probe were ordered from Integrated DNA Technologies-IDT (Coralville, IA, USA). In this article, the *N2* primer and probe will be read as *N* only for future references.

2.3. Sample Collection and Preparation

In this study, Oro-pharyngeal swabs from suspected patients were collected in Government approved virus transport medium (VTM) (Sansure Biotech. Inc., Changsha, China) at the outdoor patient department (OPD) of the DNA Solution Ltd. (DNAS), Dhaka, Bangladesh, and transported in a cool box to the laboratory for further processing. RNA extraction was carried out using QIAamp® DSP Virus Spin Kit (Qiagen, Hilden, Germany) according to the instruction manual. Briefly, 200 µL of VTM containing the oropharyngeal swab was employed as starting material for viral RNA extraction using Silica-membrane technology. The samples were lysed, binding to the silica-membrane column, washed to remove contaminants, and eluted with RNase-free elution buffer. Fifty (50) positive and fifty (50) negative SARS-CoV-2 RNA samples were selected by using as reference commercial one-step real-time COVID-19 PCR kit, Novel Coronavirus (2019-nCoV) Nucleic Acid Diagnostic Kit (Sansure Biotech Inc., Changsha, China) following manufacturer's instruction. The commercial real-time PCR kit uses PCR-Fluorescence probing technology and targets two genes, *ORF 1 ab* and conserved coding regions of the nucleocapsid protein *N* gene by Sansure Biotech kit. Positive internal control of human *RNase P*, along with positive and negative control was used to nullify the presence of PCR inhibitors.

2.4. Optimization of Bangasure™ rRT-PCR Assay

Optimization of rRT-PCR reactions of the in-house assay was carried out using four different Real-Time PCR instruments QuantStudio5 (Applied Biosystems, California, USA), BioRad CFX96, and CFX Opus 96 (Bio-Rad Laboratories, Foster City, CA, USA). The in-house assay was optimized via targeting *E* and *N* gene primer/probe published by Charité—Universitätsmedizin Berlin Institute of Virology, Berlin, Germany and CDC, USA respectively along with *RNase P* gene as an internal control [18]. The probes of *E*, *N*, and *RNase P* were labeled with FAM, VIC, and Cy5 to improve multiplexing efficiency. The cycling program was set according to the manufacturer's instruction of commercial one-step master mix (New England Biolabs, Ipswich, MA, USA). Our optimized protocol consisted of 20 μL reaction mixture containing 5 μL of 4× master mix (New England Biolabs, Ipswich, MA, USA), 2 μL of primers/probes mix, 7 μL extracted RNA or template for positive material (Integrated DNA Technologies-IDT, Coralville, IA, USA), and 6 μL of nuclease-free water (New England Biolabs, Ipswich, MA, USA) with a filter combination of FAM (*E*), VIC (*N*), and Cy5 (*RNase P*).

2.5. Limit of Detection (LoD) Determination

To determine LoD, AccuPlex™ SARS-CoV-2 Verification Panel containing replication-deficient recombinant alphaviruses incorporating the full genome of SARS-CoV-2 in known concentrations were ordered from Sera Care (Sera Care Life Sciences, Inc., Milford, MA, USA). The reference materials contained a known concentration of virus particles which were serially diluted starting from 10^5 Copies/mL to 1 Copy/mL. 5 replications of each dilution series were tested at site 1. These positive materials undergo RNA extraction in the same way as clinical specimens according to the previously described method. The LoD was determined at the lowest concentration at which assay target specific for SARS-CoV-2 was positive for all 5 replicates.

2.6. Performance Evaluation of the In-House Assay

Performance evaluation between singleplex and multiplex assay was carried out using synthetic positive control plasmids for *E*, *N*, and *RNase P* gene from IDT. The starting stock for each plasmid control was 2×10^5 copies/μL. They were serially diluted to 2000, 200, 20, and 2 copy copies/μL. Both singleplex and multiplex reactions of our *E*, *N*, and *RNase P* gene-based assay were carried out against these synthetic positive plasmids. To perform clinical evaluation, a total of 100 clinical oropharyngeal specimens were selected containing an equal number of COVID-19 positive and negative samples. The samples (positive = 50 and negative = 50) were analyzed at site 1 using an in-house assay and a commercial multiplex 1copy (1drop Inc., Gyeonggi-do, 13217, Republic of Korea) by a separate analyst and Quant StudioTM 5 real-time PCR detection system (Applied Biosystems, Foster City, CA, USA) where as a subset of those samples (positive = 30 and negative = 16) was reanalyzed using the in-house assay at site 2 by CFX OPUS 96 (Biorad, Hercules, CA, USA). In addition, the efficiency of the in-house one step SARS-CoV-2 real-time PCR assay to detect the SARS-CoV-2 variants of concerns was determined using pseudo virus specimens representing three prominent variants of concerns, i.e., B.1.1.7 (UK variant), B.1.351 (South African variant), and P.1. (Brazilian variant), along with wild type (Wuhan) variant (NC 045512) (Sera Care Life Sciences, Inc., Milford, MA, USA.) and a clinical specimen (OM574617) containing the B.1.1.529 (Omicron variant) of concern.

2.7. Accelerated Stability Testing

According to the Arrhenius equation [20], accelerated testing was done to predict stability at both sites independently. The in-house kit which includes Master mix, primers, probes, controls were stored at 4 ± 2 °C both sites and additionally −20 °C for 5 weeks at site 2 which were tested according to previously determined time points. Kits stored at 4 ± 2 °C were used to estimate the shelf life (Table S1) and kits stored at −20 °C were used to evaluate the efficiency of the kit at the actual stored temperature. A panel of specimens positive and negative for COVID-19 was stored as single separate aliquots and analyzed at each time point to determine the in-house assay efficiency. Then results of the kit at 4 ± 2 °C at both sites were compared to the results obtained for the same lot of the kit stored at −20 °C for 5 weeks in site 2.

2.8. Data Analysis

Samples were considered positive when the signal detected for *E* and/or *N* genes were detected at Ct < 40. Samples were considered negative when viral target genes had a Ct > 40 or were not detected at all along with the amplified *RP* had Ct < 40. Specimens were labeled as invalid when both *E* and *N* genes along with *RP* signals were undetermined. Nuclease-free water was also used as a no template control (NTC). Data analysis for the commercial kits was performed according to the manufacturer's instructions. The assay's sensitivity, specificity, positive predictive value, and negative predictive values were determined using the online version 20.115 of MedCalc statistical software [21].

3. Results

3.1. Multiplexing of E, N, and RP Genes for Detection of SARS-CoV-2 RNA

Various rRT-PCR reactions with different combinations and concentrations of primer and probes were carried out. Finally, an optimized multiplexing strategy targeting envelops (*E*) and nucleocapsid (*N*) gene of SARS-CoV-2 along with a primer/probe set targeting the human *RNase P* (*RP*) as the internal control was selected. The sequences of the primer/probe considered for the in-house assay are summarized in Table 1.

Table 1. Primers and probes used for in-house assay of SARS-CoV-2.

Target Gene	Primer/Probe	Oligonucleotide Sequence (5′–3′)
	E_SarbecoF_primer	ACAGGTACGTTAATAGTTAATAGCGT
E gene	E_SarbecoR_Primer	ATATTGCAGCAGTACGCACACA
	Probe_E	FAM-ACACTAGCCATCCTTACTGCGCTTCG-BHQ1
	N_cdcF_Primer	TTACAAACATTGGCCGCAAA
N gene	N_cdcFR_Primer	GCGCGACATTCCGAAGAA
	Probe_N	VIC-ACAATTTGCCCCCAGCGCTTCAG-BHQ1
	RP_F_Primer	AGATTTGGACCTGCGAGCG
RNase P	RP_R_Primer	GAGCGGCTGTCTCCACAAGT
	Probe_*RNase P*	CY5-TTCTGACCTGAAGGCTCTGCGCG-BHQ-1

The optimized combination showed noteworthy amplification for each of the target genes with the commercial one-step master mix (New England Biolabs, Ipswich, MA, USA) in both singleplex and multiplex assay. Ct values from multiplex assay were found to be increased by almost two units when compared with the singleplex assay (Figure 1). An ideal baseline along with the optimum cycle of threshold and minimum background noise was obtained in the following reaction protocol: 25 °C (30 s), 55 °C (10 min), 95 °C (1 min) followed by 45 cycles of 95 °C (10 s), 60 °C (30 s). This optimized protocol and the multiplex assay were compatible in Qunatstudio 5, BioRad CFX96, CFX Opus 96.

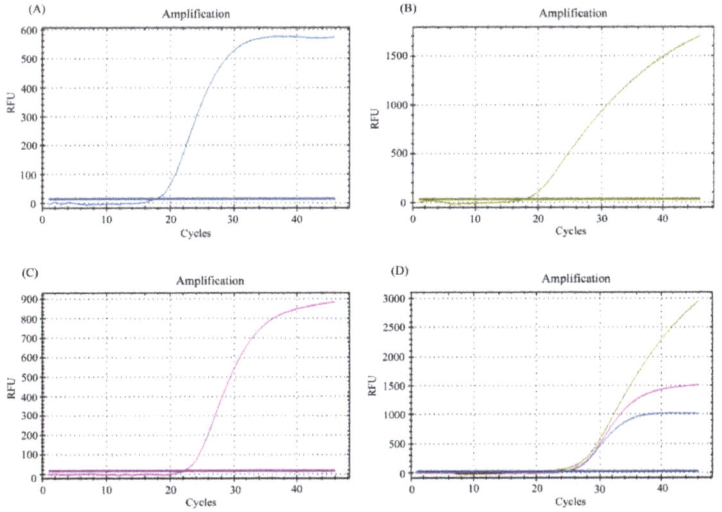

Figure 1. Amplification curves for each of the target genes in singleplex: (**A**) *E* gene, (**B**) *N* gene, (**C**) *RNase P* gene and (**D**) Multiplex assay with the optimized combination of primer-probes.

3.2. Limit of Detection (LoD) Determination of the In-House Multiplex Assay

Replication deficient alphavirus incorporating the whole genome of SARS-CoV-2 was used as reference material to determine LoD. The concentration of starting stock specimen was 10^5 copies/mL which was serially diluted to 10^4, 10^3, 10^2, 10, and 1 copy/mL. Each dilution series was replicated 5 times and tested against the in-house assay as well as the two commercial rRT-PCR COVID-19 kits considered in this study. The LoD was defined as the lowest concentration at which all replicates (five out of five) were positive for all viral assay targets. The in-house assay showed LoD at 100 copy/mL which is similar to the commercial rRT-PCR kit by Sansure Biotech Inc. However, the other commercial kit by 1drop Inc. (1copy) showed LoD at 1000 copy/mL. The data are summarized in Table 2.

Table 2. Determining the Limit of Detection (LoD) for the Bangasure™ in-house assay and the two commercial kits using specimens with known copies of replication-deficient alphaviruses incorporating the whole SARS-CoV-2 genome.

Virus Copy/mL	Bangasure™					Sansure Biotec.					1copy						
	Detection Rate, %	Target Gene				Detection Rate, %	Target Gene				Detection Rate, %	Target Gene					
		E		*N*			*ORF1ab*		*N*			*E*		*N*		*RdRp*	
		Ct Value		Ct Value			Ct Value		Ct Value			Ct Value		Ct Value		Ct Value	
		Mean	%CV	Mean	%CV		Mean	%CV	Mean	%CV		Mean	%CV	Mean	%CV	Mean	%CV
100,000	100	26.35	2.87	26.83	1.22	100	27.64	0.48	26.46	0.24	100	28.31	0.83	27.77	0.27	28.99	0.34
10,000	100	30.01	0.65	30.21	0.62	100	30.81	0.21	29.56	0.45	100	31.54	0.87	31.34	1.07	32.35	0.81
1000	100	33.52	1.29	34.48	2.40	100	34.77	0.81	33.65	1.97	100	34.99	0.82	34.90	1.63	35.43	0.96
100	100	37.49	1.34	37.71	1.59	100	38.38	1.57	37.11	1.34	0	UND	UND	UND	UND	UND	UND
10	0	UND	UND	UND	UND	0	UND	UND	UND	UND	0	UND	UND	UND	UND	UND	UND
1	0	UND	UND	UND	UND	0	UND	UND	UND	UND	0	UND	UND	UND	UND	UND	UND

UND = undetected.

3.3. Efficiency of In-House Multiplex rRT-PCR Assay

Both the singleplex and multiplex reaction of all the assay targets of the in-house assay was carried out against a 10-fold serial dilution of synthetic positive control starting from 2000 copies/µL to 2 copies/µL. The results between singleplex and multiplex showed concordant results with $R^2 > 0.99$ (Figure 2). Next, replication-deficient enveloped viruses harboring the mutation of three SARS-CoV-2 variants of concerns (B.1.1.7, B.1.351, and P.1) along with the wild type (Wuhan) variant (NC_045512) were tested with the in-house assay. A clinical specimen (OM574617) containing the variant of concern B.1.1.529 was also tested with the in-house assay. All the viral assay targets were positive against the variants of concerns, including the wild type (Figure 3).

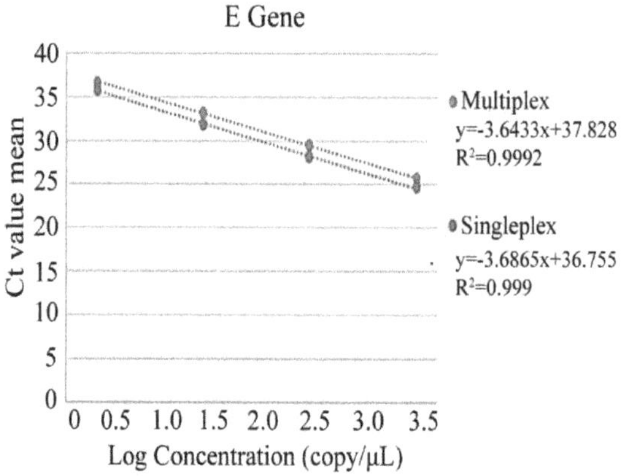

(A)

Figure 2. *Cont.*

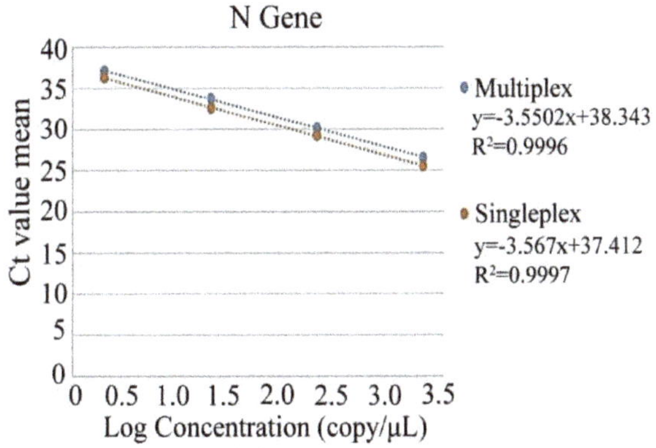

(B)

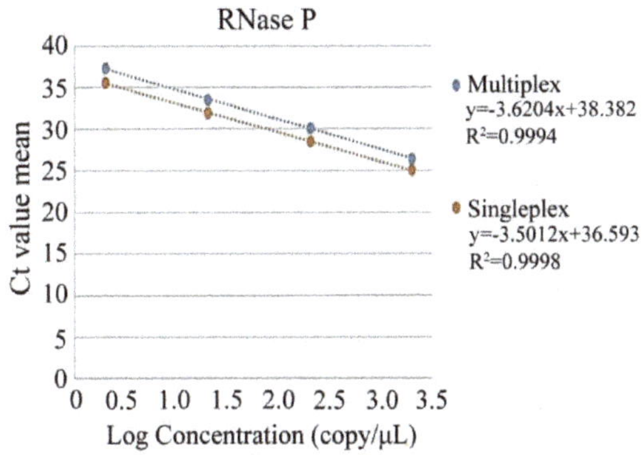

(C)

Figure 2. Calculation of calibration curves through singleplex and multiplex rRT-PCR for different copies of positive controls of *E*, *N2* and *RNase P*. (**A**) Standard curve for *E*, (**B**) Standard curve for N and (**C**) Standard curve for *RNase P*.

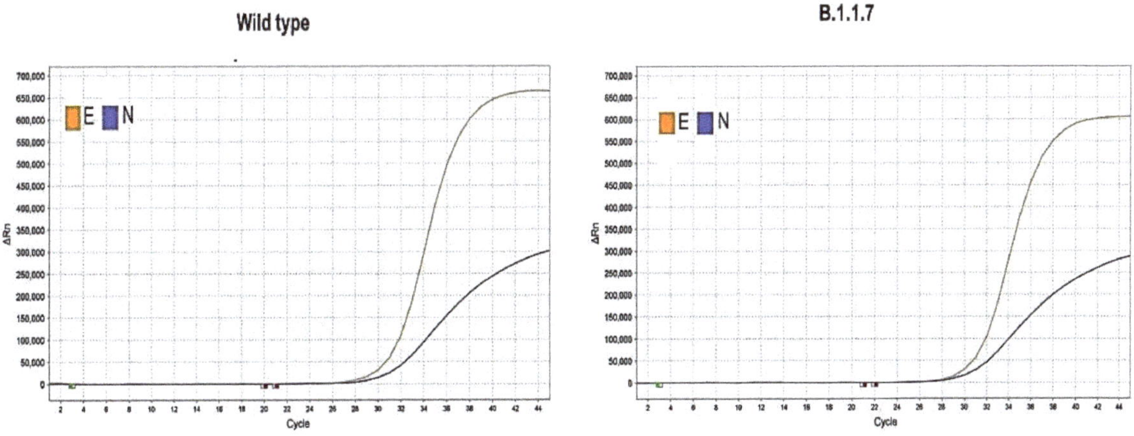

A

B

Figure 3. *Cont.*

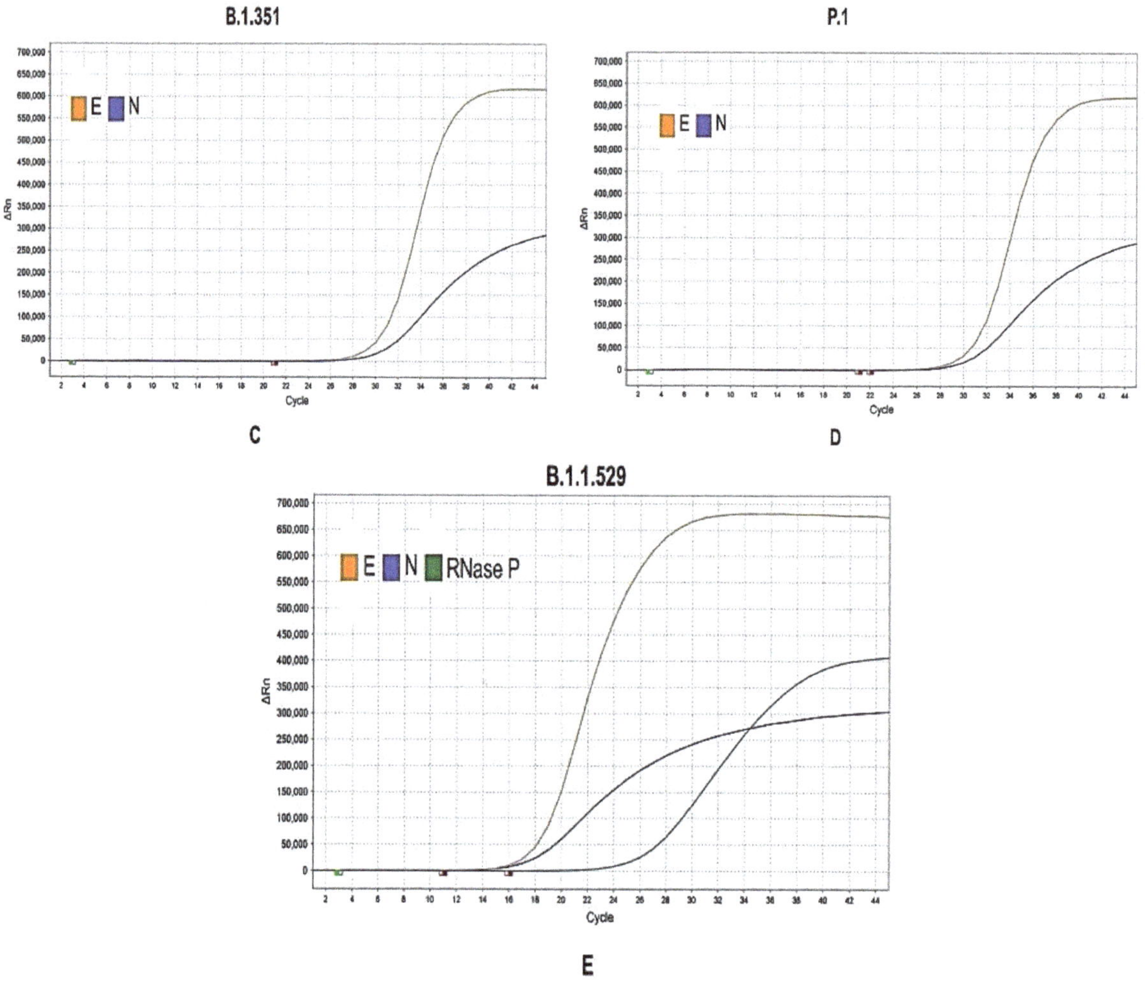

Figure 3. Detection of the SARS-CoV-2 variants of concerns by Bangasure™ multiplex rRT-PCR kit. (**A**) Wuhan variant (wild type), (**B**) UK Variant (B.1.1.7), (**C**) South African Variant (B.1.351), (**D**) Brazilian variant (P.1) and (**E**) Omicron Variant (B.1.1.529) from clinical specimen (OM574617).

3.4. Performance Evaluation of In-House Assay Using Clinical Specimens

A total of 100 (positive = 50 and negative = 50) clinical specimens (oropharyngeal swab) were considered using the Sansure Biotech PCR kit as a reference kit for the performance evaluation. Among those, at site 1 within the positive samples, 24 samples had high SARS-CoV-2 viral load (Ct < 26) while 18 and eight samples had moderate (26 < Ct ≤ 32) and low viral (32 < Ct ≤ 38) load respectively according to the Sansure COVID-19 rRT-PCR kit. At site 2, within the positive samples, 10 samples had high (Ct < 26), moderate (26 < Ct ≤ 32), and low (32 < Ct ≤ 38) viral load in each group. Besides that, the COVID-19 status of all the samples was blinded and was reanalyzed by the Bangasure™ in-house multiplex kit and 1copy COVID-19 rRT-PCR kits at site 1. The results were then compared with the Sansure data. Both the in-house assays and the 1copy kit accurately identified all the positive and negative samples for COVID-19 at both sites. Thus, in comparison to Sansure kit, the in-house assay has 100% sensitivity, specificity, accuracy, positive prediction value, and negative prediction value (Table 3A,B). The Pearson correlation analysis of *E*, *N*, and *RNase P* gene individually for both positive and negative samples at two sites with the reference kits also indicated a good relationship (Figure 4). Additionally, when compared between the two different RT PCR machines used at two different sites, we found 100% concordance, though the Ct value for each gene at site 2 was found slightly increased (Figure 5).

Table 3. Validation and performance determination of the Bangasure^{TM} RT-PCR kit against two commercially available CE-IVD and FDA approved COVID-19 qPCR diagnostic kits (**A**) in site 1 and (**B**) in site 2.

(A)

Information of Clinical Samples		Number of Samples	Tested by Bangasure^{TM} RT-PCR Kit	Tested by Sansure COVID-19 rRT-PCR Kit	Tested by 1copy 4plex Kit
Samples Tested positive, n = 50	High (Ct < 26)	24	24	24	24
	Moderate (26 < Ct ≤ 32)	18	18	18	18
	Low (32 < Ct ≤ 38)	8	8	8	8
	Total	50	50	50	50
Samples tested negative, n = 50		50	50	50	50
Sensitivity,%(95% CI)			100 (92.89–100)	100 (92.89–100)	100 (92.89–100)
Specificity,%(95% CI)			100 (92.89–100)	100 (92.89–100)	100 (92.89–100)
PPV,%			100	100	100
NPV,%			100	100	100
Accuracy,% (95% CI)			100 (96.38–100)	100 (96.38–100)	100 (96.38–100)

(B)

Information of Clinical Samples		Number of Samples	Tested by Bangasure^{TM} RT-PCR Kit	Tested by Sansure COVID-19 rRT-PCR Kit
Sample Tested positive, n = 30	High (Ct < 26)	10	10	10
	Moderate (26 < Ct ≤ 32)	10	10	10
	Low (32 < Ct ≤ 38)	10	10	10
	Total	30	30	30
Sample tested negative, n = 16		16	16	16
Sensitivity, % (95% CI)			100 (88.4–100)	100 (88.4–100)
Specificity, % (95% CI)			100 (79.4–100)	100 (79.4–100)
PPV, %			100	100
NPV, %			100	100
Accuracy, % (95%CL)			100 (92.29–100)	100 (92.29–100)

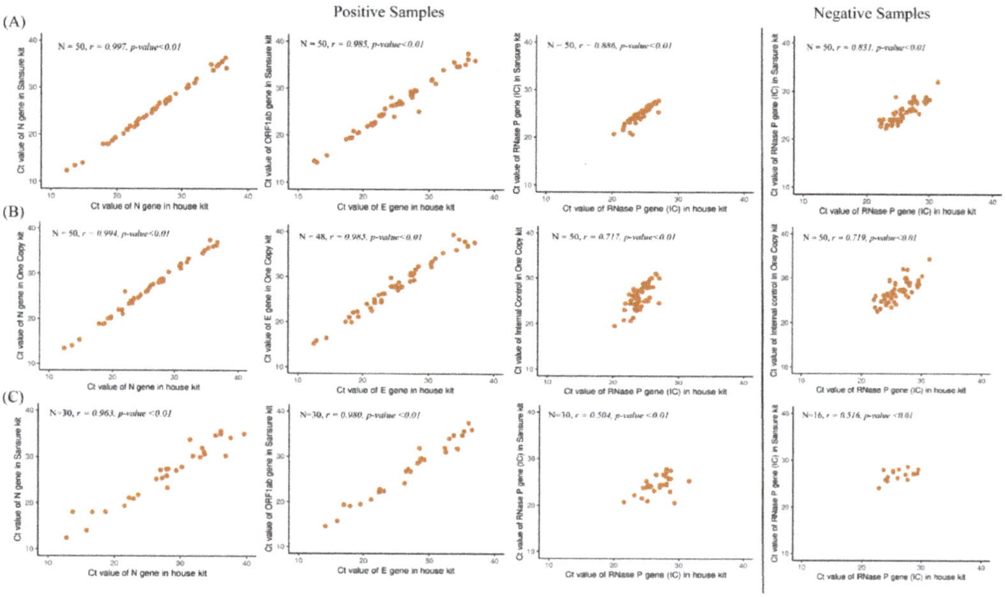

Figure 4. Pearson correlation analysis of Ct values of *E*, *N*, *RNase P* between in house kit and reference kits. (**A**) Pearson correlation between *N*, *RNase P*, *E* gene between In house and Sansure kit at site 1 (Sansure has *ORF1ab* gene instead of *E* gene), (**B**) Pearson correlation between *N*, *RNase P*, *E* gene between In house and One copy kit at site 1, (**C**) Pearson correlation between *N*, *RNase P*, *E* gene between In house and Sansure kit at site 1 (Sansure has *ORF1ab* gene instead of *E* gene).

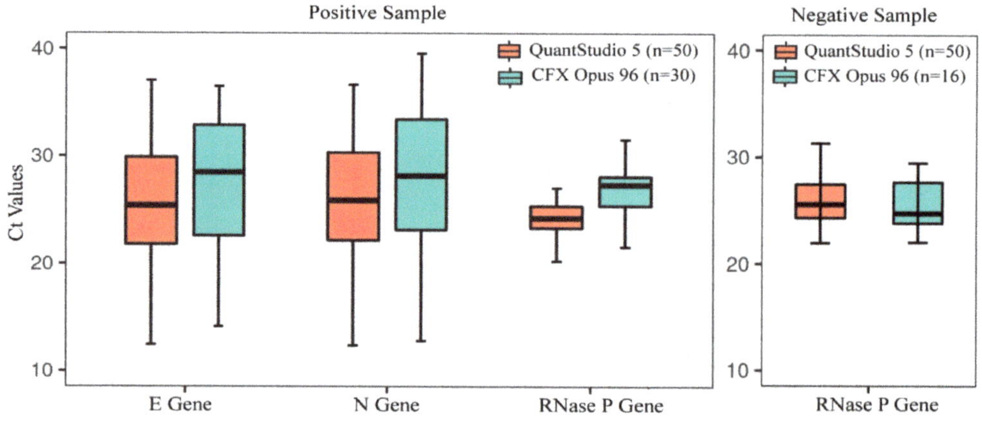

Figure 5. Ct values of individual genes included in in-house kit on two different RT machines used at two sites.

3.5. Determination of Assay Reproducibility and Stability

To determine the in-house assay reproducibility and stability, 10 clinical specimens containing five positive and five negative samples for COVID-19 were used. The specimens were aliquoted and kept at −80 °C to avoid repeated freezing and thawing. The in-house assay was kept in 4 ± 2 °C for the accelerated stability testing in both the sites and additionally −20 ± 5 °C in site 2 to mimic the practical scenario. The samples were tested for five consecutive weeks and each time the tests were replicated five times. Each time, the samples were detected with high precision with minimal deviation from the mean. Further, the coefficients of variation of the precision Ct were less than 5% in site 1 and less than 7% in site 2 at all the storage temperatures for five consecutive weeks. Further from this study, it can be predicted the in-house assay has a stability of at least five months at −20 °C. The data are summarized in Table 4.

Table 4. Reproducibility of the Bangasure™ multiplex RT-PCR kit in site 1 and site 2 over 5 week.

	Site 1			Site 2					
	Ct Values for Multiplex PCR at 4 °C			Ct Values for Multiplex PCR at 4 °C			Ct Values for Multiplex PCR at −20 °C		
	E	*N*	*RNase P*	*E*	*N*	*RNase P*	*E*	*N*	*RNase P*
Week 1	21.91	22.75	23.99	23.96	21.52	27.24	25.61	21.52	23.73
Week 2	21.44	23.73	24.42	25.068	25.35	25.54	25.35	25.35	25.63
Week 3	23.50	23.66	24.76	25.938	24.77	25.94	25.96	24.78	25.84
Week 4	22.96	24.35	23.74	26.17	25.13	25.73	26.25	24.89	25.95
Week 5	23.44	24.31	23.71	27.256	25.37	26.23	26.89	25.12	25.75
Mean (SD)	22.65 (0.93)	23.76 (0.65)	24.12 (0.45)	25.68 (1.24)	24.43 (1.64)	26.14 (0.67)	26.01(0.59)	24.33 (1.58)	25.38 (0.93)
CV (%)	4.11	2.73	1.88	4.82	6.73	2.56	2.29	6.52	3.66

4. Discussion

Since the beginning of SARS-CoV-2 pandemic, laboratories around the globe faced difficulty to expedite diagnostic tests due to a shortage of resources [22]. This was critical for developing countries that were dependent on imports for diagnostic kits and reagents. Bangladesh, a developing country in south-east Asia, is a densely populated county and was able to cover only 0.66 per 1000 of its citizen under COVID-19 diagnosis [23]. One of the major limiting factors for this poor diagnosis rate is the lack of control over the import supply chain and the quality as well the quantity of the diagnostic kits. As diagnosis is not the most important pillar of COVID-19 pandemic response, it is a critical priority to develop domestically manufactured high volume quality kits. Around the globe, various efforts are ongoing to develop accurate, reliable, and sustainable SARS-CoV-2 detection methods with good sensitivity and specificity [24].

In this study, we have reported the development of a Bangasure™ in-house multiplex rRT-PCR kit for SARS-CoV-2. Two groups of primer-probe sets (Charité/Berlin and CDC designed Primer probe sets) which are recognized globally and used in many diagnostic assays was primarily chosen to be evaluated. Evaluation of these primer probes to find an optimum combination was conducted by thoroughly reviewing the literature [25–30]. WHO recommended the Charité/Berlin assay which detects two viral targets *E* and *RdRp* gene [16]. Among these two targets, different studies revealed the sensitivity of the *E* primer-probe is much higher than the *RdRp* primer-probe set [28,30]. Ct values of amplification curves were found to be significantly higher when the *RdRp* primer-probe set was used compared to other recognized primer-probe sets used in the study [30]. On the other hand, comparing the Ct values and analytical sensitivity of *N1* and *N2* primer-probe sets, *N2* performed slightly better than the *N1* primer-probe set [28]. Moreover, the *N1* probe has a single nucleotide mismatch in more than 98% of Omicron variants which is a variant of concern and the most predominant SARS-CoV-2 variant in the world right now [26]. After analyzing all these facts and following the recommendation of Nalla et al., 2020, the *E* primer-probe of Charité/Berlin and *N2* primer-probe designed by CDC was chosen for in-house assay [28].

During the SARS-CoV-2 pandemic, testing demand increased exponentially. Singleplex reactions using various target genes demand more thermal cycler, controls, reagents, and labor which are a limiting factor in resource-poor countries. Studies showed that multiplexing through a single-tube reaction causes a negligible decrease in sensitivity compared to singleplex reaction [31]. Further, mutations are a common possibility of false-negative results. By targeting multiple SARS-CoV-2 viral assay targets, we might have reduced the possibility of false-negative results that might have been raised through any polymorphism within the primer binding site and template region. Thus, the development of a multiplex assay with high sensitivity and specificity will save time, simplify diagnosis, require less reagent, and offer increased test volume which is critical for pandemic response.

In this study, the in-house assay showed great sensitivity and specificity in detecting SARS- Cov-2 efficiently compared to two FDA-approved commercial nucleic acid amplification kits for COVID-19 at both site trials. Though the Ct values for each gene in CFX Opus 96 RT PCR machine at site 2 was found slightly increased when compared with site 1 which used Quantstudio 5 RT PCR machine this might be due to the time gap of analysis between two sites (1 week interval). However, in terms of detection, there was no discordance observed. Analytical sensitivity of the in-house kit was found to be 100 copy/mL, which indicates that samples with low viral loads can be detected efficiently by the in-house kit. The other two commercial RT-PCR kits named Sansure and 1copy showed analytical sensitivity 100 copy/mL and 1000 copy/mL respectively. The nucleic acid extraction method, primer-probe, and other reagents used in reaction might impact the sensitivity of real-time PCR, and thus optimization of an assay is necessary [32]. The linearity ($R^2 > 0.99$) we observed in the standard curve and low LoD indicates that the reaction condition used for the in-house assay might have achieved the required optimized condition. Further, all commercial RT-PCR kits along with in-house assay showed amplification in all target genes in both high and low positive samples, which demonstrates the high sensitivity of these kits in a clinical set-up.

In this study, the same set of samples was tested to be compared against all kits, and the initial volume of sample and elution volume were kept concordant for all the samples in the nucleic acid extraction procedure. The extracted RNA was allocated and stored at −80 °C to mitigate the fridge thaw cycle and prevent RNA degradation which might influence the result. These executed procedures enabled us to evaluate the performance of all kits more precisely.

The rise of various variants of concerns has increased the length of this pandemic. These variants contain different mutations in their genome, for example, the "UK Variant" B.1.1.7 contains 23 mutations in *N*, *ORF1ab*, *ORF8*, and S genes [33]. These genetic variations can affect the sensitivity of diagnostic kits by affecting primer binding sites [34]. The in-house assay was tested against different variants to evaluate the efficiency and found it 100% sensitive in detecting different variants, including B.1.1.7, B.1.351, P.1., and B.1.1.529.

As SARS-CoV-2 is a novel virus, the diagnosis is still in a developing phase and different kits show fluctuation in performance. One major aspect of the diagnostic kit is consistency [35]. To evaluate the consistency in a clinical set up, we performed an assay reproducibility and kit stability test where the in-house kit exhibited identical results for five consecutive weeks using a set of ten known samples for evaluation. The kit also showed evidence of stability at 4 °C for the five-week time period in this study, which indicates a sustainable performance of the in-house assay.

The principal feature of our developed in-house assay is that it can be performed in different real-time PCR platforms at different sites. Therefore, this kit can be used in most molecular laboratories for the diagnosis of SARS-CoV-2. Another aspect of the in-house kit is that the master mix used in this assay contains Uracil-DNA glycosylase (UDG) which contributes to eliminating carryover contamination [36]. The primer-probe used in this study is well proven to be used against SARS-CoV-2 virus assay. Hence, we might conclude that the in-house assay will be very specific with minimal chance of a false-positive result.

5. Conclusions

We developed an rRT-PCR kit to detect SARS-CoV-2 efficiently compared to kits that are recognized globally. The assay developed in our study can provide a cost-effective solution to support the mass diagnosis of SARS-CoV-2 and reduce the dependency on foreign kits which will make the health care system of Bangladesh more sustainable in during the COVID-19 pandemic.

Supplementary Materials: The following supporting information can be downloaded at: https://www.mdpi.com/article/10.3390/diagnostics12112617/s1.

Author Contributions: M.H.R. developed the research design, conducted validation study, analyzed the samples, data curation, monitored the study progress, review and edit the manuscript. Z.B.A., M.I.H., M.R.K., M.R.N. and M.A.H. optimized the method, conducted validation and stability study, analyzed the samples and review the manuscript. G.K.P. contributed to data curation. M.F.A.R. developed the research design, data curation, monitored the study progress, and wrote the original manuscript. M.M. and P.K. monitored the study progress and review the manuscript. M.K. developed the research concept and supervised the study, was a major contributor to writing the manuscript, and monitored the progress of the entire study. All authors have read and agreed to the published version of the manuscript.

Funding: This research received no external funding.

Institutional Review Board Statement: The study was conducted in accordance with the Declaration of Helsinki, and approved by the Institutional Research Ethics Committee of Bangladesh Reference Institute for Chemical Measurements (Ref No#BRiCM2206; date of approval: 5 May 2022).

Informed Consent Statement: Informed consent was obtained from all subjects involved in the study.

Data Availability Statement: All raw data are provided as Supplementary Materials.

Acknowledgments: We specially thank Honorable Minister Arct. Yeafesh Osman, Ministry of Science and Technology for his encouragement and support to develop this in-house assay kit during the pandemic situation. We also thank Rabindranath Roy Chowdhury, Additional Secretary (Rtd.), Ministry of Science and Technology and Advisor of Bangladesh Reference Institute for Chemical Measurements for his valuable suggestion and guidance to conduct this study.

Conflicts of Interest: The authors declare that RT-PCR kit production and distribution would be done by BRiCM, a statutory body under the Ministry of Science and Technology, Government of the People's Republic of Bangladesh at production cost. Hence all the authors do not have any personal competing interest.

Abbreviations

rRT-PCR (real Time Reverse Transcriptase Polymerase Chain Reaction); SARS-CoV-2 (Severe Actute Repiratory Syndrome Corona Virus-2); FDA (Food & Drug Administration); LoD (Lower limit of Detection); DNAS (DNA Solution Ltd.); BRiCM (Bangladesh Reference Institute for Chemical Measurements); Ct (Cycle Threshold); CE-IVD (Certified In Vitro Diagnosis).

References

1. Du, W.; Han, S.; Li, Q.; Zhang, Z. Epidemic update of COVID-19 in Hubei Province compared with other regions in China. *Int. J. Infect. Dis.* **2020**, *95*, 321–325. [CrossRef]
2. COVID Live Coronavirus Statistics—Worldometer n.d. Available online: https://www.worldometers.info/coronavirus/ (accessed on 19 January 2022).
3. COVID-19 Dynamic Dashboard for Bangladesh. Available online: https://dghs-dashboard.com/pages/covid19.php (accessed on 19 January 2022).
4. Ma, Q.; Liu, J.; Liu, Q.; Kang, L.; Liu, R.; Jing, W.; Wu, Y.; Liu, M. Global percentage of asymptomatic SARS-CoV-2 infections among the tested population and individuals with confirmed COVID-19 diagnosis: A systematic review and meta-analysis. *JAMA Netw. Open* **2021**, *4*, e2137257. [CrossRef] [PubMed]
5. Eis-Hübinger, A.M.; Hönemann, M.; Wenzel, J.J.; Berger, A.; Widera, M.; Schmidt, B.; Aldabbagh, S.; Marx, B.; Streeck, H.; Ciesek, S.; et al. Ad hoc laboratory-based surveillance of SARS-CoV-2 by real-time RT-PCR using minipools of RNA prepared from routine respiratory samples. *J. Clin. Virol.* **2020**, *127*, 104381. [CrossRef] [PubMed]
6. Hatcher, E.L.; Zhdanov, S.A.; Bao, Y.; Blinkova, O.; Nawrocki, E.P.; Ostapchuck, Y.; Schäffer, A.A.; Brister, J.R. Virus Variation Resource—Improved response to emergent viral outbreaks. *Nucleic Acids Res.* **2017**, *45*, D482–D490. [CrossRef] [PubMed]
7. Kucirka, L.M.; Lauer, S.A.; Laeyendecker, O.; Boon, D.; Lessler, J. Variation in false-negative rate of reverse transcriptase polymerase chain reaction–based SARS-CoV-2 tests by time since exposure. *Ann. Intern. Med.* **2020**, *173*, 262–267. [CrossRef] [PubMed]
8. Wikramaratna, P.S.; Paton, R.S.; Ghafari, M.; Lourenço, J. Estimating the false-negative test probability of SARS-CoV-2 by RT-PCR. *Eurosurveillance* **2020**, *25*, 2000568. [CrossRef] [PubMed]

9. Yu, F.; Yan, L.; Wang, N.; Yang, S.; Wang, L.; Tang, Y.; Gao, G.; Wang, S.; Ma, C.; Xie, R.; et al. Quantitative detection and viral load analysis of SARS-CoV-2 in infected patients. *Clin. Infect. Dis.* **2020**, *71*, 793–798. [CrossRef]
10. Hasan, M.M.; Rocha, I.C.N.; Ramos, K.G.; Cedeño, T.D.D.; dos Santos Costa, A.C.; Tsagkaris, C.; Billah, M.M.; Ahmad, S.; Essar, M.Y. Emergence of highly infectious SARS-CoV-2 variants in Bangladesh: The need for systematic genetic surveillance as a public health strategy. *Trop. Med. Health* **2021**, *49*, 69. [CrossRef]
11. Rahman, M.; Shirin, T.; Rahman, S.; Rahman, M.M.; Hossain, M.E.; Khan, M.H.; Rahman, M.Z.; el Arifeen, S.; Ahmed, T. The emergence of SARS-CoV-2 variants in Dhaka city, Bangladesh. *Transbound. Emerg. Dis.* **2021**, *68*, 3000–3001. [CrossRef]
12. van Dorp, L.; Acman, M.; Richard, D.; Shaw, L.P.; Ford, C.E.; Ormond, L.; Owen, C.J.; Pang, J.; Tan, C.C.S.; Boshier, F.A.T.; et al. Emergence of genomic diversity and recurrent mutations in SARS-CoV-2. *Infect. Genet. Evol.* **2020**, *83*, 104351. [CrossRef]
13. Kaushal, N.; Gupta, Y.; Goyal, M.; Khaiboullina, S.F.; Baranwal, M.; Verma, S.C. Mutational frequencies of SARS-CoV-2 genome during the beginning months of the outbreak in USA. *Pathogens* **2020**, *9*, 565. [CrossRef] [PubMed]
14. Wang, C.; Liu, Z.; Chen, Z.; Huang, X.; Xu, M.; He, T.; Zhang, Z. The establishment of reference sequence for SARS-CoV-2 and variation analysis. *J. Med. Virol.* **2020**, *92*, 667–674. [CrossRef] [PubMed]
15. Anwar, S.; Nasrullah, M.; Hosen, M.J. COVID-19 and Bangladesh: Challenges and how to address them. *Front. Public Health* **2020**, *8*, 154. [CrossRef]
16. Corman, V.M.; Landt, O.; Kaiser, M.; Molenkamp, R.; Meijer, A.; Chu, D.K.; Bleicker, T.; Brünink, S.; Schneider, J.; Schmidt, M.L.; et al. Detection of 2019 novel coronavirus (2019-nCoV) by real-time RT-PCR. *Eurosurveillance* **2020**, *25*, 2000045. [CrossRef]
17. CDC. Real-Time RT- PCR Primers and Probes for COVID-19. Available online: https://www.cdc.gov/coronavirus/2019-ncov/lab/rt-pcr-panel-primer-probes.html (accessed on 21 January 2022).
18. Zhen, W.; Berry, G.J. Design of a novel multiplex real time RT-PCR assay for SARS-CoV-2 detection. *bioRxiv* **2020**. [CrossRef]
19. Cook, R.J.; Dickens, B.M.; Fathalla, M.F. World Medical Association Declaration of Helsinki: Ethical Principles for Medical Research Involving Human Subjects. In *Reproductive Health and Human Rights*; Oxford University Press: Oxford, UK, 2003. [CrossRef]
20. Bajaj, S.; Singla, D.; Sakhuja, N. Stability testing of pharmaceutical products. *J. Appl. Pharm. Sci.* **2012**, *30*, 129–138.
21. MedCalc's Diagnostic Test Evaluation Calculator. Available online: https://www.medcalc.org/calc/diagnostic_test.php (accessed on 11 February 2022).
22. Eberle, U.; Wimmer, C.; Huber, I.; Neubauer-Juric, A.; Valenza, G.; Ackermann, N.; Sing, A. Comparison of nine different commercially available molecular assays for detection of SARS-CoV-2 RNA. *Eur. J. Clin. Microbiol. Infect. Dis.* **2021**, *40*, 1303–1308. [CrossRef]
23. Total COVID-19 Tests Per 1000 People. Available online: https://ourworldindata.org/grapher/full-list-cumulative-total-tests-per-thousand?tab=table (accessed on 11 February 2022).
24. Tombuloglu, H.; Sabit, H.; Al-Suhaimi, E.; Al Jindan, R.; Alkharsah, K.R. Development of multiplex real-time RT-PCR assay for the detection of SARS-CoV-2. *PLoS ONE* **2021**, *16*, e0250942. [CrossRef]
25. Anantharajah, A.; Helaers, R.; Defour, J.-P.; Olive, N.; Kabera, F.; Croonen, L.; Deldime, F.; Vaerman, J.; Barbée, C.; Bodéus, M.; et al. How to choose the right real-time RT-PCR primer sets for the SARS-CoV-2 genome detection? *J. Virol. Methods* **2021**, *295*, 114197. [CrossRef]
26. Cao, L.; Xu, T.; Liu, X.; Ji, Y.; Huang, S.; Peng, H.; Li, C.; Guo, D. The Impact of Accumulated Mutations in SARS-CoV-2 Variants on the qPCR Detection Efficiency. *Front. Cell. Infect. Microbiol.* **2022**, *12*. [CrossRef]
27. Freire-Paspuel, B.; Garcia-Bereguiain, M.A. Analytical sensitivity and clinical performance of a triplex RT-qPCR assay using CDC N1, N2, and RP targets for SARS-CoV-2 diagnosis. *Int. J. Infect. Dis.* **2021**, *102*, 14–16. [CrossRef] [PubMed]
28. Nalla, A.K.; Casto, A.M.; Huang, M.-L.W.; Perchetti, G.A.; Sampoleo, R.; Shrestha, L.; Wei, Y.; Zhu, H.; Jerome, K.R.; Greninger, A.L.; et al. Comparative performance of SARS-CoV-2 detection assays using seven different primer-probe sets and one assay kit. *J. Clin. Microbiol.* **2020**, *58*, e00557-20. [CrossRef] [PubMed]
29. Park, M.; Won, J.; Choi, B.Y.; Lee, C.J. Optimization of primer sets and detection protocols for SARS-CoV-2 of coronavirus disease 2019 (COVID-19) using PCR and real-time PCR. *Exp. Mol. Med.* **2020**, *52*, 963–977. [CrossRef]
30. Vogels, C.B.; Brito, A.F.; Wyllie, A.L.; Fauver, J.R.; Ott, I.M.; Kalinich, C.C.; Petrone, M.E.; Casanovas-Massana, A.M.; Muenker, C.; Moore, A.J.; et al. Analytical sensitivity and efficiency comparisons of SARS-CoV-2 RT–qPCR primer–probe sets. *Nat. Microbiol.* **2020**, *5*, 1299–1305. [CrossRef] [PubMed]
31. Noor, F.A.; Safain, K.S.; Hossain, M.W.; Arafath, K.; Mannoor, K.; Kabir, M. Development and performance evaluation of the first in-house multiplex rRT-PCR assay in Bangladesh for highly sensitive detection of SARS-CoV-2. *J. Virol. Methods* **2021**, *293*, 114147. [CrossRef] [PubMed]
32. Ishige, T.; Murata, S.; Taniguchi, T.; Miyabe, A.; Kitamura, K.; Kawasaki, K.; Nishimura, M.; Igari, H.; Matsushita, K. Highly sensitive detection of SARS-CoV-2 RNA by multiplex rRT-PCR for molecular diagnosis of COVID-19 by clinical laboratories. *Clin. Chim. Acta* **2020**, *507*, 139–142. [CrossRef]
33. Banko, A.; Petrovic, G.; Miljanovic, D.; Loncar, A.; Vukcevic, M.; Despot, D.; Cirkovic, A. Comparison and sensitivity evaluation of three different commercial real-time quantitative PCR kits for SARS-CoV-2 detection. *Viruses* **2021**, *13*, 1321. [CrossRef]
34. Wu, S.; Shi, X.; Chen, Q.; Jiang, Y.; Zuo, L.; Wang, L.; Jiang, M.; Lin, Y.; Fang, S.; Peng, B.; et al. Comparative evaluation of six nucleic acid amplification kits for SARS-CoV-2 RNA detection. *Ann. Clin. Microbiol. Antimicrob.* **2021**, *20*, 38. [CrossRef]
35. Onwuamah, C.K.; Okwuraiwe, A.P.; Salu, O.B.; Shaibu, J.O.; Ndodo, N.; Amoo, S.O.; Okoli, L.C.; Ige, F.A.; Ahmed, R.A.; Bankole, M.A.; et al. Comparative performance of SARS-CoV-2 real-time PCR diagnostic assays on samples from Lagos, Nigeria. *PLoS ONE* **2021**, *16*, e0246637. [CrossRef]

36. Tetzner, R.; Dietrich, D.; Distler, J. Control of carry-over contamination for PCR-based DNA methylation quantification using bisulfite treated DNA. *Nucleic Acids Res.* **2007**, *35*, e4. [CrossRef]

diagnostics

MDPI

Article

Determination of Diphtheria Toxin in Bacterial Cultures by Enzyme Immunoassay

Maria A. Simonova [1,†], Vyacheslav G. Melnikov [2,*,†], Olga E. Lakhtina [1], Ravilya L. Komaleva [1], Anja Berger [2,3], Andreas Sing [2,3,‡] and Sergey K. Zavriev [1,‡]

1 Shemyakin-Ovchinnikov Institute of Bioorganic Chemistry of Russian Academy of Sciences, Miklukho-Maklaya 16/10, 117997 Moscow, Russia
2 National Conciliary Laboratory on Diphtheria, Veterinaerstrasse 2, 85764 Oberschleissheim, Germany
3 Department of Public Health Microbiology, Bavarian Health and Food Safety Authority, Veterinaerstrasse 2, 85764 Oberschleissheim, Germany
* Correspondence: slavawho1@gmail.com
† These authors contributed equally to this work.
‡ These authors contributed equally to this work.

Abstract: Since diphtheria toxin (DT) is the main virulence factor of *Corynebacterium diphtheriae* and *C. ulcerans*, the detection of DT in corynebacterial cultures is of utmost importance in the laboratory diagnosis of diphtheria. The need to measure the level of DT production (LTP) arises when studying the virulence of a strain for the purpose of diphtheria agent monitoring. To determine the LTP of diphtheria agents, an immunoassay based on monoclonal antibodies (mAbs) has been developed. A pair of mAbs specific to the fragment B of DT was selected, which makes it possible to detect DT in a sandwich ELISA with a detection limit of DT less than 1 ng/mL. Sandwich ELISA was used to analyze 218 liquid culture supernatants of high-, low- and non-toxigenic strains of various corynebacteria. It was shown that the results of ELISA are in good agreement with the results of PCR and the Elek test for the *tox* gene and DT detection, respectively. The diagnostic sensitivity of the assay was approximately 99%, and specificity was 100%. It has been found that strains of *C. ulcerans*, on average, produce 10 times less DT than *C. diphtheriae*. The mAbs used in the ELISA proved to be quite discriminatory and could be further used for the design of the LFIA, a method that can reduce the labor and cost of laboratory diagnosis of diphtheria.

Keywords: *Corynebacterium diphtheriae*; *Corynebacterium ulcerans*; diphtheria toxin; ELISA; monoclonal antibodies; level of toxin production

Citation: Simonova, M.A.; Melnikov, V.G.; Lakhtina, O.E.; Komaleva, R.L.; Berger, A.; Sing, A.; Zavriev, S.K. Determination of Diphtheria Toxin in Bacterial Cultures by Enzyme Immunoassay. *Diagnostics* **2022**, *12*, 2204. https://doi.org/10.3390/diagnostics12092204

Academic Editor: Hsin-Yao Wang

Received: 13 August 2022
Accepted: 8 September 2022
Published: 11 September 2022

1. Introduction

It is easy to get to the bottom of diphtheria—the disease is all about the diphtheria toxin (DT). DT is a potent exotoxin of *Corynebacterium diphtheriae* and *C. ulcerans*, which kills susceptible cells by inhibiting protein synthesis. Specifically, DT transfers the ADP-ribose moiety of NAD to elongation factor EF-2, inactivating it. The ADP-ribosylation activity of DT is determined by the A fragment, and B fragment is required for eukaryotic cell receptor-binding. The toxin repressor (DtxR), a chromosomal regulatory protein, inhibits DT production and derepresses it when Fe^{2+} corepressor is depleted. The phage-encoded DT is the main virulence-associated factor in the disease, responsible for causing diphtheria symptoms, i.e., fever, headache, general malaise, acute tonsillitis with a pseudomembrane over the tonsils, nasopharynx, or even larynx, inflammation and swelling of the cervical lymph nodes ("bull neck"), and systemic complications, including toxin-derived damage to the myocardium, nervous system, and kidneys. Specific prevention of the disease is the vaccination of children with diphtheria toxoid, and the main route of therapy is the administration of hyperimmune equine antitoxic serum (antitoxin). Only toxigenic strains of *C. diphtheriae* and *C. ulcerans* can cause classical respiratory diphtheria, while non-toxigenic strains are not able to do so [1]. Therefore, the accelerated indication of toxin-forming corynebacteria in clinical material is of utmost importance in diphtheria laboratory-based diagnosis, both for managing the individual patient as well as for public health measures.

Laboratory diagnostic tests for toxigenicity of *C. diphtheriae*/*C. ulcerans* are based on qualitative immunological methods [1]. We set ourselves the goal of developing a sensitive and specific test to determine not only the presence, but also the amount of DT produced by the corynebacterial culture. The need to measure the concentration of DT arises when, for instance, studying a relationship between the level of toxin production (LTP) of strains of diphtheria agent, which until recently included only *C. diphtheriae*, and now also includes *C. ulcerans*, and the virulence of the strain. Thus, we found that the *C. diphtheriae* var. *gravis*, ribotype 'Sankt-Peterburg/Rossija', MLST type ST8, the diphtheria epidemic clone in Russia and other countries of the former USSR in the 1990s, caused more severe forms of infection in unvaccinated children, compared with the 1980s, when the *C. diphtheriae* var. *mitis*, ribotype 'Otchakov', MLST type ST5 was common, and also had a higher LTP. LTP studies were performed using an indirect hemagglutination test with a diagnosticum on sheep erythrocytes sensitized with diphtheria antitoxin, and the result was estimated as the maximum dilution of the liquid bacterial culture, in which hemagglutination still occurred [2]. The high level of DT production in the *C. diphtheriae* ST8 strains was explained by the fact that this epidemic clone had the GCC-> GTC (A147V) mutation in the dtxR gene, that, as shown by chemical mutagenesis studies, modified the regulatory functions of the DtxR protein [3], which, in turn, could lead to an increase in DT expression. However, another research group using the same LTP detection method found that the population of the *C. diphtheriae* ST8 clone was heterogeneous, containing both strongly and weakly toxigenic strains [4]. As can be seen from this example, studies devoted to the development of a reliable method for the determination of LTPs are of importance in assessing the pathogenic potential of corynebacteria.

ELISA remains a very robust and reliable method for the detection of various protein analytes. Previously, enzyme-linked immunosorbent and immunochromatographic methods for detecting DT were developed, the sensitivity of which varied from 0.1 to 4 ng/mL [5–7]. These tests were based on a sandwich immunoassay with equine polyclonal antibodies as binding antibodies, and mouse monoclonal antibodies (mAbs) as detecting antibodies. For the determination of LTP, we developed a sensitive immunoassay based only on mAbs, since they have constant properties and, therefore, such a test is easier to standardize.

In addition, we set out to determine whether the mAbs used in ELISA are discriminatory enough to be used in the Lateral Flow Immunoassay (LFIA), a method that can reduce labour and cost of laboratory diagnosis of diphtheria.

2. Materials and Methods

2.1. Bacterial Strains

A total of 218 strains of corynebacteria for this study (listed in Table S1 in Supplementary Materials) were obtained from the German Conciliary Laboratory on Diphtheria (GCLoD) culture collection. They were both of human and animal origin and isolated in Germany in 2011–2022. The presence of the toxin gene and the DT production were detected by RT-PCR and the Elek test, respectively [8]. The bacterial strains were grown on Columbia Blood Agar (Oxoid, Basingstoke, UK) for 24 h prior to testing.

2.2. Sample Preparation

ELISA testing was performed between February 2021 and January 2022. For ELISA testing bacterial strains were cultured on Elek broth [6,7] for 6 h at 37 °C, after which the bacterial cells were removed by filtration through a 0.22-µm-pore-size membrane (Merck Millipore, Burlington, MA, USA). The culture supernatants were stored at −20 °C prior to analysis in the ELISA.

2.3. mAb Production and Purification

Cells of mAb-producing hybridomas were used to generate mAbs [9]. Briefly, the producing cells were introduced into BALB/C mice, and preparative amounts of the antibodies were isolated from the ascitic fluids of these mice. The mAbs from the ascitic fluids were purified by affinity chromatography on protein-A-Sepharose (GE Healthcare, Chicago, IL, USA). The ascitic fluid was diluted by four times with the starting buffer (1.5 M glycine and 3 M NaCl, pH 8.9) and applied onto a column that was filled with the affinity sorbent and equilibrated with the same buffer. The mAbs were eluted with a 0.1 M citrate buffer with pH 4.0. The mAb-containing fractions were dialyzed against phosphate buffered saline (PBS). The purity of the mAbs was defined by SDS-PAGE. The mAbs antigen-binding activity was confirmed by indirect ELISA as described previously [9].

2.4. Sandwich ELISA

Purified mAbs were biotinylated using the EZ-Link Sulfo-NHS-LC-Biotin reagent (ThermoFisher, Waltham, MA, USA) according to the manufacturer's instructions. For ELISA, binding antibodies (10 μg/mL in PBS) were adsorbed overnight at 4 °C in the wells (100 μL per well) of a 96-well polystyrene high-binding plate (Costar-Corning, NY, USA). Next, the plate washed 3 times with PBS with 0.05% tween-20 (PBST). Solutions of DT (Sigma-Aldrich, St. Louis, MO, USA) were prepared in PBST with 1% BSA (PBST-BSA) or in Elek broth at various concentrations and added by 100 μL to the wells of the plate with adsorbed antibodies. PBST-BSA or Elek broth without the addition of toxin were used as negative controls. The plate was incubated for 1 h at room temperature on a shaker. Then, the plate was washed 3 times with PBST, 100 μL of a solution of detecting biotinylated mAbs (1 μg/mL in PBST-BSA) was added to each well and incubated for 1 h at room temperature on a shaker. After washing the plate 3 times with PBST, a solution of horseradish peroxidase-labeled streptavidin (BD Biosciences, Franklin Lakes, NJ, USA) in PBST-BSA at a working dilution of 100 μL per well was added and incubated 1 h at room temperature on a shaker. At the end of the incubation, the plate was washed as described above, and 100 μL of the peroxidase substrate, ortho-phenylenediamine (Sigma-Aldrich, St. Louis, MO, USA), was added to each well at a concentration of 1 mg/mL in 1% citrate buffer, pH 4.5, containing 0.05% hydrogen peroxide. The reaction was stopped by adding 50 μL of 2 M sulfuric acid to each well and the color intensity recorded spectrophotometrically (>Packard SpectraCount BS10000, PerkinElmer, Waltham, MA, USA) by determining the optical absorbance at 490 nm.

For detection of DT production in cultures of corynebacteria, culture supernatants were added to the wells of the plate with adsorbed binding antibodies, 100 μL per well. To quantify DT in culture supernatants, samples were diluted 2–100 times with PBST-BSA. The analysis was then carried out as described above. Each sample of the culture supernatant was analyzed in at least duplicates.

2.5. Statistical Analysis

Statistical data processing was carried out using the R software environment [10] and specialized packages. The *drc* extension package was used to construct calibration curves and determine DT concentration in culture supernatants [11]. The limit of detection of DT was calculated using the calibration curves and was defined as the concentration of DT corresponding to an optical absorbance value two times higher than the average optical absorbance value of the repeated (at least 10 times) negative control. Differences between samples were tested using the Mann–Whitney U-test and considered statistically significant at $p < 0.05$. ROC analysis by the pROC and ROCR packages was used for the assessment of the accuracy of the method for detecting the toxin, as well as the determination of the threshold of sensitivity of the toxin in bacterial cultures [12,13]. Accuracy, sensitivity, and specificity of qualitative test at each threshold was defined by the formulas: (TP+TN)/(P+N), TP/P, and TN/N, respectively, where P—positive samples, N—negative samples, TP—true positives, TN—true negatives [12].

3. Results

3.1. Selection of Diagnostic Pair of mAbs

Purified anti-DT mAbs for this study were obtained using hybridoma-producing mAb cells. The purity of mAbs preparations was at least 95% according to the data of SDS-PAGE electrophoresis, and all the mAbs were active in indirect ELISA (data not shown).

The search of diagnostic pairs of mAbs for detection of DT in the sandwich ELISA was carried out. For this, all mAbs were biotinylated and used as detecting antibodies (labeled "biot"). Purified DT manufactured by Sigma was used as a standard. Only mAbs C2G5 and E6B9 worked as a diagnostic pair in the sandwich ELISA. In the C2G5-E6B9biot configuration, the detection limit for DT was 0.4 ± 0.1 ng/mL, so this pair of diagnostic antibodies was used in further studies. It should be noted that both mAbs included in the diagnostic pair were specific for the receptor-binding (B) fragment of DT (Table 1).

Table 1. Characteristics of monoclonal antibodies to diphtheria toxin (DT).

mAb ID	Isotype	DT Fragment Specificity
C2G5	IgG_1	B
C12E5	IgG_{2b}	A
E4C4	IgG_{2a}	A
E6B9	IgG_1	B
G2D9	IgG_{2a}	A
H10B3	n/d	A

n/d—not determined.

3.2. Detection of DT in Elek Broth

Since the purpose of this work was to determine the DT in liquid bacterial culture, we further studied the effect of the cultivation medium on the results of the analysis of DT. The purified DT was diluted in a standard buffer and Elek broth, and the dose–response curves were analyzed (Figure 1). The detection limit of DT in Elek broth was 0.3 ± 0.1 ng/mL. Background signals in the buffer and Elek medium were not statistically different ($p = 0.22$). Thus, Elek broth did not significantly affect the analysis parameters compared to the buffer.

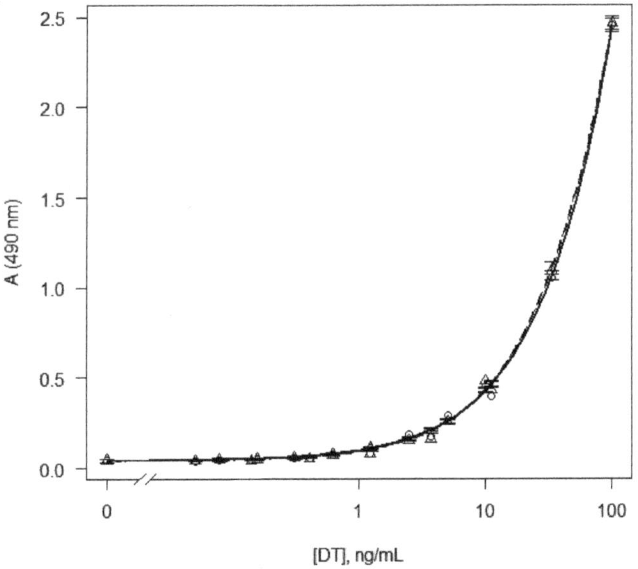

Figure 1. Dose–response curves obtained as results of sandwich ELISA of DT in buffer (circles, solid line) and Elek broth (triangles, dashed line). Model-based standard errors are also shown.

3.3. *Sandwich ELISA for Determination of the DT in Bacterial Cultures*

Further, we performed the ELISA for detection of the DT in liquid corynebacterial cultures (Table S1 in Supplementary Materials). To determine the background value of the optical absorbance, the average value of the optical absorbance in the samples of the non-inoculated Elek broth was calculated (at least eight replications for each analyzed plate). Next, the ratios of the optical absorbance in the analyzed samples to the background value of the optical absorbance were calculated. Based on the calculated values, as well as the presence of the DT gene and the Elek test results, ROC analysis was performed to determine the predictive ability of the assay, as well as the optimal threshold value of the signal/background ratio. The calculated AUC value was 0.99 (95% confidence interval (CI): 0.97–1.00), which indicates a high predictive ability of the test (Figure S1A in Supplementary Materials). The maximum signal/background ratio, which provides more than 99% accuracy of the qualitative determination of the toxin, was 2.3 (Figure S1B in Supplementary Materials). Thus, the samples for which the signal/background ratio was less than 2.3 were classified as negative, the rest of the samples were classified as positive. For positive samples, a quantitative analysis of DT was performed using calibration curves similar to the curve on Figure 1 (Table S1 in Supplementary Materials).

As can be seen from Table 2, the developed enzyme immunoassay made it possible to detect DT with high accuracy in 218 corynebacterial cultures. At threshold 2.3, the diagnostic sensitivity of the assay was approximately 99%, and specificity was 100%. For all strains, except for one (*C. ulcerans* KL 1902, Table S1 in Supplementary Materials), the results of the ELISA coincided with the results of PCR and the Elek test. All strains producing DT in the Elek test, except for *C. ulcerans* KL 1902 (Table S1 in Supplementary Materials), were ELISA-positive. The KL 1902 strain was *tox*+ and DT-positive, but ELISA-negative. DT-gene-negative *C. diphtheriae*, *C. ulcerans*, and *C. pseudotuberculosis* (diphtheria clade), along with cultures of non-diphtheria corynebacteria, as expected, were found ELISA-negative. Non-toxigenic *tox*-gene positive (NTTB) *C. diphtheriae* and *C. silvaticum* strains were also ELISA-negative.

Table 2. Confusion matrix for the results of qualitative DT detection by sandwich ELISA in corynebacterial cultures.

Total Samples: 218	ELISA: Negative	ELISA: Positive	
Negative samples *:	TN = 114	FP = 0	Total: 114
Positive samples **:	FN = 1	TP = 103	Total: 104
	Total: 115	Total: 103	

FN—false negative; FP—false positive; TN—true negative; TP—true positive. The evaluation was carried out at a threshold signal/background ratio of 2.3. Note: the presence of the toxin gene was detected by RT-PCR; in the absence of the *tox* gene, DT production in most cases was not determined, and strain was considered as negative (*). In the presence of the *tox* gene, DT production was confirmed by the Elek test (**), and if toxin production was not detected in the Elek test, then the strain was considered as negative (*).

The average concentrations of DT determined in ELISA-positive *C. ulcerans* cultures (excluding a strain *C. ulcerans* M06-759) were significantly (10 times) lower than the concentrations of DT in cultures of *C. diphtheriae*: 85.0 and 894.0 ng/mL, respectively ($p < 0.001$). *C. ulcerans* M06-759, compared to other strains of *C. ulcerans*, is unique in that it produces an increased amount of DT (2514.8 ng/mL). The reasons for this phenomenon require further study.

4. Discussion

The results of this study indicate the high efficiency of the developed ELISA. The only discrepancy was the strain *C. ulcerans* KL 1902, which was producing DT by the Elek test but not by the ELISA. This strain needs to be studied in detail, including by performing whole genome sequencing. It might be speculated that there are some mutations in the toxin gene that disrupt the folding of the toxin molecule and thereby prevent mAbs from binding to the toxin.

Among the 218 strains from GCLoD culture collection used in our study, 21 strains of *C. ulcerans* were *tox* gene positive but initially negative in the Elek test and therefore classified as NTTBs, which are known to circulate worldwide [1,2,4,8,14]. At the same time, all of these 21 strains appeared weakly positive in ELISA. It has been suggested that the current Elek test may not detect the toxin in low-toxigenic strains of *C. ulcerans*. Such observations were first made about 20 years ago [15] by the author of this study (A.S.). The clinical isolate *C. ulcerans* A6361 possessed the DT gene and was Elek test negative. However, the ability of the isolate A6361 to express DT was disclosed using a highly sensitive immunochromatographic strip (ICS) test, which was developed to replace the Elek test [7]. As shown by external quality assessments of the European Diphtheria Surveillance Network (EDSN), most of the laboratories participating in the study also had difficulty testing low-toxigenic strains of *C. ulcerans* with the Elek method [16]. We have made some changes to the immunoprecipitation Elek method (namely, type and concentration of antitoxin, inoculum distance from the antitoxin disk, shape of the bacterial plaques, and position of control strains) and developed a protocol for the optimised Elek test with the capacity to detect all the toxigenic corynebacteria in our study, including those 21 strains with low toxin production [17]. It should be noted that using the previous (less sensitive) modification of the Elek test [8], it was possible to detect every single toxigenic strain of *C. diphtheriae*, even the weakly toxigenic reference strain NCTC 3984. Our study makes this result understandable. The "weakly toxigenic" reference strain of *C. diphtheriae* NCTC 3984 expresses only 4 times less toxin than the control toxigenic strain *C. diphtheriae* NCTC 10648 (878.4 vs. 3370.0 ng/mL), while 21 true weakly toxigenic strains of *C. ulcerans* have average level of toxin production 110 times (!) lower than that of *C. diphtheriae* NCTC 10648 (30.5 vs. 3370.0 ng/mL). It can be concluded that some strains of *C. ulcerans* produce low levels of DT, which were not previously detected by the Elek test and therefore were erroneously classified as non-toxigenic. Hence, ELISA can be used as a reference method to identify isolates with questionable toxin production.

C. silvaticum (a recently described species of the diphtheria corynebacteria [18] with a non-expressing DT gene) strains were ELISA-negative. Since the toxigenicity of these GCLoD collection's *C. silvaticum* cultures was assessed using the previous modification of the Elek test, and that the genetic reason for the non-expression of the DT gene was not revealed even by sequencing, the results of our study proved to be very useful, confirming the lack of ability of *C. silvaticum* to produce a DT. It should be remembered that both ELISA and Elek testing are in vitro methods, therefore, labeling *C. ulcerans* and *C. silvaticum* strains as "poorly toxigenic" or "non-toxigenic" reflects only in vitro data; it cannot be excluded, however, that they are able to produce a significant amount of DT when grown in vivo.

Given that toxigenic *C. ulcerans* were recently recognized as an emerging zoonotic pathogen causing diphtheria-like infections in humans [1,8], the use of sensitive methods for assessing DT production in weakly toxigenic *C. ulcerans* is now of importance. Despite the fact that at present *C. ulcerans* do not cause either severe forms of infection or diphtheria outbreaks, the pathogenetic role of corynebacteria with a low level of toxin production should not be underestimated. The toxin is lethal for susceptible animals as well as unvaccinated humans at doses of 100 ng/kg or less [19].

Moreover, in our recent study 18 allelic variants of the *tox* gene were found across the 291 *tox*+ *C. diphtheriae* isolates. Of these 18 allelic types, 8 contained non-synonymous SNP changes, estimated to be of medium to high structural impact [20]. *C. ulcerans* have a much higher level of *tox* gene variability. They carry about 30 non-synonymous mutations [15] that significantly affect the molecular structure of *C. ulcerans* DT (data not shown). The continually increasing toxin diversity does forecast a real possibility of vaccine escape and antitoxin treatment failure in future. Thus, even if *C. ulcerans* strains are weak toxin producers, mutated strains may become capable of causing disease in people vaccinated against diphtheria.

To conclude, the ELISA is a suitable method for monitoring diphtheria agents by determining LTP. However, using this method in routine practice to detect DT is quite laborious. Thus, there is an urgent need for a simple and reliable test for the rapid indication of toxigenic corynebacteria that can be used in the conventional laboratory. This will significantly reduce the diagnostic time, since it will no longer be necessary to send the clinical specimen or cultures isolated from the patient to the diphtheria reference laboratory. Such a method, for example, can be LFIA based on a pair of mAbs that performed well in this ELISA study.

Supplementary Materials: The following supporting information can be downloaded at: https://www.mdpi.com/article/10.3390/diagnostics12092204/s1, Figure S1: ROC-curve (A) and threshold-accuracy dependence curve (B) obtained as results of ROC analysis of ELISA results. AUC, 95% CI for AUC, as well as the signal/background ratio threshold at maximal accuracy are shown. CI—confidence interval. Table S1: The results of the detection of diphtheria toxin by sandwich ELISA in corynebacterial cultures.

Author Contributions: M.A.S., V.G.M., O.E.L. and R.L.K. conducted research; M.A.S. and V.G.M. drafted the manuscript, M.A.S., V.G.M. and A.B. evaluated the data, all authors participated in the interpretation of data as well as critical revisions of the manuscript. A.S. and S.K.Z. supervised the study. All authors have read and agreed to the published version of the manuscript.

Funding: This project has received funding from the European Union's Horizon 2020 research and innovation programme under grant agreement No. 843405-DIFTERIA-H2020-MSCA-IF-2018.

Institutional Review Board Statement: The animal study protocol was approved by the Ethics Committee of the Shemyakin–Ovchinnikov Institute of Bioorganic Chemistry of RAS, Moscow, Russia (protocol code 325 dated 14 June 2021).

Informed Consent Statement: Not applicable.

Data Availability Statement: All relevant data are within the manuscript.

Conflicts of Interest: The authors declare no conflict of interest.

References

1. Sharma, N.C.; Efstratiou, A.; Mokrousov, I.; Mutreja, A.; Das, B.; Ramamurthy, T. Diphtheria. *Nat. Rev. Dis. Prim.* **2019**, *5*, 81. [CrossRef] [PubMed]
2. Mazurova, I.K.; Kombarova SYu Borisova OYu Melnikov, V.G.; Maximova, N.M.; Gadua, N.T.; Naumov, L.S.; Volozhantsev, N.V. Monitoring of Corynebacterium diphtheriae strains. *Russ. J. Epidemiol. Vaccin.* **2009**, *46*, 17–22. Available online: https://cyberleninka.ru/article/n/monitoring-vozbuditelya-difteriynoy-infektsii (accessed on 7 September 2022).
3. Wang, Z.; Schmitt, M.P.; Holmes, R.K. Characterization of mutations that inactivate the diphtheria toxin repressor gene (dtxR). *Infect. Immun.* **1994**, *62*, 1600–1608. [CrossRef] [PubMed]
4. Titov, L.; Kolodkina, V.; Dronina, A.; Grimont, F.; Grimont, P.A.D.; Lejay-Collin, M.; de Zoysa, A.; Andronescu, C.; Diaconescu, A.; Marin, B.; et al. Genotypic and Phenotypic Characteristics of Corynebacterium diphtheriae Strains Isolated from Patients in Belarus during an Epidemic Period. *J. Clin. Microbiol.* **2003**, *41*, 1285–1288. [CrossRef] [PubMed]
5. Mazurova, I.K.; Potemkina, E.E.; Sviridov, V.V.; Zaitsev, E.M. Detection of toxin and evaluation of the degree of toxin-formation of Corynebacterium diphtheriae using immunoenzyme analysis. *Zhurnal Mikrobiol. Epidemiol. I Immunobiol.* **1989**, *6*, 66–70. Available online: https://pubmed.ncbi.nlm.nih.gov/2508377/ (accessed on 7 September 2022).
6. Engler, K.H.; Efstratiou, A. A rapid enzyme immunoassay for the detection of diphtheria toxin among clinical isolates of Corynebacterium spp. *J. Clin. Microbiol.* **2000**, *38*, 1385–1389. [CrossRef] [PubMed]
7. Engler, K.H.; Efstratiou, A.; Norn, D.; Kozlov, R.S.; Selga, I.; Glushkevich, T.G.; Tam, M.; Melnikov, V.; Mazurova, I.K.; Kim, V.E.; et al. Immunochromatographic Strip Test for Rapid Detection of Diphtheria Toxin: Description and Multicenter Evaluation in Areas of Low and High Prevalence of Diphtheria. *J. Clin. Microbiol.* **2002**, *40*, 80–83. [CrossRef] [PubMed]
8. *WHO Laboratory Manual for the Diagnosis of Diphtheria and Other Related Infections*; World Health Organization: Geneva, Switzerland, 2021. Available online: https://apps.who.int/iris/bitstream/handle/10665/352275/9789240038059-eng.pdf (accessed on 7 September 2022).
9. Valyakina, T.I.; Lakhtina, O.E.; Komaleva, R.L.; Simonova, M.A.; Samokhvalova, L.V.; Shoshina, N.S.; Kalinina, N.A.; Rubina, A.Y.; Filippova, M.A.; Vertiev, Y.V.; et al. Production and characteristics of monoclonal antibodies to the diphtheria toxin. *Russ. J. Bioorganic Chem.* **2009**, *35*, 556–565. [CrossRef] [PubMed]
10. R Core Team. *R: A Language and Environment for Statistical Computing*; R Foundation for Statistical Computing: Vienna, Austria, 2013. Available online: https://www.R-project.org/ (accessed on 7 September 2022).
11. Ritz, C.; Baty, F.; Streibig, J.C.; Gerhard, D. Dose-Response Analysis Using R. *PLoS ONE* **2015**, *10*, e0146021. [CrossRef] [PubMed]

12. Robin, X.; Turck, N.; Hainard, A.; Tiberti, N.; Lisacek, F.; Sanchez, J.-C.; Müller, M. pROC: An open-source package for R and S+ to analyze and compare ROC curves. *BMC Bioinform.* **2011**, *12*, 77. [CrossRef] [PubMed]
13. Sing, T.; Sander, O.; Beerenwinkel, N.; Lengauer, T. ROCR: Visualizing classifier performance in R. *Bioinformatics* **2005**, *21*, 3940–3941. [CrossRef] [PubMed]
14. Zakikhany, K.; Neal, S.; Efstratiou, A. Emergence and molecular characterisation of non-toxigenic tox gene-bearing Corynebacterium diphtheriae biovar mitis in the United Kingdom, 2003–2012. *Eurosurveillance* **2014**, *19*, 20819. [CrossRef] [PubMed]
15. Sing, A.; Hogardt, M.; Bierschenk, S.; Heesemann, J. Detection of differences in the nucleotide and amino acid sequences of diphtheria toxin from Corynebacterium diphtheriae and Corynebacterium ulcerans causing extrapharyngeal infections. *J. Clin. Microbiol.* **2003**, *41*, 4848–4851. [CrossRef] [PubMed]
16. Both, L.; Neal, S.; De Zoysa, A.; Mann, G.; Czumbel, I.; Efstratiou, A. European Diphtheria Surveillance Network. External quality assessments for microbiologic diagnosis of diphthe-ria in Europe. *J. Clin. Microbiol.* **2014**, *52*, 4381–4384. [CrossRef]
17. Melnikov, V.G.; Berger, A.; Sing, A. Detection of diphtheria toxin production by toxigenic corynebacteria using an optimized Elek test. *Infection* **2022**, 1–5. [CrossRef]
18. Dangel, A.; Berger, A.; Rau, J.; Eisenberg, T.; Kampfer, P.; Margos, G.; Contzen, M.; Busse, H.-J.; Konrad, R.; Peters, M.; et al. *Corynebacterium silvaticum* sp. nov., a unique group of NTTB corynebacteria in wild boar and roe deer. *Int. J. Syst. Evol. Microbiol.* **2020**, *70*, 3614–3624. [CrossRef] [PubMed]
19. Pappenheimer, A.M., Jr. Diphtheria Toxin. *Annu. Rev. Biochem.* **1977**, *46*, 69–94. [CrossRef] [PubMed]
20. Will, R.C.; Ramamurthy, T.; Sharma, N.C.; Veeraraghavan, B.; Sangal, L.; Haldar, P.; Pragasam, A.K.; Vasudevan, K.; Kumar, D.; Das, B.; et al. Spatiotemporal persistence of multiple, diverse clades and toxins of Corynebacterium diphtheriae. *Nat. Commun.* **2021**, *12*, 1500. [CrossRef] [PubMed]

diagnostics

MDPI

Review

Antibiotic Resistance Diagnosis in ESKAPE Pathogens—A Review on Proteomic Perspective

Sriram Kalpana [1], Wan-Ying Lin [2], Yu-Chiang Wang [3,4], Yiwen Fu [5], Amrutha Lakshmi [6] and Hsin-Yao Wang [1,*]

1 Department of Laboratory Medicine, Linkou Chang Gung Memorial Hospital, Taoyuan 333423, Taiwan
2 Syu Kang Sport Clinic, Taipei 112053, Taiwan
3 Department of Medicine, Harvard Medical School, Boston, MA 02115, USA
4 Department of Medicine, Brigham and Women's Hospital, Boston, MA 02115, USA
5 Department of Medicine, Kaiser Permanente Santa Clara Medical Center, Santa Clara, CA 95051, USA
6 Department of Biochemistry, University of Madras, Guindy Campus, Chennai 600025, India
* Correspondence: mdhsinyaowang@gmail.com

Abstract: Antibiotic resistance has emerged as an imminent pandemic. Rapid diagnostic assays distinguish bacterial infections from other diseases and aid antimicrobial stewardship, therapy optimization, and epidemiological surveillance. Traditional methods typically have longer turn-around times for definitive results. On the other hand, proteomic studies have progressed constantly and improved both in qualitative and quantitative analysis. With a wide range of data sets made available in the public domain, the ability to interpret the data has considerably reduced the error rates. This review gives an insight on state-of-the-art proteomic techniques in diagnosing antibiotic resistance in ESKAPE pathogens with a future outlook for evading the "imminent pandemic".

Keywords: antibiotic resistance; bacterial resistance; ESKAPE; MALDI-TOF; mass spectrometry; proteomics

Citation: Kalpana, S.; Lin, W.-Y.; Wang, Y.-C.; Fu, Y.; Lakshmi, A.; Wang, H.-Y. Antibiotic Resistance Diagnosis in ESKAPE Pathogens—A Review on Proteomic Perspective. *Diagnostics* **2023**, *13*, 1014. https://doi.org/10.3390/diagnostics13061014

Academic Editor: Mario Cruciani

Received: 7 February 2023
Revised: 26 February 2023
Accepted: 28 February 2023
Published: 7 March 2023

1. Introduction

Bacterial antimicrobial resistance (AMR) has emerged as a leading public health hazard, and the World Health Organization (WHO) has acknowledged an estimated 10 million people being killed annually by 2050 [1]. A synchronized action plan is needed to address the "imminent pandemic" of AMR. The US Centers for Disease Control and Prevention (CDC) reported 18 AMR threats, and the European Union and the European Economic Area reported 16 AMR threats in the estimated burden of eight pathogens. The foremost challenge is the multidrug resistance burden of six pathogens [2] prioritized by the WHO, namely *Escherichia coli*, *Staphylococcus aureus*, *Klebsiella pneumoniae*, *Acinetobacter baumannii*, *Pseudomonas aeruginosa*, and *Enterobacter* (ESKAPE), that contribute to the burden of AMR [3]. The ESKAPE pathogens are also listed by the Global Action Plan on AMR, the UN Interagency Coordination Group, and the One Health Global Leaders Group [4]. More attention is needed in funding research and development in understanding the drug resistance in each of the ESKAPE pathogens. Limitations in developing new and effective antibiotic treatments arise from the lack of a coordinated global assessment of bacterial AMR.

Bacterial AMR burden increases with increased antibiotic usage in high-resource settings and is a function of bacterial resistance and acute infections. Other factors include the lack of microbiological testing to prevent inappropriate antibiotic use, inadequate guidelines, and the easy procurement of antibiotics [5]. The AMR burden increases primarily from the inadequate availability of second- and third-line antibiotics, the availability of fake or inferior antibiotic drugs [6–8], and the lack of sanitation and hygiene [9–11]. The AMR pattern varies globally, with the existence of pathogen variants and variations in pathogen–drug interactions. Antibiotic stewardship is an integrated approach in controlling the spread of AMR. Limiting access to antibiotics is not viable in life-saving situations particularly when second-line antibiotics are unavailable [7].

Several innovative approaches are available to improve antibiotic use [12]. Logically the most effective way would be to allow the choice of narrow-spectrum antibiotics, reducing the intensity of the selection of a broad spectrum of antibiotics and reserving them for situations that are in real need which can be accomplished by the early detection of bacterial susceptibility [13]. Resistance diagnosis enables the "search and destroy" tactics to combat potentially dangerous pathogen strains [14–16]. A targeted infection control measure such as "search and destroy" may be possible from a rapid and accurate identification. This review comprehensively describes the proteomic profile of resistance diagnosis with a special focus on ESKAPE pathogens AST including the state-of-the-art techniques available, their roles ranging from typing to drug selection, and their advantages despite their limitations.

2. Antibiotic Resistance and Resilience

Antibiotic resistance is the clinical stance resulting from the insensitivity to an antibiotic drug and is categorized in terms of the minimum inhibitory concentration (MIC) in µg/mL, which is the lowest concentration of the drug that inhibits bacterial growth [17]. Microorganisms with an MIC beyond the normal distribution are resistant. According to EUCAST, a Susceptible (S) organism has therapeutic success with a standard dosing regimen, a Susceptible (I) organism has therapeutic success requiring increased exposure, and a Resistant (R) organism has therapeutic failure even with increased exposure.

Antibiotic resilience is the ability of the organism to recover from antibiotic stress and is expressed as the minimum duration for killing (MDK). By definition, it is the time needed for 50% of the total biomass to recover after antibiotic treatment. Resilience is described by a range of aspects such as bacterial tolerance, persistence, recalcitrance, adaptation, etc. These aspects reflect the diverse machinery prevailing in the bacteria to withstand antibiotic treatments and any of the related disturbances [18]. Identifying the determinants of bacterial resistance and resilience is crucial for understanding the response and strategy development. For instance, the resistance–resilience analysis framework has helped in the identification of the phenotypic signatures of extended-spectrum β-lactamase (ESBL) bacteria and has been used as a guide in combination treatments [19].

3. Methods of Resistance Profiling and Diagnosis

Many mechanisms are involved in bacterial antibiotic resistance [20]. Antibiotic resistance is exhibited on a genetic or mechanistic basis. Genetic basis includes mutational resistance that modifies antimicrobial targets such as decreasing drug uptake, activating drug efflux, or modulating regulatory networks. Mutations in genes arise from the acquisition of antibiotic resistance genes by horizontal gene transfer by a variety of mechanisms chiefly involving conjugation in which mobile genetic elements (MGEs) notably plasmids and transposons are mobilized. MGEs are crucial in the development and dissemination of antimicrobial resistance among clinically relevant organisms.

Mechanistically, bacteria acquire resistance by modifications of the antibiotic (chemical alteration or destruction), decreased penetration and efflux of the antibiotic, change in the target site (modification/mutation/bypass), and resistance due to global cell adaptations. Resistance is also induced by virulence factors such as biofilm formation associated with desiccation [21,22].

Profiling microbial resistance has come a long way. Primarily, microbial-culture-based methods identify the bacterial phenotype, whereas bacterial strain and species identification requires biochemical assays [23]. The evaluation of antimicrobial resistance based on the disk diffusion or broth dilution methods quantitatively evaluates resistance in terms of MICs [24] based on the protocols prescribed by the Clinical and Laboratory Standards Institute (CLSI) and the European Committee on Antimicrobial Susceptibility Testing

(EUCAST) as the "gold standard" [25]. These growth-based tests have limitations of longer turn-around times of 12 to 72 h [25,26]. The bacterial cultivation adds further 18 to 24 h for biochemical characterization [27]. The disadvantages of culturing methods include collection conditions and specific growth media requirements that generate errors leading to a lack of sensitivity [28,29]. In addition, routine bacterial culture methods are not practically applicable to non-cultivable pathogens [30,31]. Automated AST systems such as the Vitek 2, Phoenix, and MicroScan WalkAway perform in a simplified workflow and reduced time to results compared to traditional methods but still need bacterial culturing [32]. Therefore, the highly specific and sensitive molecule-based approach has also been used in the bacterial identification of resistance [33].

Molecular-based approaches amplify or hybridize genetic sequences encoding specific resistance determinants using conventional polymerase chain reactions (PCRs), quantitative real-time polymerase chain reactions (RT-PCRs), or DNA-micro-arrays with more sensitivity, specificity, and shorter turn-around times [23,34,35] which is not possible in culture-based methods [36]. However, these methods require detectable levels of DNA in conditions of low-abundance genes and heteroresistance [25]. Culture-independent methods are limited with variable clinical sensitivities [37]. Digital PCR systems detect low-abundance targets and heteroresistance analysis immediately without requiring prior culture enrichment [38]. Pitfalls with the molecular-based techniques are results with false-positive outcomes due to the amplification of silent genes or pseudogenes and false-negative outcomes due to mutations in the primer binding sites. Conventional PCRs also fail to detect hypervariable organisms and rapidly changing mechanisms, particularly in the detection of Gram-negative bacteria, including ESBL strains and carbapenem-resistant *Enterobacteriaceae* (CREs) with single-nucleotide polymorphisms (SNPs) [39]. Certain resistance markers detected by the PCR do not correlate with phenotypic resistance [40].

Culture-independent techniques termed nucleic acid testing (NAT) perform quicker diagnosis with higher sensitivity [41] but require prior information on the pathogen under test and its nucleic acid sequences [26]. The methods include molecular methods such as the PCR, RT-PCR, loop-mediated isothermal amplification (LAMP), nucleic acid sequence-based amplification (NASNBA), transcription-mediated amplification (TMA), and strand displacement amplification (SDA) [42]. Highly multiplexed PCR panels simultaneously detect bacterial pathogens that commonly cause specific clinical syndromes [37]. The other non-targeted methods that do not require prior nucleic acid information include next-generation sequencing (NGS) technologies [43,44] which in combination with bioinformatics provide accurate detection and characterization of pathogens and predict the strains evading vaccines [36]. Metagenomics NGS (mNGS) provides accurate data on the composition of microbial communities that are impossible to culture [45].

Clinical microbiology has also focused on applying genomics for AST. Whole-genome sequencing (WGS) is the primary genomic approach that predicts strains of all prevalent resistant phenotypes accurately and consistently. It ascertains the simultaneous identification of antibiotic-resistant phenotypes from the entire genome by screening multiple loci. The data from the genome sequence are stored digitally and are independent of primer specificity reducing false-negative results [46]. With a huge availability of data in the public domain, antimicrobial resistance determinants are readily identifiable with both the whole-genome and NGS technologies [39]. As a primer-independent method, it detects antibiotic resistance rapidly but is capable of detecting only previously documented mechanisms [47,48].

Around the mid-2000s, innovations in sequencing technology helped develop second-generation instruments based on Illumina sequencing that provided short-sequence ($\leq$300 bp) reads and paired ends at reduced costs. From about 2010, third-generation sequencing innovations helped develop Oxford Nanopore Technologies (ONT) and Pacific Biosciences (PacBio) technologies that produce longer reads > 2 Mb [13] with fewer gaps allowing tandem repeats and nested insertions [49], but they have higher error rates than Illumina [50]. Hybrid assemblies achieve accurate results by combining the accuracy of Illumina as well as using the longer reads of ONT/PacBio to overcome the shortcomings of both technologies. As new approaches emerge, clinical sequencing constantly shifts for cost effectiveness. The minimum cost is around 80 USD/genome which is expensive for routine use in clinical laboratories, although results are obtained within less than 24 h. Although the ONT Flongle disposable flow cells are less expensive, sequencing problems prevail in prediction as false positives are introduced from sequencing errors and DNA contamination from other organisms [46].

4. Proteomic Tools in Antibiotic Resistance

Proteomic analysis provides more functionally or clinically relevant information than genetic/genomic testing as protein levels indicate the actual functional status of the cell. Proteomic studies are capable of analyzing the protein—expression, post-translational modifications, and turnover rates [51]. Bacterial proteomics utilize both gel-based and non-gel-based techniques. Preliminary analysis involves a two-dimensional gel electrophoresis (2-DE) followed by the analysis of the gel image. The differential expression of protein is analyzed by a differential-in-gel electrophoresis (DIGE) technique using a fluorescent dye [52]. With the advancement of technologies, mass spectrometric analysis directly quantifies the protein as well as its functional status [53]. The bacterial proteomics have emerged on par with the proteomic tools developed (Figure 1).

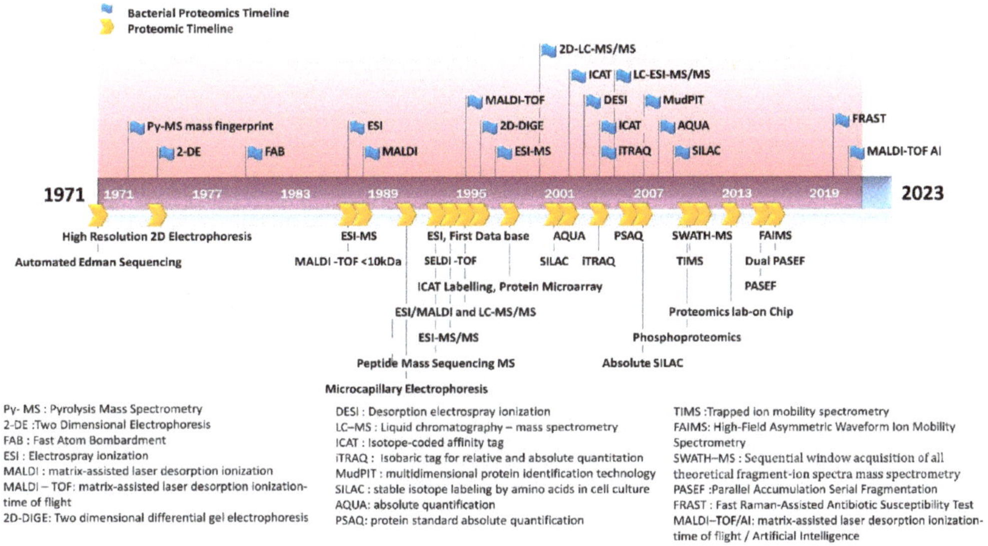

Figure 1. Emergence of bacterial proteomics in line with proteomics milestone. The figure shows the application of proteomic tools in bacterial testing.

Mass spectrometry (MS) analyzes ionized samples separated on the basis of the mass-to-charge (m/z) ratio and detects as a mass spectrum. Ionization techniques namely electrospray (ESI) and matrix-assisted laser desorption/ionization (MALDI) ionize analytes in a solution and a dry, crystalline matrix, respectively. Mass analyzers are of four types: ion trap, time-of-flight (TOF), quadrupole, and Fourier transform ion cyclotron (FT-MS). Time-of-flight (TOF) instruments analyze complex peptide mixtures [54], with a high acquisition rate permitting coupling with ion mobility spectrometry (IMS) [55]. In IMS, ion separation is size- and shape-based or based on the collisional cross section (CCS) [56]. TOF analyzes the emerging ions in a ms or sub-ms time frame. IMS nested between LC and MS or any additional dimension of separation is referred to as IMS-MS [57,58]; it increases the speed of analysis and selectivity [59] in highly complex proteomics samples and adds to the fourth dimension of proteomic analysis [60,61].

Relative quantification in MS is of two types: label and label-free methods. Label-free quantification uses MS signal intensity or spectral counting which is directly proportional to the peptide concentration. In the label method, the protein/peptide is labeled with a stable isotope tag chemically, metabolically, or enzymatically. Stable isotopes exhibit slight mass differences compared to their unlabeled counterparts that produce distinguishable signals in MS. In vivo protein is labeled by growing the cells in isotopically labeled amino acids—13C or 15N—referred to as the stable isotope labeling by amino acids in cell culture (SILAC) method [62].

Proteins/peptides are also tagged chemically with isobaric mass tags known as tandem mass tags (TMTs), which on fragmentation yield reporter ions of differing mass that is quantified. The isobaric tags for relative and absolute quantitation (iTRAQ) method quantitates the relative protein levels from different sources in a single experiment. The workflow is that the isobaric label is covalently attached to peptides after protein digestion, and samples are pooled, fractionated by LC, and analyzed in a tandem mass spectrometer (MS/MS). The relative quantification of the protein is obtained from the combined ratios of proteins/peptides. iTRAQ combined with MALDI or ESI-MS/MS provides accurate information on the relative protein concentration.

In the absolute quantification (AQUA) method, internal standard peptides are labeled and added to the sample during proteolytic digestion. The relative protein concentration is quantitated from both isotope-labeled AQUA peptides and unlabeled native peptides and measured by selected reaction monitoring (LC-SRM). From the known amount of the internal standard, the MS determines the ratio between the internal standard and analyte [63]. It provides the relative quantity of protein and information on the post-translational modifications.

In trapped ion mobility spectrometry (TIMS), the ions are rested in an ion tunnel device and balanced in a stream of gas at a low electrical potential [64]. The time-resolved ions are released into the mass analyzer downstream [65]. Another MS-based approach is parallel accumulation–serial fragmentation (PASEF) [66] which synchronizes the MS/MS precursor selection with TIMS separation. TIMS scan acquires more than one precursor, and peptides are continually selected for sequencing. Typical DDA measurements are performed after a survey scan, and the N-highest abundant precursor ions are targeted for MS/MS analysis [67]. The MS/MS spectrum quality is improved from the fast acquisition speed (50–200 ms for a full scan) and the repeated re-targeting of low-abundance precursors.

In the bio-orthogonal noncanonical amino acid tagging (BONCAT) method, non-canonical amino acid (ncAA) is incorporated into protein, conjugated to an affinity tag, and enriched. The enriched proteins are identified and quantified by LC-MS/MS [68,69]. Its advantage is that labeled proteins are separated physically from the remaining proteome [70]. The ncAA pulse time is only a few minutes in bacteria and thus quantifies dynamic processes. Extended pulse times identify proteins synthesized at extremely low rates under anaerobic conditions such as in the survival of *Pseudomonas aeruginosa* [71]. ncAA incorporation uses a mutant aminoacyl-tRNA synthetase and is expressed according to the target cell [72] or specific cell state condition [73].

Raman spectroscopy is an optical technique, where the sample is irradiated, and the scattered light is analyzed. The shift between the frequency of incident and scattered light is the Raman effect. This shift is induced by molecular vibrations in the sample which are distinct for a bacterial cell based on protein, lipids, and DNA and are the "chemical fingerprint". Based on Raman spectroscopy, a single-cell Raman spectrum (SCRS) is used in the identification of microbes at a single-cell level as it provides a spatial resolution of $<1\ \mu m^3$. Like FACS, a laser beam is applied on a single cell, and the Raman spectrum is obtained. On the basis of a shift in the spectra, cell type and phenotypic changes in bacteria are characterized [74,75]. When labeling with stable isotopes such as 13C, 15N, and

2 H(D), bacteria also display a characteristic Raman spectrum shift due to heavy isotopic atom replacement with biomolecules. For instance, labeling with D_2O incorporates D into biomolecules forming carbon-deuterium (C-D) bonds that show a distinguishable Raman band (2000–2300 cm^{-1}) shifted from C-H vibration [76].

Raman-based bacterial identification distinguishes bacteria susceptibility from the absence of a Raman band in resistant bacteria which is referred to as an "antibiotic effect signature" [77–80]. Employing the same principle, the fast Raman-assisted antibiotic susceptibility test (FRAST) method was developed. The clinical protocol includes steps of Raman-based single-cell GS classification, two-step antibiotic inhibition, D_2O labeling, SCRS acquisition, and data analysis [81–83] from subtle variations in SCRS.

Raman spectroscopy distinguishes bacterial strains [84–86]. Surface-enhanced Raman spectroscopy (SERS) analysis of bacteria discriminates Gram-positive and Gram-negative strains, and the classification is based on linear discriminant analysis (LDA) [87]. Classical Gram staining requires 16–24 h, delaying the rapid diagnosis. However, in the FRAST, Gram classification is obtained within a few hours, and its accuracy reaches 100% when >90% of single cells have been Gram classified. The dual-mode detection—Gram classification antibiotic susceptibly detection by the FRAST—makes a stand-alone automatic Raman infection diagnostic system possible.

In another latest development, the direct-on-target microdroplet growth assay (DOT-MGA) measures bacterial growth on the MALDI-TOF MS directly by incubating with and without the indicator antibiotic in the microdroplet nutrient broth. It is based on the principle of the broth microdilution method, with a modification in which the bacteria are incubated on the MS target plate, and bacterial growth is determined at the breakpoint concentration based on MS identification scores. By assessing the growth in the presence of various antibiotics, the potential sensitivity mechanisms of drug resistance are analyzed. It is superior to the broth microdilution method and the direct-from-blood-culture disk-diffusion method in terms of speed and easy operation. Nix et al., 2020 employed the DOT-MGA in the rapid detection of pathogens in the blood culture of methicillin-resistant *Staphylococcus aureus* (MRSA) patients [88] producing reliable results within 4 h incubation in determining carbapenemase resistance in *K. pneumoniae, E. cloacae, E. aerogenes, P. mirabilis,* and *K. aerogenes* [89].

The emergence of bacterial proteomics on par with the proteomic technologies is illustrated in Figure 1.

Top-Down versus Bottom-Up Proteomics

Proteomics has evolved from simple gel-based (2-DE or 1-DE gel-LC-MS/MS) to gel-free methods. Proteomic analysis is categorized as "top-down" and "bottom-up". "Top-down" proteomic analysis encompasses intact proteins, whereas "bottom-up" analyses involving proteolytically digested protein are categorized into three types: "shotgun" or untargeted proteomics that is MS-operated in a data-dependent acquisition (DDA) mode; targeted proteomics carried out by multiple reaction monitoring (MRM); and the data-independent acquisition (DIA) method [90].

In top-down proteomics, intact protein analysis enables the analysis of protein isoforms and the stoichiometry of post-translational modifications (PTM). In the bottom-up approach, digested proteins are separated by LC and ionized and mass-analyzed with a mass spectrometer in full scans (MS), and fragments are selected in N consecutive MS/MS scans. Targeted proteomics detect and quantify a predetermined set of peptides by selected reaction monitoring (SRM) which is multiple reaction monitoring (MRM) from a set comprehensive protein database [62].

The "data-independent acquisition" (DIA) method is unbiased and involves cyclic recording in the entire LC time range and the fragment ion spectra contained in predetermined isolation windows. A combination of the DIA method with a targeted data extraction strategy is the "sequential isolation window acquisition theoretical mass spectra" (SWATH

MS) in which the user-defined m/z window is fragmented and correlated to previously generated query parameters and scored [91].

The advantages of a gel-free/label-free proteomic technique with the potential application of proteomics in bacterial pathogen studies including comparative proteomics and differential protein expression in response to antibiotic treatment clearly explain the superiority of proteomic technologies (Figure 2).

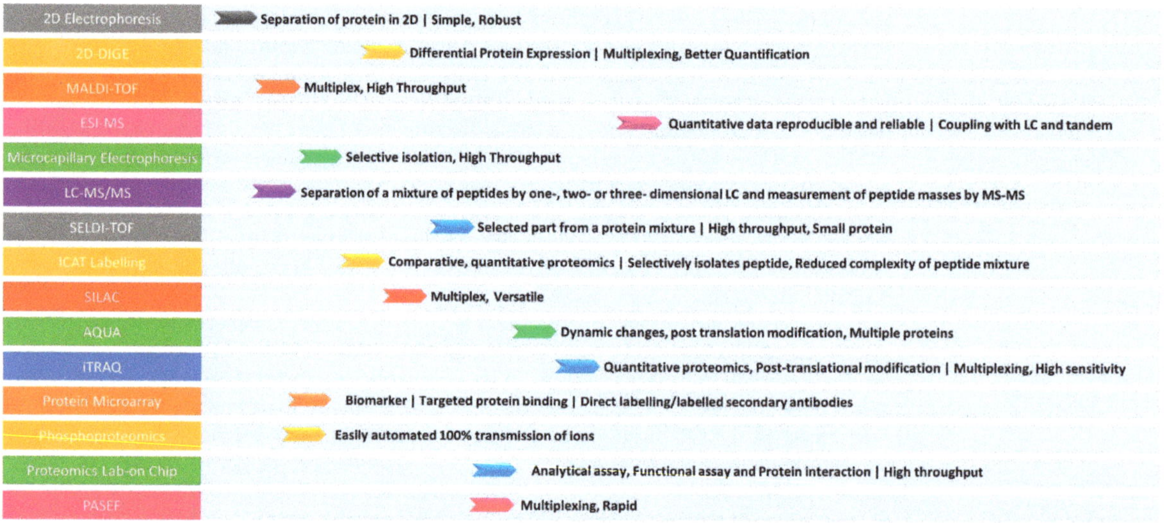

Figure 2. Summary of the advantages for various proteomic tools in AMR detection. The (**left**) panel indicates the techniques. The (**right**) panel indicates the application and its advantage.

5. ESKAPE Pathogens

Recently, an extensive review described the antibiotic resistance mechanisms identified in pathogens given priority status, i.e., ESKAPE (*Enterococcus* spp., *Staphylococcus aureus*, *Klebsiella pneumoniae*, *Acinetobacter baumannii*, *Pseudomonas aeruginosa*, and *Enterobacter* spp.) [92]. In ESKAPE pathogens, resistance develops through genetic mutations and the acquisition of MGEs [93]. ESKAPE pathogens are resistant to oxazolidinones, lipopeptides, macrolides, fluoroquinolones, tetracyclines, β-lactams, β-lactam–β-lactamase inhibitor combinations, and last-line antibiotics including carbapenems, glycopeptides, and polymyxins [94]. Therefore, preclinical and clinical trials encompassed many treatment options including vaccine development to control the burden. Unfortunately, no vaccines are available for ESKAPE infections [5].

Both in clinical settings and at the community level, ESKAPE pathogens serve as the model organism for resistance. Despite their heterogeneity, the overall mechanisms involved in the emergence and persistence are shared by all ESKAPE pathogens individually. ESKAPE pathogens are highly prevalent in the clinical setting due to their ability to form a biofilm on abiotic and biotic surfaces. Apart from drug development, inappropriate use of antibiotics, and sustained stewardship, improved diagnosis is essential to control ESKAPE AMR burden.

One Health Approach in ESKAPE Management

In 2017, the European Union implemented the "One Health" approach to combat antibiotic resistance [95] recognizing the need for safeguarding human health by protecting animal and environmental health as well as related fields [96]. ESKAPE bacteria with AMR are widely distributed into the environment and ecosystem [97]. Among the ESKAPE pathogens, *Pseudomonas* and *Acinetobacter* are enteric bacteria and soil commensals that are ubiquitous in livestock animals and slaughterhouse wastewater discharges. Outbreaks in veterinary hospitals are relevant to the isolation of MRSA, vancomycin-resistant *Enterococcus* (VRE), and ESBL, producing *Escherichia coli*, *Klebsiella pneumoniae*, and *Acinetobacter baumannii* strains from humans, livestock, and contaminated food [98]. Most ESKAPE isolates are multidrug-resistant (MDR) with the highest risk of mortality. The consequences of AMR-related infections are related to iatrogenic disease states in which treatment of the infection results in co-morbidities [99]. Therefore, the key aspect of the One Health concept may be addressed from the early and rapid diagnosis of resistance.

6. Proteomic Studies on ESKAPE Resistance

6.1. *Enterococcus spp.*

Enterococci are Gram-positive cocci, facultatively anaerobic, inhabiting the gastrointestinal tract, and cause a variety of infections including urinary tract infections, bacteremia, intra-abdominal infections, and endocarditis [100]. *Enterococci* develop antibiotic resistance both intrinsically and by acquisition. They develop resistance to cephalosporins, aminoglycosides, lincosamides, and streptogramins intrinsically [101] and thus acquire added resistance from MGEs [102]. The malleability of genomes and the disseminating determinants are attributed to their adaptation to harsh environments. Thus, both the microbial and host factors convert the second-rate pathogen into a first-rate clinical problem [103].

Aminoglycoside resistance in *Enterococci* is acquired from the plasmid-borne resistance factor [104] and also by aminoglycoside-modifying enzymes from the mobile elements [105]. β-lactamase activity in *Enterococci* compromises combination therapy [106]. A comprehensive proteomic study on vancomycin-resistant the *Enterococci faecalis* strain revealed the proteins vital for antibiotic resistance [107]. It included the pheromone-binding proteins involved in the conjugative plasmid transfer [108], the detection of which could aid in antibiotic cross selection. An LC-ESI/MS-based proteomic study predicted the functions of pheromone precursors, pheromone/peptide-binding components of ABC transporters, and basic membrane proteins [109].

MALDI-TOF MS spectra with artificial intelligence (AI) discriminated the proteomic patterns of VRE from the vancomycin-susceptible *Enterococci faecium* (VSE) [110,111]. The proteomic profile of VRE revealed the elongation factor EF-Tu in the cytoplasm and elongation factor G (EF-G) in the membrane [107] that moonlights the link with target receptors from host cell membranes and paves the way for colonization [112]. These data predict the timing of the introduction of prodrugs affecting Ef-Tu and regulating bacterial elongation.

Of the several stress factors in *Enterococci faecalis* [113], the antiphagocytic factor Cold shock protein A (CspA) encoded by the *csp* operon is the virulence factor induced by temperature changes [114,115] which was involved in bacterial evasion [107]. The identification of CspA sheds light on its involvement in the regulation of bile resistance in *Enterococci faecalis*.

Another MALDI-TOF-MS-based proteomic study of *E. faecalis* reported the upregulation of proteins involved in biofilm formation such as LutC, RsmH, and RRF protein and the downregulation of RepN, ScpA, PrsA, and PurM after antibiotic treatment indicating a decrease in proteins associated with cell division and metabolism during biofilm formation [116].

A nano-LC/MSE (at elevated energy)/(Q/TOF-MS) study reported the upregulation of protein related to glycolysis, amino acid biosynthesis, and biofilm formation. Besides the basic survival pathways, LuxS-mediated quorum sensing, arginine metabolism, rhamnose biosynthesis, and pheromone- and adhesion-associated proteins were upregulated during biofilm formation [117]. Various oxidative stress response proteins and transcriptional regulators correlating with oxidative stress are involved in the pathogenesis of enterococcal infections [107]. The most significant was the identification of peroxide regulator PerR as a ferric uptake regulator-like protein involved in iron homeostasis and OhrR, a transcriptional repressor that senses oxidants [107]. This provides insights into oxidative sensitive targets in *E. faecalis* death with antimicrobial drug intervention.

In *Enterococci*, the expression of Opu, the osmoprotectant uptake transport system, correlates to better survival of bacteria and confers responses to heat shock or other stress factors [118]. This shows that the salt-stress adaptation of *E. faecalis* rather than general stress protection contributes to *E. faecalis* resistance.

The MDR in *Enterococci* is acquired by plasmid pCF10 with pheromone-inducible genes that mediate adhesion and virulence functions through surface proteins amongst which PrgA, B, and C are the main contributor. PrgB is an aggregation factor in biofilm development and virulence enhancement, whereas PrgA is required for *Enterococci* in order to bind to abiotic surfaces, and PrgC's presence facilitates PrgA function [119].

Raman spectroscopy was also used to analyze the interaction between vancomycin and vancomycin-sensitive *Enterococcus faecalis* strains within a span of 90 min. The effect of the drug was evident from characteristic spectral changes visualized and analyzed with a multivariate statistical model that predicted the impact of vancomycin treatment. The robustness was evident from classification accuracies of >90% at lower concentrations of vancomycin. The Raman spectroscopy methods characterized the drug–pathogen interactions in a label-free and fast method [81]. Vancomycin sensitivity could be noted on the basis of spectral changes with accuracies >90% marking it as a potential tool in diagnosis.

The cellular changes in *E. faecalis* alter the central metabolism and membrane permeability at a low pH. The integration of quantitative proteomic data with a genomic model from SWATH-MS was useful to contextualize these proteomic data [120]. This finding suggests that *E. faecalis* survival is reduced at alkalinity by the blockage of the proton pump.

6.2. *Staphylococcus aureus*

Staphylococcus aureus is a Gram-positive cocci, a normal human flora inhabitant, and a nosocomial and community-associated pathogen, causing diverse infections ranging from superficial skin and soft tissue infections to life-threatening infections [121]. Methicillin-resistant *Staphylococcus aureus* (MRSA) strain infections are associated with high morbidity and mortality. Therefore, identifying MRSA is important in targeted hospital infection control measures and the detection of outbreaks [122]. *Staphylococcus aureus* protein A (Spa) typing, multilocus sequence typing (MLST), and pulsed-field gel electrophoresis (PFGE) [123] are the commonly used methods in the detection.

From a proteomics approach, the MALDI-TOF-based MRSA typing scheme has differentiated the major MRSA clonal complexes. It validated a hospital-acquired MRSA (HA-MRSA) typing scheme requiring an average of 2.5 h compared to 3–6 days for the PFGE typing method [124]. The whole-cell MALDI-TOF is also useful in MRSA strain typing [125,126].

An LC-MS/MS study based on iTRAQ reported changes both in the upregulation and downregulation of proteins involved in antimicrobial resistance, stress response, mismatch repair, and cell-wall synthesis. The immunodominant antigen B (IsaB) protein for binding [127] was upregulated in MRSA compared to MSSA. The upregulation of cell-wall-associated fibronectin-binding protein Ebh (for ECM-binding protein homologue) complements resistance in MRSA by altering cell size [128].

However, in one MALDI-TOF-MS-based study, the MRSA and MSSA strains failed to identify a reproducible diagnostic peak but yielded a high discriminative peak with the deployment of artificial intelligence [129,130]. In situations of limited sample availability, the coupling of MALDI-TOF with PBP2a latex agglutination offers a solution for the MRSA assay [131].

The Raman approach discriminated MRSA and MSSA strains in an SCRS at 532 nm excitation and achieved 87.5% accuracy in differentiation. Excitation directly on the bacterial colonies at 785 nm differentiated MRSA and MSSA based on prominent staphyloxanthin bands. A high-intensity band is noted in MRSA strains compared to MSSA, although staphyloxanthin is not linked to antimicrobial resistance mechanisms [132]. The direct application of Raman spectroscopy on bacterial colonies grown on a Mueller–Hinton agar plate yielded 100% accuracy in MRSA detection confirming its potential use in routine clinical diagnostics [133].

The cell size and biochemical features of *Staphylococcus aureus* pose several challenges in their detection. The antibiotic effect signature by SCRS analysis in three cefoxitin-resistant *Staphylococcus aureus* strains and two susceptible strains revealed a weaker *Staphylococcus aureus* spectrum than that previously detected with bacteria–drug combinations and was highly variable. The phenotype correlated with the spectra confirming SCRS can be extended to *Staphylococcus aureus* and introduced into the diagnostic system [134].

Raman microspectroscopy, where Raman spectrometry is coupled to a microscope, had the ability to distinguish between *Streptococcus agalactiae* and *Staphylococcus aureus*. Isogenic variants of *Staphylococcus aureus* strains lacking or expressing antibiotic resistance determinants were also identified and marked as spectral biomarkers. Raman microspectroscopy has the ability to distinguish distinct forms of a single bacterial species *in situ* and thus in detecting antibiotic-resistant strains of bacteria [132].

In addition, a SWATH-based quantitative study in combination with scanning electron microscopy (SEM) and transmission electron microscopy (TEM) validated resistance mechanisms in MRSA [135].

6.3. *Klebsiella pneumoniae*

Klebsiella are Gram-negative, encapsulated, non-motile, rod-shaped, and oxidase-negative bacteria [136] classified under the *Enterobacteriaceae* family with a wide diversity of species, including *K. pneumoniae* and others—*K. indica, K. terrigena, K. spallanzanii, K. huaxiensis, K. oxytoca, K. grimontii, K. pasteurii*, and *K. michiganensis*. *K. pneumoniae* accounts for both community- and hospital-acquired infections [137]. *K. pneumoniae* are resistant to third-generation cephalosporins and ESBL strains and are susceptible to carbapenems but account for significant mortality and morbidity [138] as well for the dramatic surge of pan resistance of *Klebsiella pneumoniae* [139,140]. However, recent studies have shown emerging resistance to carbapenems [141].

A high-throughput mass spectrometric analysis of ESBL strains and non-ESBL strains of *Klebsiella pneumoniae* unraveled the pathogenicity determinants. The proteomic analysis identified fimbrial adhesins type 1 and type 3 related to cell invasion [142] and that type 1 fimbrial adhesive proteins facilitate adherence and biofilm formation on abiotic surfaces [143]. The detection of these adhesive structures has paved the way for the development of alternative non-antibiotic strategies targeting the adhesive factors. A shotgun proteomic analysis identified a capsule assembly of Wzi family protein and a capsule in *Klebsiella pneumoniae*, which are critical in bacterial resistance [144] and induce the capacity of the bacteria to enter the bloodstream causing bacteremia and pneumonia in the host [145].

The study by Enany et al., 2020, identified with nano LC-MS different stress response proteins such as the ElaB protein, Lon protease, and universal stress proteins G and A. ESBL strains exhibited unique stress proteins—oxidative stress defense proteins and EntB proteins—with isochorismatase activity, whereas non-ESBL strains had general stress proteins. These proteins facilitate the bacteria to acquire iron and adapt to variable ranges of oxygen levels, for example, hypoxia in the human colon, microoxia at different sites, and hyperoxia in external media. The exploitation of siderophores by bacteria in exhibiting resistance has led to siderophore–drug conjugates and synthetic analogues with therapeutic potential in treatment.

Other unique proteins solely identified in the ESBL-producing *Klebsiella pneumoniae* proteome were the OsmC and general stress protein. OsmC has a critical role in peroxide metabolism and against oxidative stress [146] and general stress protein in the stress resistance response [147].

Clinical studies show that carbapenem-resistant *Klebsiella pneumoniae* (CRKP) account for 70–90% of carbapenem-resistant *Enterobacteriaceae* (CRE) and usually are multidrug-resistant (MDR) [148] with a mortality rate > 50% even after appropriate antibiotic treatment [141]. Colistin is the "last resort" for CRKP infections, and the suboptimal use of it has given rise to colistin-resistant CRKP which are extensively drug-resistant (XDR) strains [149]. A TMT-labeled proteomic technique on both MDR and XDR strains identified DEPs related to drug resistance namely ArnT, ArnD, ArnA, ArnC, ArnB, PmrD, YddW, and OmpK36 in both strains. Notable among them were four β-lactamases, namely, KPC-2, CTX-M-14, SHV-11, and TEM-1, in all the resistant strains. A distinct upregulation of efflux pumps—KexD and AcrA—was noted. The enrichment of WecH, Bm3R1, OppC, OppA, and OppF had the same DEPs in the MDR and XDR strains.

The colistin-resistant XDR strains have a robust biofilm-forming ability and are more resistant [150]. Defects in porins OmpK35 and OmpK36 reduce sensitivity to carbapenems [151,152]. Proteomic analysis detected decreases in the expression of OmpK36 in XDR strains and OmpN in colistin-resistant XDR strains, and the sensitivity to several antibiotics was enhanced with the overexpression of OmpN [153]. The DEPs between the MDR and XDR strains were mainly enriched in cationic antimicrobial peptide (CAMP) resistance and the two-component system—PhoP/PhoQ and PmrA/PmrB [154]. In the CAMP resistance pathway, ArnBCADT, PmrD, and YddW were highly expressed in the colistin-resistant XDR strains, which indicated that lipid A modification persisted as the primary mechanism of colistin resistance in *Klebsiella pneumoniae*.

The two-component system comprises a sensor kinase and a response regulator that maintains bacterial homeostasis including nutrition and antibiotic exposure [155]. The proteomic analysis identified KdpB, OmpK36, PfeA, NasR, NarJ, and ArnB in the two-component system pathway with KdpB being a subunit of K+ transporting ATPase. Among these, Omp 36 is a porin protein important for iron homeostasis [156], PfeA is a ferric enterobactin receptor [157], NasR is a regulator of nitrate/nitrite respiration and assimilation [158], and NarJ is a system-specific chaperone for the respiratory nitrate reductase complex [159].

A comparative proteomic study introduced MICs of a single antibiotic and revealed the role of nutrient modulation in reducing resistance in single-antibiotic-resistant *Klebsiella pneumoniae* [160,161] with a total of nine metabolic pathway proteins (Gar K, UxaC, ExuT, HpaB, FhuA, KPN_01492, FumA, HisC, AroE) being differentially expressed. Similarly, a comprehensive investigation of the proteomes of polymyxin-resistant and polymyxin-susceptible strains of *Klebsiella pneumoniae* revealed that bacterial metabolism plays a crucial role in mediating resistance. For example, the upregulation of the arginine biosynthesis flux after colistin treatment increases the arginine-biosynthetic enzymes ArgABCDE, ArgI, ArgG, and ArgH in colistin-treated *Acinetobacter baumannii* [162] and in gentamicin-treated *Staphylococcus aureus* [163]. Arginine metabolism in *Klebsiella pneumoniae* moderates hydroxyl-radical-induced damage via ammonia production [164].

One study reported the impact of colistin in decreasing the expression of the maltose transporter LamB, a porin involved in the influx of antibiotics and the class A β lactamases—TEM, SHV-11, and SHV-4 [165]. Comparative proteomic analysis of polymyxin-susceptible *Klebsiella pneumoniae* validated the role of *crrB*-mediated colistin resistance in which lipid A profiles presented the addition of one or two L-Ara4N molecules and palmitoylation with elevations in CrrAB, PmrAB, and ArnBCADT levels. The multidrug efflux pump KexD and the GNAT family N-acetyltransferase were highly expressed in the crrB mutant. Thus, the proteomic study confirmed the role of *crrB* mutation in colistin resistance [164].

UV resonance Raman (UVRR) spectroscopy applied for the differentiation of *Klebsiella pneumoniae* outperformed Raman microspectroscopy with 92% accuracy in species classification [166].

6.4. *Acinetobacter baumannii*

Acinetobacter baumannii are Gram-negative, round, rod-shaped bacteria (coccobacillus) that predominantly cause nosocomial infections primarily, such as ventilator-associated pneumonia (VAP) [21,167]. Carbapenem-resistant *Acinetobacter baumannii* (CRAB) is ranked as a number-one-priority organism by the WHO. For multidrug-resistant strains of *Acinetobacter baumannii* (MDR-AB), carbapenem is the preferred treatment drug [168]. However, prior use of carbapenem increases resistance to carbapenem [169]. The alternate treatment options for MDR-AB are polymyxins [170,171]. *Acinetobacter baumannii* strains resistant to three or more classes of antimicrobials (penicillins and cephalosporins—including inhibitor combinations, fluoroquinolones, aminoglycosides, and carbapenems) are classified as extensive drug-resistant strains (XDR-AB), and XDR-AB strains resistant to polymyxins and tigecycline are pandrug-resistant (PDR-AB) [172,173].

In the MDR strain, the upregulation of antibiotic-resistant proteins β-lactamases (AmpC, Oxa-23 carbapenemase, and TEM), outer membrane proteins (OmpA, a CarO homolog, OmpW, NlpE homolog involved in copper resistance), drug-modifying enzymes (aminoglycoside acetyltransferases, aminoglycoside 3′, phosphotransferase, nitroreductase DrgA), and drug transporters (a homolog of the ABC transporter HlyD; the AcrB-AdelJK cation/multidrug efflux pump) were noted. Host defense proteins, CRISPR-associated proteins (Csy3 and Csy1), LexA-like regulator (SOS response), and cell surface porin DcaP-like protein for biofilm formation, have been noted.

A TMT labeling and label-free proteomic study identified metal-dependent hydrolase-related proteins and β-lactamase-related proteins upregulated in MDR strains. Aminoglycoside-modifying AphA1b was uniquely expressed in MDR strains. Antibiotic-resistant protein DacD (D-alanyl-D-alanine carboxypeptidase), a PBP6b, and cell division protein ZapA, involved in β-lactam resistance, were also upregulated. The ABC transporter, MFS transporter, and RND transporter were upregulated. Stress-response-related proteins—Trigger factor (TF), Heavy-metal-associated (HMA), Rhodanese-Like Domain (RHD), Universal stress protein (Usp), AldA, and CysK—were upregulated.

A 2D-DIGE, MALDI-TOF/TOF, and iTRAQ/SCX-LC-MS/MS study identified the unique biofilm capability of *Acinetobacter baumannii* [174]. A 2DE and LC-MS/MS study noted the overexpression of proteins involved in iron storage, the metabolic process, and lipid biosynthesis while an iron-deficient condition leads to the overexpression of proteins involved in iron acquisition [175]. Quantitative phosphoproteomics identified the phosphorylation sites in *Acinetobacter baumannii* by LTQ-Orbitrap MS enriched by SCX-TiO_2 chromatography [176].

A comparison of the spectral difference in *Acinetobacter* strains by Raman spectroscopy emphasizes its advantages and the rapidity of the discriminative power compared to MS. Further, the performance of Raman spectroscopy was superior in *Acinetobacter baumannii* strain differentiation as it contained whole-cell information [177].

6.5. *Pseudomonas aeruginosa*

Pseudomonas aeruginosa are Gram-negative, aerobic–facultatively anaerobic, rod-shaped bacteria that frequently establish bacteremia in neutropenic patients causing high morbidity and mortality rates [178,179]. It is a model organism in understanding biofilm physiology and antibiotic tolerance. It is the primary causative organism of chronic infections in chronic cystic fibrotic lungs by forming biofilms that are refractory to the host immune system and antimicrobial therapies [180]. *Pseudomonas aeruginosa* accounts for >5% of infectious exacerbations in chronic obstructive pulmonary disease (COPD) patients and associated mortality [181].

The resistance mechanisms exhibited by *Pseudomonas aeruginosa* are intrinsic, acquired, and adaptive. Intrinsic resistance results from low outer membrane permeability and expression of the efflux pump. It acquires resistance either by horizontal gene transfer or from mutations in resistance genes [182]. Adaptive resistance is marked by the formation of a biofilm that serves as a diffusion barrier [183]. In addition, multidrug-tolerant cells form a biofilm as is the case with cystic fibrosis patients [184].

Virulence factors are not expressed constitutively but are cell-density-dependent and sensed by a diffusible molecule such as N-acyl homoserine lactone (AHL), in a process known as quorum sensing [185–187]. In *Pseudomonas aeruginosa*, quorum sensing is regulated by the *las* and *rhl* system that is interrelated. *las* mediates transcriptional activator LasR and LasI and an AHL synthase to synthesize N-3-oxo-dodecanoyl-homoserine lactone (3-oxo-C12-HSL). The *rhl* system mediates RhlR and RhlI for the synthesis of N-butanoyl homoserine lactone (C4-HSL). The *las* system is an activator of rhlR and rhlI. Mutations in the quorum sensing circuitry lower virulence [188–190]. Proteomic analysis of post-translational modifications in *Pseudomonas aeruginosa* PAO1 quorum-sensing (QS) system revealed differentially expressed proteins partly rescued only by a medium containing AHL signal molecules [191]. Another study also revealed that the inactivation of the QS system termed "quorum quenching" results in the reduced expression of many extracellular virulence factors, including proteases, chitinase, and lipases [192,193] and the downregulation of the type II Xcp secretion system [194]. The outer membrane hemin-binding receptor PhuR was positively regulated by AHL, demonstrating that the *has* system (haem acquisition system) and the Phu Haem acquisition system are regulated by the *las*I *rhl*I QS circuitry.

The LC-ESI MS/MS study identified DEPs that correspond with porins OprD, OprE, OprF, OprH, and Opr86, LPS assembly protein, and A-type flagellin. Significant downregulation of flagellin A protein, OprF, and OprD and the upregulation and modification of OprH, OprE, Opr86, and LptD are noted in tolerant strains reflecting the adaptability of bacteria in conditions in which porins play an important role.

Proteomic studies by iTRAQ revealed the involvement of biofilm formation in antibiotic resistance mediated by proteins ArcA and IscU. Antibiotic resistance alterations by drugs also showed changes in the expression of the proteins PhzA, PhzB, PhzM, MetQ1, ArcA, IscU, lpsJ, and PilA involved individually or synergistically in the regulation of PA quorum sensing, the bacterial secretion system, bacterial biofilm formation, and CAMP resistance [195].

Detection of carbapenemases activity is challenging which has been simplified by a modified MALDI-TOF MS assay that detects the β-lactam ring and its degradation products. B-lactamases disrupt the central β-lactam ring of drugs by hydrolysis, and this hydrolysis corresponds to a mass shift of +18 Da that is easily detected by MALDI-TOF MS. This method has validated β-lactamase activity in *Acinetobacter baumannii* [196]. In the case of assays involving meropenem, the visualization of degradation products by MALDI-TOF MS is difficult due to their binding to cell lysate components. The modified method detects degradation products and has been validated with NDM-1-, VIM-1-, KPC-2-, KPC-3-, and OXA-48/-162-producing members of the *Enterobacteriaceae* and NDM-1-producing *Acinetobacter baumannii* isolates [197–199].

By convention, carbapenemase strains are identified by phenotypic methods such as the modified Hodge test. Carbapenems in combination with different inhibitors (e.g., cloxacillin, EDTA, or 3-aminophenyl boronic acid (APB)) are used to differentiate among AmpC, metallo-β-lactamases (MBLs), and *Klebsiella pneumoniae* carbapenemase (KPC). The MBLs are identified by inhibition with EDTA, for differentiating between MBL and other carbapenemases in *Enterobacteriaceae* and *Pseudomonas* spp. in a MALDI-TOF platform [200].

Pseudomonas aeruginosa adapt to low-oxygen environments, and the protein involved in this adaptation was investigated by both SWATH MS and data-dependent SPS-MS3 of TMT-labeled peptides. Under hypoxic stress ($O_2 < 1\%$), both aerobic (Cbb3-1 and Cbb3-2 terminal oxidases) and anaerobic denitrification and arginine fermentation proteins were increased [201]. Another proteomic analysis using iTRAQ technology identified DEPs associated with resistance mechanisms such as quorum sensing, bacterial biofilm formation, and active pumping [195].

6.6. *Enterobacter spp.*

Enterobacter are Gram-negative, rod-shaped bacteria in the *Enterobacteriaceae* family. *Enterobacter aerogenes* and *Enterobacter cloacae* are clinically significant species that are opportunistic, nosocomial pathogens originating from intensive care units especially on mechanical ventilation [202]. Colistin, a cationic lipopeptide, is administered to treat multidrug-resistant (MDR) *Enterobacter* infections [203], including ESBL strains and/or resistant to carbapenems [173]. Cell membrane electronegativity is lowered by modifying lipid A, which decreases the binding affinity of colistin [204]. The classical methods of testing colistin susceptibility are challenging [205], due to the lack of reproducibility, inconsistencies [206], and limitations and due to inaccurate MICs resulting from the adherence of colistin to the testing wells [207]. Moreover, limitations exist in the protein-based MALDI-TOF MS detection of *Enterobacter* infections and a modified lipid-based MS platform [208].

The lipid-based MS is the fast lipid analysis technique (FLAT) on a MALDI-TOF/MS platform that rapidly identifies Gram-negative and Gram-positive bacteria [209,210]. FLAT-MS is a highly sensitive method in identifying CRE and *K. aerogenes* [211]. The modifications in the terminal phosphates of lipid A with phosphoethanolamine, L-amino-4-arabinose (Ara4N), or galactosamine confer colistin resistance [212] but are detected by MALDI-TOF.

MALDI-TOF clustering confirmed the existence of a preferential way of transmission for Gram-negative bacteria from the invasive procedure employed. LC-MS/MS identified potentially pathogenic factor OmpX as the most abundant protein in *Enterobacter cloacae* OMVs with hydrolase enzymes, that cause cell interaction [213] and enhance immune tolerance [214] and the passage of microbial molecules through the tight junction of the gut [215]. The OMVs assist in the formation of biofilm, as indicated by the presence of OmpX.

Finally, a specific robust method to comprehensively detect ESKAPE pathogens at a single-cell level uses Raman microspectroscopy. The spectral features were distinct for each of the pathogenic bacteria and thus facilitated the identification [216]. Raman scattering microscopy was also useful for the rapid identification and AST of pathogens in urine [217] and notable in its ability to classify on a Gram-staining basis and AST results within ~3 h drawing attention for clinical applications.

7. Summary and Perspective on the Role of Proteomics in Microbial Resistance Diagnosis

A number of proteomic tools have been used in the detection of AMR for ESKAPE pathogens. To be practical and useful in the routine practice of clinical microbiology labs, the proteomic tool should be accurate, rapid, and cost-effective. Modern microbiology has attempted to introduce technology into laboratories that includes MALDI-TOF MS "profiling" or "biotyping" as the first-line identification method as it involves a very simple sample preparation. The workflow illustrates the direct smearing of a bacterial sample onto the MALDI target, a short chemical extraction classically after overnight cultivation, covered by a simple layer of one of the standard matrices, which is followed by the acquisition of a suitable number of profile spectra from randomly chosen locations of the sample spot. In "fingerprinting", the peak list extracted from an averaged profile spectrum is compared to the reference spectra peak lists. This has developed into a routine tool for microbial identification transforming clinical microbiology. The rapid success of MALDI-TOF-MS is attributable to the accuracy of identification, speed of analysis enabling earlier implementation of therapy, and significant cost effectiveness, thus outperforming earlier clinical routine tests based on biochemical reactions. Further, it has excellent performance data on the accuracy of identification including those difficult to analyze by traditional methods as in the case of Gram-negative non-fermenting bacteria.

MALDI-TOF profiling has comparative accuracy comparable to DNA-based methods. For instance, in cystic fibrotic patients, biotyping for the identification of Gram-negative, non-fermenting bacilli improves treatment outcomes, as they are life-threatening organisms. It has also been useful in identifying anaerobic bacteria which are generally difficult to identify by traditional clinical microbiological methods such as *Clostridium*, *Bacteroides*, *Prevotella*, etc. A simple MALDI-TOF profiling approach has a chance of identifying bacteria that are rare and difficult to culture and highly pathogenic bacteria, such as *Francisella tularensis*, *Brucella* spp., *Burkholderia mallei*, and *Burkholderia pseudomallei*.

Prior inactivation has to be applied to highly pathogenic microorganisms before analyzing them in a MALDI-TOF mass spectrometer to prevent any contamination of the instrument and avoid health risks for the users. A comparison with partial 16S rRNA gene sequencing for difficult-to-analyze bacteria revealed correct identification (85.9%) in the MALDI-TOF MS profiling, with the misidentification resulting from laboratory errors rather than the failure of method.

The MALDI-TOF-MS-based species identification of bacteria provides results reproducible within 10 min without any substantial costs for consumables. The MALDI protocol is able to identify 1.45 days earlier on average. Incorporation of the MALDI protocol significantly reduces reagent and labor costs together with a remarkable decrease in waste disposal as well. In ESKAPE pathogens, proteomic antibiotic resistance detection has been noted predominantly involving MALDI-based technologies.

The proteomic profiling of ESKAPE pathogens involving various technologies and their relevance to antibiotic resistance is summarized in Table 1.

Table 1. Proteomic techniques for ESKAPE resistance.

Pathogen	Proteomic Technique	Physiological Effect	Reference
Enterococcus	2DE/MALDI-TOF/MS	Resistance—VanA, VanB, Heat shock response—CspA	[107]
	LC-MS	Peptidoglycan synthesis— d-Ala-d-Ala	[218]
	TIMS-TOF	Multidrug resistance—EfrA, EfrB	[219]
	Nano-LC MS	OptrA protein, Esp protein Surface exclusion protein—Sea1 Conjugal transfer protein—TraB Replication protein—RepA XRE—transcription regulator protein	[220]
	MALDI-TOF	Typing VanB positive	[116,221]
	MS/MS	LPxTG—Ace, Acm, Scm Pili—Ebp, PilA, PilB	[222]
	iTRAQ	Biofilm formation—strong and weak biofilm forming	[223]
	Raman spectroscopy	Vancomycin resistance detection	[81]
	SWATH-MS	PFL, LDH1	[120]
Staphylococcus aureus	MALDI-TOF	PBP2a	[129,224]
	Tandem MS	β-lactam resistance, BORSA, MODSA	[225,226]
	SWATH-MS	MRSA mechanism	[135]
	Raman spectroscopy	Coagulase strain identification	[227,228]
	MALDI-TOF/MS	Typing MRSA vs. MSSA	[125,229,230]
	LC-MS	Endogenous peptides for differentiation	[231]
	2DE	Alkali shock protein 23—Asp23, Cold-shock protein—CspABC Virulence regulator—SarA	[232]
	iTRAQ-LC-MS/MS iTRAQ/MS	Ftsh, AtpA, AtpC, AtpD, AtpH, GlyA β-lactam resistance—PBP2′, bifunctional autolysin—Atl, FmtA, PBP2, peptidoglycan elongation protein MurA2, transglycosylase domain protein—Mgt, teicoplanin resistance TcaA, LCP domain-containing proteins—MsrR	[233,234]

Table 1. *Cont.*

Pathogen	Proteomic Technique	Physiological Effect	Reference
Klebsiella pneumoniae	1D-LC MS/MS	Porins—LamB, CirA, FepA, OmpC	[235]
	iTRAQ/LC-MS/MS	Colistin resistance—CrrAB, PmrAB, PhoPQ, ArnBCADT, PagP Multidrug efflux pump—KexD	[164]
	iTRAQ	Capsule production proteins—Wza, Wzb, Wzc, Wzi, Gnd, Ugd, Wca, CpsB, CpsG, GalF in ESBL+ TreA, Wza, Gnd, RmlA, RmlC, RmlD, GalE, AceE, SucD Porins—OmpK35, OmpK36	[236]
	LC-MS	Carbapenemase activity	[237]
	MALDI-TOF	Differentiates carbapenemase vs. metallo β lactamases Carbapenemase Carbapenemases—KPC-1, GES-5, NDM-1, VIM-1, VIM-2, IMP-1, GIM-1, SPM-1, OXA-48, OXA-162	[238–240]
	SILAC	CRKP outer membrane	[241]
	Raman Spectroscopy	Differentiate *K. pneumoniae* strains	[166]
Acinetobacter baumannii	2DE/MS-MS 1D/LC/MS-MS	Antibiotic stress proteins— $OmpA_{38}$, CarO, OmpW	[242]
	2DE	AmpC, Cpn60 chaperonin, ATP synthase, OmpA	[243]
	2DIGE	Omp A, CarO, CsuA/B Inner membrane fraction	[244] [245]
	TMT-LC-MS	B-lactamase—Oxa23	[246]
	MALDI-TOF	MDR—biotyping Carbapenemase detection	[247] [248,249]
	Raman spectroscopy	Epidemiological analysis	[250]
	MALDI-TOF/MS	MDR proteins Quorum sensing—AHL	[251] [252]
	iTRAQ	OmpW	[253,254]
	TRAQ/SCX-LC-MS/MS	Biofilm—CsuABABCDE chaperone	[174]
Pseudomonas aeruginosa	MALDI-TOF	Quorum sensing Antibiotic resistance proteins—OprG, OprF, MexA, OprD, OmpH	[255] [256]
	MALDI-TOF/MS	Metallo β lactamases	[238,257]
	LC-ESI MS/MS	OprE, OprH, Opr86	[258]
	BONCAT	Biofilm	[70]
	2DGE/MALDI TOF	Quorum sensing protein—PhuR, HasAp	[259]
	2DGE/XCT MS	Adaptive resistance—porins (OprF and OprG) and lipoproteins (OprL and OprI)	[260]
	SWATH-MS	Cbb3-1, Cbb3-2 terminal oxidases NarG, NarH, NarI nitrate oxidases ArcA, ArcB, ArcC, PchA-G, FpvA, FpvB, FptA, PhuR, HasR, PutA, KatG, KatE, Dps	[201]
	Raman Spectroscopy	Quorum sensing	[261]
	iTRAQ	Biofilm—ArcA, IscU	[195]
Enterobacter spp.	DIGE/LC-MS/MS	ESBL	[262]
	LC-MS	OMPV	[263]
	MALDI-TOF-MS	MDR—carbapenem resistance	[264]

8. Pros and Cons of Proteomics in AMR

Antibiotic resistance is a serious problem. Proteomic studies in their detection has provided vital information as it provides the entire protein profile after exposure of the resistant, intermediate, and susceptible bacteria to sublethal antibiotic concentrations. The response to antibiotics involves proteins related to almost the entire metabolic processes such as energy, nitrogen metabolism, nucleic acid synthesis, glucan biosynthesis, and stress response. Usually, proteomic expression profiles are confirmed with a genomic and/or transcriptome analysis including post-transcriptional modifications. The major pros are that the proteomic tools are more functionally and phenotypically relevant than genetic/genomic assays. In the era of massive nucleic acid sequencing, proteomic tools are promising to mitigate the gap between nucleic acid sequencing and AMR. The advantage of providing more phenotypically relevant information in AMR is crucial because there is still a considerable discrepancy between nucleic acid sequencing and AMR. Harnessing proteomic tools in AMR is needed in the investigation of AMR.

The major cons are that most proteomic tools are expensive, labor-intensive, and time-consuming. While the cost of nucleic acid sequencing has dropped significantly over the past two years and will continue to drop in the near future, the cost of proteomics tools does not appear to be decreasing in the near term. More importantly, most proteomic tools are labor-intensive and lack automation. This would have a significant impact on their widespread use in clinical microbiology while addressing the massive clinical testing demands. Due to a lot of manual processes, proteomic tools are relatively time-consuming. When the flaws are not significantly improved, proteomic tools can be used only for research but are not possible to be widely used in clinical microbiology.

Proteomic tools are more functionally and phenotypically relevant than genetic/genomic assays. Among the proteomic tools, MALDI-TOF MS is only one proteomic tool that is rapid and accurate. Thus, easy sample preparation and short turn-around time make MALDI-TOF a practical tool that has been widely used in clinical microbiology labs. Some studies have reported successful AMR detection based on the MALDI-TOF MS spectra. However, the wide application of MALDI-TOF MS in AMR detection has not met a general agreement yet. The reason could be that results reported from various countries and teams were still significantly different.

The difference in prevailing local strains can be the possible mechanism explaining the performance discordance. One of the possible solutions is using a more sophisticated AI algorithm to build a more robust MALDI-TOF AI model, so the AI model can be generalized to every local region. By contrast, another solution is to train a locally useful MALDI-TOF AI model based on locally relevant MS data. In the methodology, the idea of one-fits-all generalization is abandoned. Instead, a locally tailored MALDI-TOF AI model is the focus. Further investigations addressing the issue are still on the way.

9. Conclusions

In conclusion, proteomics plays a critical role in providing functionally relevant information in the study of bacterial resistance diagnostics. From simple two-dimensional gel electrophoresis to mass spectrometry, current proteomics methods used for microbial studies are reliable. With the combined capabilities of top-down and bottom-up approaches, proteomics can pursue studies ranging from the quantification of gene expression to host–pathogen interactions. As evidenced by the recent pandemic, it is noteworthy that proteomic advances can aid in the diagnosis of ESKAPE resistance and prevent the next impending pandemic of antibiotic resistance. Moreover, the cost of proteomic techniques is effective when considering the laborious bacterial culture techniques. Together with genomics, advances in proteomic tools promise to provide a more comprehensive view of antibiotic resistance mechanisms and diagnostics.

Author Contributions: Conceptualization, H.-Y.W.; methodology, S.K.; software, S.K. and H.-Y.W.; validation, S.K., W.-Y.L., Y.-C.W. and H.-Y.W.; formal analysis, S.K., W.-Y.L., Y.-C.W., A.L. and H.-Y.W.; investigation, S.K., W.-Y.L., Y.-C.W. and H.-Y.W.; resources, H.-Y.W.; data curation, S.K. and H.-Y.W.; writing—original draft preparation, S.K. and H.-Y.W.; writing—review and editing, S.K., W.-Y.L., Y.-C.W., Y.F. and H.-Y.W.; visualization, S.K. and H.-Y.W.; supervision, H.-Y.W.; project administration, H.-Y.W.; funding acquisition, H.-Y.W. All authors have read and agreed to the published version of the manuscript.

Funding: This research was funded by Linkou Chang Gung Memorial Hospital, grant number CMRPG3M0851, CMRPG3L1011; and funded by Ministry of Science and Technology, Taiwan, grant number 111-2320-B-182A-002-MY2.

Institutional Review Board Statement: Not applicable.

Data Availability Statement: Data sharing not applicable.

Conflicts of Interest: The authors declare no conflict of interest.

References

1. WHO: Antimicrobial Resistance. 2021. Available online: https://www.who.int/news-room/fact-sheets/detail/antimicrobial-resistance (accessed on 6 February 2023).
2. CDC. *Antibiotic Resistance Threats in the United States, 2019*; CDC: Atlanta, GA, USA, 2019.
3. WHO. *Global Priority List of Antibiotic-Resistant Bacteria to Guide Research, Discovery, and Development of New Antibiotics*; WHO: Geneva, Switzerland, 2017.
4. WHO. *Global Leaders Group on Antimicrobial Resistance*; WHO: Geneva, Switzerland, 2021.
5. Jansen, K.U.; Knirsch, C.; Anderson, A.S. The role of vaccines in preventing bacterial antimicrobial resistance. *Nat. Med.* **2018**, *24*, 10–11. [CrossRef] [PubMed]
6. Morgan, D.J.; Okeke, I.N.; Laxminarayan, R.; Perencevich, E.N.; Weisenberg, S. Non-prescription antimicrobial use worldwide: A systematic review. *Lancet Infect. Dis.* **2011**, *11*, 692–701. [CrossRef] [PubMed]
7. Laxminarayan, R.; Duse, A.; Wattal, C.; Zaidi, A.K.; Wertheim, H.F.; Sumpradit, N.; Vlieghe, E.; Hara, G.L.; Gould, I.M.; Goossens, H.; et al. Antibiotic resistance—The need for global solutions. *Lancet Infect. Dis.* **2013**, *13*, 1057–1098. [CrossRef]
8. Pozsgai, K.; Szűcs, G.; Kőnig-Péter, A.; Balázs, O.; Vajda, P.; Botz, L.; Vida, R.G. Analysis of pharmacovigilance databases for spontaneous reports of adverse drug reactions related to substandard and falsified medical products: A descriptive study. *Front. Pharmacol.* **2022**, *13*, 964399. [CrossRef]
9. Collignon, P.; Beggs, J.J.; Walsh, T.R.; Gandra, S.; Laxminarayan, R. Anthropological and socioeconomic factors contributing to global antimicrobial resistance: A univariate and multivariable analysis. *Lancet Planet Health* **2018**, *2*, e398–e405. [CrossRef]
10. Ramay, B.M.; Caudell, M.A.; Cordón-Rosales, C.; Archila, L.D.; Palmer, G.H.; Jarquin, C.; Moreno, P.; McCracken, J.P.; Rosenkrantz, L.; Amram, O.; et al. Antibiotic use and hygiene interact to influence the distribution of antimicrobial-resistant bacteria in low-income communities in Guatemala. *Sci. Rep.* **2020**, *10*, 13767. [CrossRef]
11. Hendriksen, R.S.; Munk, P.; Njage, P.; van Bunnik, B.; McNally, L.; Lukjancenko, O.; Röder, T.; Nieuwenhuijse, D.; Pedersen, S.K.; Kjeldgaard, J.; et al. Global monitoring of antimicrobial resistance based on metagenomics analyses of urban sewage. *Nat. Commun.* **2019**, *10*, 1124. [CrossRef] [PubMed]
12. Sunde, M.; Nygaard, M.M.; Høye, S. General Practitioners' Attitudes toward Municipal Initiatives to Improve Antibiotic Prescribing—A Mixed-Methods Study. *Antibiotics* **2019**, *8*, 120. [CrossRef]
13. Hay, A.D. Point-of-care tests to inform antibiotic prescribing. *BMJ* **2021**, *374*, n2253. [CrossRef]
14. Cunha, C.B.; Opal, S.M. Antibiotic Stewardship: Strategies to Minimize Antibiotic Resistance While Maximizing Antibiotic Effectiveness. *Med. Clin. North Am.* **2018**, *102*, 831–843. [CrossRef]
15. Rice, L.B. Antimicrobial Stewardship and Antimicrobial Resistance. *Med. Clin. North Am.* **2018**, *102*, 805–818. [CrossRef]
16. Septimus, E.J. Antimicrobial Resistance: An Antimicrobial/Diagnostic Stewardship and Infection Prevention Approach. *Med. Clin. North Am.* **2018**, *102*, 819–829. [CrossRef]
17. Meredith, H.R.; Srimani, J.K.; Lee, A.J.; Lopatkin, A.J.; You, L. Collective antibiotic tolerance: Mechanisms, dynamics and intervention. *Nat. Chem. Biol.* **2015**, *11*, 182–188. [CrossRef]
18. Nimmo, D.G.; Mac Nally, R.; Cunningham, S.C.; Haslem, A.; Bennett, A.F. Vive la résistance: Reviving resistance for 21st century conservation. *Trends Ecol. Evol.* **2015**, *30*, 516–523. [CrossRef] [PubMed]
19. Carvalho, G.; Forestier, C.; Mathias, J.-D. Antibiotic resilience: A necessary concept to complement antibiotic resistance? *Proc. R. Soc. B: Biol. Sci.* **2019**, *286*, 20192408. [CrossRef] [PubMed]
20. Munita, J.M.; Arias, C. Mechanisms of Antibiotic Resistance. *Microbiol. Spectr.* **2016**, *4*, 481–511. [CrossRef] [PubMed]
21. Peleg, A.Y.; Seifert, H.; Paterson, D.L. *Acinetobacter baumannii*: Emergence of a Successful Pathogen. *Clin. Microbiol. Rev.* **2008**, *21*, 538–582. [CrossRef] [PubMed]

22. Roca, I.; Espinal, P.; Vila-Farrés, X.; Vila, J. The *Acinetobacter baumannii* Oxymoron: Commensal Hospital Dweller Turned Pan-Drug-Resistant Menace. *Front. Microbiol.* **2012**, *3*, 148. [CrossRef] [PubMed]
23. Tsalik, E.L.; Bonomo, R.A.; Fowler, V.G., Jr. New Molecular Diagnostic Approaches to Bacterial Infections and Antibacterial Resistance. *Ann. Rev. Med.* **2018**, *69*, 379–394. [CrossRef] [PubMed]
24. Reller, L.B.; Weinstein, M.; Jorgensen, J.H.; Ferraro, M.J. Antimicrobial Susceptibility Testing: A Review of General Principles and Contemporary Practices. *Clin. Infect. Dis.* **2009**, *49*, 1749–1755.
25. van Belkum, A.; Bachmann, T.T.; Lüdke, G.; Lisby, J.G.; Kahlmeter, G.; Mohess, A.; Becker, K.; Hays, J.P.; Woodford, N.; Mitsakakis, K.; et al. Developmental roadmap for antimicrobial susceptibility testing systems. *Nat. Rev. Microbiol.* **2019**, *17*, 51–62. [CrossRef] [PubMed]
26. Yang, S.; Rothman, R.E. PCR-based diagnostics for infectious diseases: Uses, limitations, and future applications in acute-care settings. *Lancet Infect. Dis.* **2004**, *4*, 337–348. [CrossRef] [PubMed]
27. Tenover, F.C. The role for rapid molecular diagnostic tests for infectious diseases in precision medicine. *Expert Rev. Precis. Med. Drug Dev.* **2018**, *3*, 69–77. [CrossRef]
28. Miao, Q.; Ma, Y.; Wang, Q.; Pan, J.; Zhang, Y.; Jin, W.; Yao, Y.; Su, Y.; Huang, Y.; Wang, M.; et al. Microbiological Diagnostic Performance of Metagenomic Next-generation Sequencing When Applied to Clinical Practice. *Clin. Infect. Dis.* **2018**, *67*, S231–S240. [CrossRef] [PubMed]
29. Özenci, V.; Patel, R.; Ullberg, M.; Strålin, K. Demise of Polymerase Chain Reaction/Electrospray Ionization-Mass Spectrometry as an Infectious Diseases Diagnostic Tool. *Clin. Infect. Dis.* **2017**, *66*, 452–455. [CrossRef]
30. Chen, C.-y.; Clark, C.G.; Langner, S.; Boyd, D.A.; Bharat, A.; McCorrister, S.J.; McArthur, A.G.; Graham, M.R.; Westmacott, G.R.; Van Domselaar, G. Detection of Antimicrobial Resistance Using Proteomics and the Comprehensive Antibiotic Resistance Database: A Case Study. *Proteom. Clin. Appl.* **2020**, *14*, 1800182. [CrossRef]
31. Lecuit, M.; Eloit, M. The potential of whole genome NGS for infectious disease diagnosis. *Expert Rev. Mol. Diagn.* **2015**, *15*, 1517–1519. [CrossRef]
32. Khan, A.; Arias, C.A.; Abbott, A.; Dien Bard, J.; Bhatti, M.M.; Humphries, R.M. Evaluation of the Vitek 2, Phoenix, and MicroScan for Antimicrobial Susceptibility Testing of Stenotrophomonas maltophilia. *J. Clin. Microbiol.* **2021**, *59*, e0065421. [CrossRef]
33. Li, Y.; Yang, X.; Zhao, W. Emerging Microtechnologies and Automated Systems for Rapid Bacterial Identification and Antibiotic Susceptibility Testing. *SLAS Technol.* **2017**, *22*, 585–608. [CrossRef]
34. Maugeri, G.; Lychko, I.; Sobral, R.; Roque, A.C.A. Identification and Antibiotic-Susceptibility Profiling of Infectious Bacterial Agents: A Review of Current and Future Trends. *Biotechnol. J.* **2019**, *14*, 1700750. [CrossRef]
35. Hicks, A.L.; Wheeler, N.; Sánchez-Busó, L.; Rakeman, J.L.; Harris, S.R.; Grad, Y.H. Evaluation of parameters affecting performance and reliability of machine learning-based antibiotic susceptibility testing from whole genome sequencing data. *PLoS Comput. Biol.* **2019**, *15*, e1007349. [CrossRef]
36. Maljkovic Berry, I.; Melendrez, M.C.; Bishop-Lilly, K.A.; Rutvisuttinunt, W.; Pollett, S.; Talundzic, E.; Morton, L.; Jarman, R.G. Next Generation Sequencing and Bioinformatics Methodologies for Infectious Disease Research and Public Health: Approaches, Applications, and Considerations for Development of Laboratory Capacity. *J. Infect. Dis.* **2019**, *221*, S292–S307. [CrossRef]
37. Young, B.A.; Hanson, K.E.; Gomez, C.A. Molecular Diagnostic Advances in Transplant Infectious Diseases. *Curr. Infect. Dis. Rep.* **2019**, *21*, 52. [CrossRef] [PubMed]
38. Boolchandani, M.; D'Souza, A.W.; Dantas, G. Sequencing-based methods and resources to study antimicrobial resistance. *Nat. Rev. Genet.* **2019**, *20*, 356–370. [CrossRef]
39. Pereckaite, L.; Tatarunas, V.; Giedraitiene, A. Current antimicrobial susceptibility testing for beta-lactamase-producing Enterobacteriaceae in clinical settings. *J. Microbiol. Methods* **2018**, *152*, 154–164. [CrossRef]
40. Gajic, I.; Kabic, J.; Kekic, D.; Jovicevic, M.; Milenkovic, M.; Mitic Culafic, D.; Trudic, A.; Ranin, L.; Opavski, N. Antimicrobial Susceptibility Testing: A Comprehensive Review of Currently Used Methods. *Antibiotics* **2022**, *11*, 427. [CrossRef]
41. Nilsson, A.C.; Björkman, P.; Persson, K. Polymerase chain reaction is superior to serology for the diagnosis of acute Mycoplasma pneumoniae infection and reveals a high rate of persistent infection. *BMC Microbiol.* **2008**, *8*, 93. [CrossRef] [PubMed]
42. Niemz, A.; Ferguson, T.; Boyle, D. Point-of-care nucleic acid testing for infectious diseases. *Trends Biotechnol.* **2011**, *29*, 240–250. [CrossRef]
43. Boers, S.A.; Jansen, R.; Hays, J. Understanding and overcoming the pitfalls and biases of next-generation sequencing (NGS) methods for use in the routine clinical microbiological diagnostic laboratory. *Eur. J. Clin. Microbiol. Infect. Dis.* **2019**, *38*, 1059–1070. [CrossRef] [PubMed]
44. Khodakov, D.; Wang, C.; Zhang, D.Y. Diagnostics based on nucleic acid sequence variant profiling: PCR, hybridization, and NGS approaches. *Adv. Drug Deliv. Rev.* **2016**, *105*, 3–19. [CrossRef] [PubMed]
45. Goldberg, B.; Sichtig, H.; Geyer, C.; Ledeboer, N.; Weinstock, G.M. Making the Leap from Research Laboratory to Clinic: Challenges and Opportunities for Next-Generation Sequencing in Infectious Disease Diagnostics. *mBio* **2015**, *6*, e01888-15. [CrossRef] [PubMed]
46. Su, M.; Satola, S.W.; Read, T.D. Genome-Based Prediction of Bacterial Antibiotic Resistance. *J. Clin. Microbiol.* **2019**, *57*, e01405-18. [CrossRef] [PubMed]

47. McDermott, P.F.; Tyson, G.H.; Kabera, C.; Chen, Y.; Li, C.; Folster, J.P.; Ayers, S.L.; Lam, C.; Tate, H.P.; Zhao, S. Whole-Genome Sequencing for Detecting Antimicrobial Resistance in Nontyphoidal Salmonella. *Antimicrob. Agents Chemother.* **2016**, *60*, 5515–5520. [CrossRef]
48. Gordon, N.C.; Price, J.R.; Cole, K.; Everitt, R.; Morgan, M.; Finney, J.; Kearns, A.M.; Pichon, B.; Young, B.; Wilson, D.J.; et al. Prediction of Staphylococcus aureus Antimicrobial Resistance by Whole-Genome Sequencing. *J. Clin. Microbiol.* **2014**, *52*, 1182–1191. [CrossRef] [PubMed]
49. Giordano, F.; Aigrain, L.; Quail, M.A.; Coupland, P.; Bonfield, J.K.; Davies, R.M.; Tischler, G.; Jackson, D.K.; Keane, T.M.; Li, J.; et al. De novo yeast genome assemblies from MinION, PacBio and MiSeq platforms. *Sci. Rep.* **2017**, *7*, 3935. [CrossRef]
50. Lu, H.; Giordano, F.; Ning, Z. Oxford Nanopore MinION Sequencing and Genome Assembly. *Genom. Proteom. Bioinform.* **2016**, *14*, 265–279. [CrossRef]
51. Gupta, N.; Tanner, S.; Jaitly, N.; Adkins, J.N.; Lipton, M.; Edwards, R.; Romine, M.; Osterman, A.; Bafna, V.; Smith, R.D.; et al. Whole proteome analysis of post-translational modifications: Applications of mass-spectrometry for proteogenomic annotation. *Genome Res.* **2007**, *17*, 1362–1377. [CrossRef]
52. Unlü, M.; Morgan, M.E.; Minden, J.S. Difference gel electrophoresis: A single gel method for detecting changes in protein extracts. *Electrophoresis* **1997**, *18*, 2071–2077. [CrossRef]
53. Coldham, N.G.; Woodward, M.J. Characterization of the Salmonella typhimurium proteome by semi-automated two dimensional HPLC-mass spectrometry: Detection of proteins implicated in multiple antibiotic resistance. *J. Proteome Res.* **2004**, *3*, 595–603. [CrossRef]
54. Han, X.; Aslanian, A.; Yates, J.R., III. Mass spectrometry for proteomics. *Curr. Opin. Chem. Biol.* **2008**, *12*, 483–490. [CrossRef]
55. Cumeras, R.; Figueras, E.; Davis, C.E.; Baumbach, J.I.; Gràcia, I. Review on ion mobility spectrometry. Part 2: Hyphenated methods and effects of experimental parameters. *Analyst* **2015**, *140*, 1391–1410. [CrossRef] [PubMed]
56. Eiceman, G.A.; Karpas, Z.; Hill, H.H., Jr. *Ion Mobility Spectrometry*; CRC Press: Boca Raton, FL, USA, 2013.
57. Valentine, S.J.; Counterman, A.E.; Hoaglund, C.S.; Reilly, J.P.; Clemmer, D.E. Gas-phase separations of protease digests. *J. Am. Soc. Mass Spectrom.* **1998**, *9*, 1213–1216. [CrossRef] [PubMed]
58. Ewing, M.A.; Glover, M.S.; Clemmer, D.E. Hybrid ion mobility and mass spectrometry as a separation tool. *J. Chromatogr. A* **2016**, *1439*, 3–25. [CrossRef] [PubMed]
59. Lanucara, F.; Holman, S.W.; Gray, C.J.; Eyers, C.E. The power of ion mobility-mass spectrometry for structural characterization and the study of conformational dynamics. *Nat. Chem.* **2014**, *6*, 281–294. [CrossRef] [PubMed]
60. Helm, D.; Vissers, J.P.; Hughes, C.J.; Hahne, H.; Ruprecht, B.; Pachl, F.; Grzyb, A.; Richardson, K.; Wildgoose, J.; Maier, S.K.; et al. Ion mobility tandem mass spectrometry enhances performance of bottom-up proteomics. *Mol. Cell Proteom.* **2014**, *13*, 3709–3715. [CrossRef]
61. Cumeras, R.; Figueras, E.; Davis, C.E.; Baumbach, J.I.; Gràcia, I. Review on ion mobility spectrometry. Part 1: Current instrumentation. *Analyst* **2015**, *140*, 1376–1390. [CrossRef]
62. Suna, G.; Mayr, M. Proteomics. In *Encyclopedia of Cardiovascular Research and Medicine*; Vasan, R.S., Sawyer, D., Eds.; Elsevier: Oxford, UK, 2018; pp. 166–180.
63. Brönstrup, M. Absolute quantification strategies in proteomics based on mass spectrometry. *Expert Rev. Proteom.* **2004**, *1*, 503–512. [CrossRef]
64. Ridgeway, M.E.; Lubeck, M.; Jordens, J.Z.; Mann, M.; Park, M.A. Trapped ion mobility spectrometry: A short review. *Int. J. Mass Spectrom.* **2018**, *425*, 22–35. [CrossRef]
65. Fernandez-Lima, F.A.; Kaplan, D.A.; Park, M.A. Note: Integration of trapped ion mobility spectrometry with mass spectrometry. *Rev. Sci. Instrum.* **2011**, *82*, 126106. [CrossRef]
66. Meier, F.; Brunner, A.D.; Koch, S.; Koch, H.; Lubeck, M.; Krause, M.; Goedecke, N.; Decker, J.; Kosinski, T.; Park, M.A.; et al. Online Parallel Accumulation-Serial Fragmentation (PASEF) with a Novel Trapped Ion Mobility Mass Spectrometer. *Mol. Cell Proteom.* **2018**, *17*, 2534–2545. [CrossRef]
67. Michalski, A.; Cox, J.; Mann, M. More than 100,000 Detectable Peptide Species Elute in Single Shotgun Proteomics Runs but the Majority is Inaccessible to Data-Dependent LC−MS/MS. *J. Proteome Res.* **2011**, *10*, 1785–1793. [CrossRef]
68. Dieterich, D.C.; Link, A.J.; Graumann, J.; Tirrell, D.A.; Schuman, E.M. Selective identification of newly synthesized proteins in mammalian cells using bioorthogonal noncanonical amino acid tagging (BONCAT). *Proc. Natl. Acad. Sci. USA* **2006**, *103*, 9482–9487. [CrossRef] [PubMed]
69. Dieterich, D.C.; Lee, J.J.; Link, A.J.; Graumann, J.; Tirrell, D.A.; Schuman, E.M. Labeling, detection and identification of newly synthesized proteomes with bioorthogonal non-canonical amino-acid tagging. *Nat. Protoc.* **2007**, *2*, 532–540. [CrossRef]
70. Babin, B.M.; Atangcho, L.; Eldijk, M.B.V.; Sweredoski, M.J.; Moradian, A.; Hess, S.; Tolker-Nielsen, T.; Newman, D.K.; Tirrell, D.A. Selective Proteomic Analysis of Antibiotic-Tolerant Cellular Subpopulations in *Pseudomonas aeruginosa*. Biofilms. *mBio* **2017**, *8*, e01593-17. [CrossRef] [PubMed]
71. Babin, B.M.; Bergkessel, M.; Sweredoski, M.J.; Moradian, A.; Hess, S.; Newman, D.K.; Tirrell, D.A. SutA is a bacterial transcription factor expressed during slow growth in *Pseudomonas aeruginosa*. *Proc. Natl. Acad. Sci. USA* **2016**, *113*, E597–E605. [CrossRef]
72. Grammel, M.; Dossa, P.D.; Taylor-Salmon, E.; Hang, H.C. Cell-selective labeling of bacterial proteomes with an orthogonal phenylalanine amino acid reporter. *Chem. Commun.* **2012**, *48*, 1473–1474. [CrossRef]

73. Ngo, J.T.; Babin, B.M.; Champion, J.A.; Schuman, E.M.; Tirrell, D.A. State-Selective Metabolic Labeling of Cellular Proteins. *ACS Chem. Biol.* **2012**, *7*, 1326–1330. [CrossRef] [PubMed]
74. Huang, W.E.; Ferguson, A.; Singer, A.C.; Lawson, K.; Thompson, I.P.; Kalin, R.M.; Larkin, M.J.; Bailey, M.J.; Whiteley, A.S. Resolving genetic functions within microbial populations: In situ analyses using rRNA and mRNA stable isotope probing coupled with single-cell raman-fluorescence in situ hybridization. *Appl. Env. Microbiol.* **2009**, *75*, 234–241. [CrossRef]
75. Wang, Y.; Song, Y.; Tao, Y.; Muhamadali, H.; Goodacre, R.; Zhou, N.-Y.; Preston, G.M.; Xu, J.; Huang, W.E. Reverse and Multiple Stable Isotope Probing to Study Bacterial Metabolism and Interactions at the Single Cell Level. *Anal. Chem.* **2016**, *88*, 9443–9450. [CrossRef]
76. Berry, D.; Mader, E.; Lee, T.K.; Woebken, D.; Wang, Y.; Zhu, D.; Palatinszky, M.; Schintlmeister, A.; Schmid, M.C.; Hanson, B.T.; et al. Tracking heavy water (D2O) incorporation for identifying and sorting active microbial cells. *Proc. Natl. Acad. Sci. USA* **2014**, *112*, E194–E203.
77. Tao, Y.; Wang, Y.; Huang, S.; Zhu, P.; Huang, W.E.; Ling, J.; Xu, J. Metabolic-Activity-Based Assessment of Antimicrobial Effects by D(2)O-Labeled Single-Cell Raman Microspectroscopy. *Anal. Chem.* **2017**, *89*, 4108–4115. [CrossRef] [PubMed]
78. Yang, K.; Li, H.-Z.; Zhu, X.; Su, J.-Q.; Ren, B.; Zhu, Y.-G.; Cui, L. Rapid Antibiotic Susceptibility Testing of Pathogenic Bacteria Using Heavy-Water-Labeled Single-Cell Raman Spectroscopy in Clinical Samples. *Anal. Chem.* **2019**, *91*, 6296–6303. [CrossRef]
79. Hong, W.; Karanja, C.W.; Abutaleb, N.S.; Younis, W.; Zhang, X.; Seleem, M.N.; Cheng, J.-X. Antibiotic Susceptibility Determination within One Cell Cycle at Single-Bacterium Level by Stimulated Raman Metabolic Imaging. *Anal. Chem.* **2018**, *90*, 3737–3743. [CrossRef]
80. Zhang, M.; Hong, W.; Abutaleb, N.S.; Li, J.; Dong, P.T.; Zong, C.; Wang, P.; Seleem, M.N.; Cheng, J.X. Rapid Determination of Antimicrobial Susceptibility by Stimulated Raman Scattering Imaging of D(2)O Metabolic Incorporation in a Single Bacterium. *Adv. Sci.* **2020**, *7*, 2001452. [CrossRef] [PubMed]
81. Assmann, C.; Kirchhoff, J.; Beleites, C.; Hey, J.; Kostudis, S.; Pfister, W.; Schlattmann, P.; Popp, J.; Neugebauer, U. Identification of vancomycin interaction with Enterococcus faecalis within 30 min of interaction time using Raman spectroscopy. *Anal. Bioanal. Chem.* **2015**, *407*, 8343–8352. [CrossRef] [PubMed]
82. Novelli-Rousseau, A.; Espagnon, I.; Filiputti, D.; Gal, O.; Douet, A.; Mallard, F.; Josso, Q. Culture-free Antibiotic-susceptibility Determination From Single-bacterium Raman Spectra. *Sci. Rep.* **2018**, *8*, 3957. [CrossRef]
83. Kirchhoff, J.; Glaser, U.; Bohnert, J.A.; Pletz, M.W.; Popp, J.; Neugebauer, U. Simple Ciprofloxacin Resistance Test and Determination of Minimal Inhibitory Concentration within 2 h Using Raman Spectroscopy. *Anal. Chem.* **2018**, *90*, 1811–1818. [CrossRef]
84. Colniță, A.; Dina, N.E.; Leopold, N.; Vodnar, D.C.; Bogdan, D.; Porav, S.A.; David, L. Characterization and Discrimination of Gram-Positive Bacteria Using Raman Spectroscopy with the Aid of Principal Component Analysis. *Nanomaterials* **2017**, *7*, 248. [CrossRef]
85. Tang, M.; McEwen, G.D.; Wu, Y.; Miller, C.D.; Zhou, A. Characterization and analysis of mycobacteria and Gram-negative bacteria and co-culture mixtures by Raman microspectroscopy, FTIR, and atomic force microscopy. *Anal. Bioanal. Chem.* **2013**, *405*, 1577–1591. [CrossRef]
86. Kloss, S.; Kampe, B.; Sachse, S.; Rösch, P.; Straube, E.; Pfister, W.; Kiehntopf, M.; Popp, J. Culture independent Raman spectroscopic identification of urinary tract infection pathogens: A proof of principle study. *Anal. Chem.* **2013**, *85*, 9610–9616. [CrossRef]
87. Prucek, R.; Ranc, V.; Kvítek, L.; Panáček, A.; Zbořil, R.; Kolář, M. Reproducible discrimination between gram-positive and gram-negative bacteria using surface enhanced Raman spectroscopy with infrared excitation. *Analyst* **2012**, *137*, 2866–2870. [CrossRef] [PubMed]
88. Nix, I.D.; Idelevich, E.A.; Storck, L.M.; Sparbier, K.; Drews, O.; Kostrzewa, M.; Becker, K. Detection of Methicillin Resistance in Staphylococcus aureus From Agar Cultures and Directly from Positive Blood Cultures Using MALDI-TOF Mass Spectrometry-Based Direct-on-Target Microdroplet Growth Assay. *Front. Microbiol.* **2020**, *11*, 232. [CrossRef] [PubMed]
89. Idelevich, E.A.; Storck, L.M.; Sparbier, K.; Drews, O.; Kostrzewa, M.; Becker, K. Rapid Direct Susceptibility Testing from Positive Blood Cultures by the Matrix-Assisted Laser Desorption Ionization–Time of Flight Mass Spectrometry-Based Direct-on-Target Microdroplet Growth Assay. *J. Clin. Microbiol.* **2018**, *56*, e00913-18. [CrossRef] [PubMed]
90. Aebersold, R.; Mann, M. Mass-spectrometric exploration of proteome structure and function. *Nature* **2016**, *537*, 347–355. [CrossRef] [PubMed]
91. Collins, B.C.; Hunter, C.L.; Liu, Y.; Schilling, B.; Rosenberger, G.; Bader, S.L.; Chan, D.W.; Gibson, B.W.; Gingras, A.C.; Held, J.M.; et al. Multi-laboratory assessment of reproducibility, qualitative and quantitative performance of SWATH-mass spectrometry. *Nat. Commun.* **2017**, *8*, 291. [CrossRef] [PubMed]
92. Oliveira, D.M.P.D.; Forde, B.M.; Kidd, T.J.; Harris, P.N.A.; Schembri, M.A.; Beatson, S.A.; Paterson, D.L.; Walker, M.J. Antimicrobial Resistance in ESKAPE Pathogens. *Clin. Microbiol. Rev.* **2020**, *33*, e00181-19. [CrossRef] [PubMed]
93. Beatson, S.A.; Walker, M.J. Tracking antibiotic resistance. *Science* **2014**, *345*, 1454–1455. [CrossRef] [PubMed]
94. Naylor, N.R.; Atun, R.; Zhu, N.; Kulasabanathan, K.; Silva, S.; Chatterjee, A.; Knight, G.M.; Robotham, J.V. Estimating the burden of antimicrobial resistance: A systematic literature review. *Antimicrob. Resist. Infect. Control.* **2018**, *7*, 58. [CrossRef]
95. Dafale, N.A.; Srivastava, S.; Purohit, H.J. Zoonosis: An Emerging Link to Antibiotic Resistance Under "One Health Approach". *Indian J. Microbiol.* **2020**, *60*, 139–152. [CrossRef]

96. Garvey, M. Bacteriophages and the One Health Approach to Combat Multidrug Resistance: Is This the Way? *Antibiotics* **2020**, *9*, 414. [CrossRef]
97. Savin, M.; Bierbaum, G.; Hammerl, J.A.; Heinemann, C.; Parcina, M.; Sib, E.; Voigt, A.; Kreyenschmidt, J. ESKAPE Bacteria and Extended-Spectrum-β-Lactamase-Producing Escherichia coli Isolated from Wastewater and Process Water from German Poultry Slaughterhouses. *Appl. Environ. Microbiol.* **2020**, *86*, e02748-19. [CrossRef] [PubMed]
98. Argudín, M.A.; Deplano, A.; Meghraoui, A.; Dodémont, M.; Heinrichs, A.; Denis, O.; Nonhoff, C.; Roisin, S. Bacteria from Animals as a Pool of Antimicrobial Resistance Genes. *Antibiotics* **2017**, *6*, 12. [CrossRef] [PubMed]
99. Spiller, R.C. Hidden Dangers of Antibiotic Use: Increased Gut Permeability Mediated by Increased Pancreatic Proteases Reaching the Colon. *Cell. Mol. Gastroenterol. Hepatol.* **2018**, *6*, 347–348.e1. [CrossRef] [PubMed]
100. Kristich, C.J.; Rice, L.; Arias, C. *Enterococcal Infection—Treatment and Antibiotic Resistance, in Enterococci: From Commensals to Leading Causes of Drug Resistant Infection*; Gilmore, M.S., Ed.; Massachusetts Eye and Ear Infirmary: Boston, MA, USA, 2014.
101. Hollenbeck, B.L.; Rice, L.B. Intrinsic and acquired resistance mechanisms in enterococcus. *Virulence* **2012**, *3*, 421–433. [CrossRef]
102. Taur, Y.; Xavier, J.B.; Lipuma, L.; Ubeda, C.; Goldberg, J.; Gobourne, A.; Lee, Y.J.; Dubin, K.A.; Socci, N.D.; Viale, A.; et al. Intestinal domination and the risk of bacteremia in patients undergoing allogeneic hematopoietic stem cell transplantation. *Clin. Infect. Dis.* **2012**, *55*, 905–914. [CrossRef]
103. Ramos, S.; Silva, V.; Dapkevicius, M.d.L.E.; Igrejas, G.; Poeta, P. Enterococci, from Harmless Bacteria to a Pathogen. *Microorganisms* **2020**, *8*, 1118. [CrossRef] [PubMed]
104. Basker, M.J.; Slocombe, B.; Sutherland, R. Aminoglycoside-resistant enterococci. *J. Clin. Pathol.* **1977**, *30*, 375–380. [CrossRef]
105. Hegstad, K.; Mikalsen, T.; Coque, T.M.; Werner, G.; Sundsfjord, A. Mobile genetic elements and their contribution to the emergence of antimicrobial resistant Enterococcus faecalis and Enterococcus faecium. *Clin. Microbiol. Infect.* **2010**, *16*, 541–554. [CrossRef]
106. Murray, B.E. Beta-lactamase-producing enterococci. *Antimicrob. Agents Chemother.* **1992**, *36*, 2355–2359. [CrossRef]
107. Pinto, L.; Torres, C.; Gil, C.; Santos, H.M.; Capelo, J.L.; Borges, V.; Gomes, J.P.; Silva, C.; Vieira, L.; Poeta, P.; et al. Multiomics Substrates of Resistance to Emerging Pathogens? Transcriptome and Proteome Profile of a Vancomycin-Resistant Enterococcus faecalis Clinical Strain. *Omics* **2020**, *24*, 81–95. [CrossRef]
108. Clewell, D.B.; An, F.Y.; Flannagan, S.E.; Antiporta, M.; Dunny, G.M. Enterococcal sex pheromone precursors are part of signal sequences for surface lipoproteins. *Mol. Microbiol.* **2000**, *35*, 246–247. [CrossRef] [PubMed]
109. Benachour, A.; Morin, T.; Hébert, L.; Budin-Verneuil, A.; Le Jeune, A.; Auffray, Y.; Pichereau, V. Identification of secreted and surface proteins from Enterococcus faecalis. *Can. J. Microbiol.* **2009**, *55*, 967–974. [CrossRef] [PubMed]
110. Wang, H.Y.; Chung, C.R.; Chen, C.J.; Lu, K.P.; Tseng, Y.J.; Chang, T.H.; Wu, M.H.; Huang, W.T.; Lin, T.W.; Liu, T.P.; et al. Clinically Applicable System for Rapidly Predicting Enterococcus faecium Susceptibility to Vancomycin. *Microbiol. Spectr.* **2021**, *9*, e0091321. [CrossRef] [PubMed]
111. Wang, H.-Y.; Hsieh, T.-T.; Chung, C.-R.; Chang, H.-C.; Horng, J.-T.; Lu, J.-J.; Huang, J.-H. Efficiently Predicting Vancomycin Resistance of Enterococcus Faecium From MALDI-TOF MS Spectra Using a Deep Learning-Based Approach. *Front. Microbiol.* **2022**, *13*, 821233. [CrossRef] [PubMed]
112. Widjaja, M.; Harvey, K.L.; Hagemann, L.; Berry, I.J.; Jarocki, V.M.; Raymond, B.B.A.; Tacchi, J.L.; Gründel, A.; Steele, J.R.; Padula, M.P.; et al. Elongation factor Tu is a multifunctional and processed moonlighting protein. *Sci. Rep.* **2017**, *7*, 11227. [CrossRef]
113. Michaux, C.; Hartke, A.; Martini, C.; Reiss, S.; Albrecht, D.; Budin-Verneuil, A.; Sanguinetti, M.; Engelmann, S.; Hain, T.; Verneuil, N.; et al. Involvement of Enterococcus faecalis small RNAs in stress response and virulence. *Infect. Immun.* **2014**, *82*, 3599–3611. [CrossRef]
114. He, Q.; Hou, Q.; Wang, Y.; Li, J.; Li, W.; Kwok, L.Y.; Sun, Z.; Zhang, H.; Zhong, Z. Comparative genomic analysis of Enterococcus faecalis: Insights into their environmental adaptations. *BMC Genom.* **2018**, *19*, 527. [CrossRef]
115. Keto-Timonen, R.; Hietala, N.; Palonen, E.; Hakakorpi, A.; Lindström, M.; Korkeala, H. Cold Shock Proteins: A Minireview with Special Emphasis on Csp-family of Enteropathogenic Yersinia. *Front. Microbiol.* **2016**, *7*, 1151. [CrossRef]
116. Ozma, M.A.; Khodadadi, E.; Rezaee, M.A.; Kamounah, F.S.; Asgharzadeh, M.; Ganbarov, K.; Aghazadeh, M.; Yousefi, M.; Pirzadeh, T.; Kafil, H.S. Induction of proteome changes involved in biofilm formation of Enterococcus faecalis in response to gentamicin. *Microb. Pathog.* **2021**, *157*, 105003. [CrossRef]
117. Suryaletha, K.; Narendrakumar, L.; John, J.; Radhakrishnan, M.P.; George, S.; Thomas, S. Decoding the proteomic changes involved in the biofilm formation of Enterococcus faecalis SK460 to elucidate potential biofilm determinants. *BMC Microbiol.* **2019**, *19*, 146. [CrossRef]
118. Laport, M.S.; Dos Santos, L.L.; Lemos, J.A.; do Carmo, F.B.M.; Burne, R.A.; Giambiagi-Demarval, M. Organization of heat shock dnaK and groE operons of the nosocomial pathogen Enterococcus faecium. *Res. Microbiol.* **2006**, *157*, 162–168. [CrossRef]
119. Bhatty, M.; Cruz, M.R.; Frank, K.L.; Gomez, J.A.; Andrade, F.; Garsin, D.A.; Dunny, G.M.; Kaplan, H.B.; Christie, P.J. Enterococcus faecalis pCF10-encoded surface proteins PrgA, PrgB (aggregation substance) and PrgC contribute to plasmid transfer, biofilm formation and virulence. *Mol. Microbiol.* **2015**, *95*, 660–677. [CrossRef] [PubMed]
120. Großeholz, R.; Koh, C.C.; Veith, N.; Fiedler, T.; Strauss, M.; Olivier, B.; Collins, B.C.; Schubert, O.T.; Bergmann, F.; Kreikemeyer, B.; et al. Integrating highly quantitative proteomics and genome-scale metabolic modeling to study pH adaptation in the human pathogen Enterococcus faecalis. *NPJ Syst. Biol. Appl.* **2016**, 2, 16017. [CrossRef]

121. Monteiro, R.; Vitorino, R.; Domingues, P.; Radhouani, H.; Carvalho, C.; Poeta, P.; Torres, C.; Igrejas, G. Proteome of a methicillin-resistant Staphylococcus aureus clinical strain of sequence type ST398. *J. Proteom.* **2012**, *75*, 2892–2915. [CrossRef] [PubMed]
122. Struelens, M.J.; Hawkey, P.M.; French, G.L.; Witte, W.; Tacconelli, E. Laboratory tools and strategies for methicillin-resistant Staphylococcus aureus screening, surveillance and typing: State of the art and unmet needs. *Clin. Microbiol. Infect.* **2009**, *15*, 112–119. [CrossRef] [PubMed]
123. Hallin, M.; Deplano, A.; Denis, O.; De Mendonça, R.; De Ryck, R.; Struelens, M.J. Validation of pulsed-field gel electrophoresis and spa typing for long-term, nationwide epidemiological surveillance studies of Staphylococcus aureus infections. *J. Clin. Microbiol.* **2007**, *45*, 127–133. [CrossRef]
124. Murchan, S.; Kaufmann, M.E.; Deplano, A.; de Ryck, R.; Struelens, M.; Zinn, C.E.; Fussing, V.; Salmenlinna, S.; Vuopio-Varkila, J.; El Solh, N.; et al. Harmonization of pulsed-field gel electrophoresis protocols for epidemiological typing of strains of methicillin-resistant Staphylococcus aureus: A single approach developed by consensus in 10 European laboratories and its application for tracing the spread of related strains. *J. Clin. Microbiol.* **2003**, *41*, 1574–1585.
125. Kim, J.M.; Kim, I.; Chung, S.H.; Chung, Y.; Han, M.; Kim, J.S. Rapid Discrimination of Methicillin-Resistant Staphylococcus aureus by MALDI-TOF MS. *Pathogens* **2019**, *8*, 214. [CrossRef]
126. Wang, H.-Y.; Lee, T.-Y.; Tseng, Y.-J.; Liu, T.-P.; Huang, K.-Y.; Chang, Y.-T.; Chen, C.-H.; Lu, J.-J.; Wang, H.-Y.; Lee, T.-Y.; et al. A new scheme for strain typing of methicillin-resistant Staphylococcus aureus on the basis of matrix-assisted laser desorption ionization time-of-flight mass spectrometry by using machine learning approach. *PLoS ONE* **2018**, *13*, e0194289. [CrossRef]
127. Lindsay, J.A.; Moore, C.E.; Day, N.P.; Peacock, S.J.; Witney, A.A.; Stabler, R.A.; Husain, S.E.; Butcher, P.D.; Hinds, J. Microarrays reveal that each of the ten dominant lineages of Staphylococcus aureus has a unique combination of surface-associated and regulatory genes. *J. Bacteriol.* **2006**, *188*, 669–676. [CrossRef]
128. Xu, Z.; Chen, J.; Vougas, K.; Shah, A.; Shah, H.; Misra, R.; Mkrtchyan, H.V. Comparative Proteomic Profiling of Methicillin-Susceptible and Resistant Staphylococcus aureus. *Proteomics* **2020**, *20*, e1900221. [CrossRef] [PubMed]
129. Wang, H.Y.; Chung, C.R.; Wang, Z.; Li, S.; Chu, B.Y.; Horng, J.T.; Lu, J.J.; Lee, T.Y. A large-scale investigation and identification of methicillin-resistant Staphylococcus aureus based on peaks binning of matrix-assisted laser desorption ionization-time of flight MS spectra. *Brief Bioinform.* **2021**, *22*, bbaa138. [CrossRef]
130. Weis, C.; Cuénod, A.; Rieck, B.; Dubuis, O.; Graf, S.; Lang, C.; Oberle, M.; Brackmann, M.; Søgaard, K.K.; Osthoff, M.; et al. Direct antimicrobial resistance prediction from clinical MALDI-TOF mass spectra using machine learning. *Nat. Med.* **2022**, *28*, 164–174. [CrossRef] [PubMed]
131. Song, Z.; Liu, X.; Zhu, M.; Tan, Y.; Wu, K. Using MALDI-TOF-MS to test Staphylococcus aureus-infected vitreous. *Mol. Vis.* **2017**, *23*, 407–415. [PubMed]
132. Ayala, O.D.; Wakeman, C.A.; Pence, I.J.; Gaddy, J.A.; Slaughter, J.C.; Skaar, E.P.; Mahadevan-Jansen, A. Drug-Resistant Staphylococcus aureus Strains Reveal Distinct Biochemical Features with Raman Microspectroscopy. *ACS Infect. Dis.* **2018**, *4*, 1197–1210. [CrossRef]
133. Rebrošová, K.; Bernatová, S.; Šiler, M.; Uhlirova, M.; Samek, O.; Ježek, J.; Holá, V.; Růžička, F.; Zemanek, P. Raman spectroscopy—A tool for rapid differentiation among microbes causing urinary tract infections. *Anal. Chim. Acta* **2022**, *1191*, 339292. [CrossRef]
134. Rousseau, A.N.; Faure, N.; Rol, F.; Sedaghat, Z.; Le Galudec, J.; Mallard, F.; Josso, Q. Fast Antibiotic Susceptibility Testing via Raman Microspectrometry on Single Bacteria: An MRSA Case Study. *ACS Omega* **2021**, *6*, 16273–16279. [CrossRef] [PubMed]
135. Kang, S.; Kong, F.; Liang, X.; Li, M.; Yang, N.; Cao, X.; Yang, M.; Tao, D.; Yue, X.; Zheng, Y. Label-Free Quantitative Proteomics Reveals the Multitargeted Antibacterial Mechanisms of Lactobionic Acid against Methicillin-Resistant Staphylococcus aureus (MRSA) using SWATH-MS Technology. *J. Agric. Food Chem.* **2019**, *67*, 12322–12332. [CrossRef]
136. Brisse, S.; Grimont, F.; Grimont, P.A.D. The Genus Klebsiella. In *The Prokaryotes: A Handbook on the Biology of Bacteria Volume 6: Proteobacteria: Gamma Subclass*; Dworkin, M., Ed.; Springer: New York, NY, USA, 2006; pp. 159–196.
137. Spagnolo, A.M.; Orlando, P.; Panatto, D.; Perdelli, F.; Cristina, M. An overview of carbapenem-resistant Klebsiella pneumoniae: Epidemiology and control measures. *Rev. Res. Med. Microbiol.* **2014**, *25*, 7–14. [CrossRef]
138. Schwaber, M.J.; Carmeli, Y. Mortality and delay in effective therapy associated with extended-spectrum β-lactamase production in Enterobacteriaceae bacteraemia: A systematic review and meta-analysis. *J. Antimicrob. Chemother.* **2007**, *60*, 913–920. [CrossRef]
139. Gharrah, M.M.; El-Mahdy, A.M.; Barwa, R. Association between Virulence Factors and Extended Spectrum Beta-Lactamase Producing Klebsiella pneumoniae Compared to Nonproducing Isolates. *Interdiscip. Perspect. Infect. Dis.* **2017**, *2017*, 7279830. [CrossRef] [PubMed]
140. Surgers, L.; Boersma, P.; Girard, P.M.; Homor, A.; Geneste, D.; Arlet, G.; Decré, D.; Boyd, A. Molecular epidemiology of ESBL-producing E. coli and K. pneumoniae: Establishing virulence clusters. *Infect. Drug Resist.* **2019**, *12*, 119–127. [CrossRef] [PubMed]
141. Cassini, A.; Högberg, L.D.; Plachouras, D.; Quattrocchi, A.; Hoxha, A.; Simonsen, G.S.; Colomb-Cotinat, M.; Kretzschmar, M.E.; Devleesschauwer, B.; Cecchini, M.; et al. Attributable deaths and disability-adjusted life-years caused by infections with antibiotic-resistant bacteria in the EU and the European Economic Area in 2015: A population-level modelling analysis. *Lancet Infect. Dis.* **2019**, *19*, 56–66. [CrossRef]
142. Sahly, H.; Navon-Venezia, S.; Roesler, L.; Hay, A.; Carmeli, Y.; Podschun, R.; Hennequin, C.; Forestier, C.; Ofek, I. Extended-spectrum beta-lactamase production is associated with an increase in cell invasion and expression of fimbrial adhesins in Klebsiella pneumoniae. *Antimicrob. Agents Chemother.* **2008**, *52*, 3029–3034. [CrossRef] [PubMed]

143. Hennequin, C.; Robin, F.; Cabrolier, N.; Bonnet, R.; Forestier, C. Characterization of a DHA-1-producing Klebsiella pneumoniae strain involved in an outbreak and role of the AmpR regulator in virulence. *Antimicrob. Agents Chemother.* **2012**, *56*, 288–294. [CrossRef]
144. Williams, P.; Smith, M.A.; Stevenson, P.; Griffiths, E.; Tomas, J.M.T. Novel Aerobactin Receptor in Klebsiella pneumoniae. *Microbiology* **1989**, *135*, 3173–3181. [CrossRef]
145. Neilands, J.B. Siderophores: Structure and Function of Microbial Iron Transport Compounds. *J. Biol. Chem.* **1995**, *270*, 26723–26726. [CrossRef]
146. Saikolappan, S.; Das, K.; Sasindran, S.J.; Jagannath, C.; Dhandayuthapani, S. OsmC proteins of Mycobacterium tuberculosis and Mycobacterium smegmatis protect against organic hydroperoxide stress. *Tuberculosis* **2011**, *91*, S119–S127. [CrossRef]
147. de Souza, C.S.; Torres, A.G.; Caravelli, A.; Silva, A.; Polatto, J.M.; Piazza, R.M.F. Characterization of the universal stress protein F from atypical enteropathogenic Escherichia coli and its prevalence in Enterobacteriaceae. *Protein Sci.* **2016**, *25*, 2142–2151. [CrossRef]
148. Falagas, M.E.; Kasiakou, S.K.; Saravolatz, L.D. Colistin: The Revival of Polymyxins for the Management of Multidrug-Resistant Gram-Negative Bacterial Infections. *Clin. Infect. Dis.* **2005**, *40*, 1333–1341. [CrossRef]
149. Jousset, A.B.; Bonnin, R.A.; Rosinski-Chupin, I.; Girlich, D.; Cuzon, G.; Cabanel, N.; Frech, H.; Farfour, E.; Dortet, L.; Glaser, P.; et al. A 4.5-Year Within-Patient Evolution of a Colistin-Resistant Klebsiella pneumoniae Carbapenemase–Producing K. pneumoniae Sequence Type 258. *Clin. Infect. Dis.* **2018**, *67*, 1388–1394. [CrossRef]
150. Vuotto, C.; Longo, F.; Pascolini, C.; Donelli, G.; Balice, M.P.; Libori, M.F.; Tiracchia, V.; Salvia, A.; Varaldo, P.E. Biofilm formation and antibiotic resistance in Klebsiella pneumoniae urinary strains. *J. Appl. Microbiol.* **2017**, *123*, 1003–1018. [CrossRef] [PubMed]
151. Hamzaoui, Z.; Ocampo-Sosa, A.; Fernandez Martinez, M.; Landolsi, S.; Ferjani, S.; Maamar, E.; Saidani, M.; Slim, A.; Martinez-Martinez, L.; Boutiba-Ben Boubaker, I. Role of association of OmpK35 and OmpK36 alteration and blaESBL and/or blaAmpC genes in conferring carbapenem resistance among non-carbapenemase-producing Klebsiella pneumoniae. *Int. J. Antimicrob. Agents* **2018**, *52*, 898–905. [CrossRef] [PubMed]
152. Ngbede, E.O.; Adekanmbi, F.; Poudel, A.; Kalalah, A.; Kelly, P.; Yang, Y.; Adamu, A.M.; Daniel, S.T.; Adikwu, A.A.; Akwuobu, C.A.; et al. Concurrent Resistance to Carbapenem and Colistin Among Enterobacteriaceae Recovered from Human and Animal Sources in Nigeria Is Associated with Multiple Genetic Mechanisms. *Front. Microbiol.* **2021**, *12*, 740348. [CrossRef] [PubMed]
153. Cai, R.; Deng, H.; Song, J.; Zhang, L.; Zhao, R.; Guo, Z.; Zhang, X.; Zhang, H.; Tian, T.; Ji, Y.; et al. Phage resistance mutation triggered by OmpC deficiency in Klebsiella pneumoniae induced limited fitness costs. *Microb. Pathog.* **2022**, *167*, 105556. [CrossRef] [PubMed]
154. Chen, F.J.; Lauderdale, T.L.; Huang, W.C.; Shiau, Y.R.; Wang, H.Y.; Kuo, S.C. Emergence of mcr-1, mcr-3 and mcr-8 in clinical Klebsiella pneumoniae isolates in Taiwan. *Clin. Microbiol. Infect.* **2021**, *27*, 305–307. [CrossRef] [PubMed]
155. Bhagirath, A.Y.; Li, Y.; Patidar, R.; Yerex, K.; Ma, X.; Kumar, A.; Duan, K. Two Component Regulatory Systems and Antibiotic Resistance in Gram-Negative Pathogens. *Int. J. Mol. Sci.* **2019**, *20*, 1781. [CrossRef]
156. Gerken, H.; Vuong, P.; Soparkar, K.; Misra, R. Roles of the EnvZ/OmpR Two-Component System and Porins in Iron Acquisition in *Escherichia coli*. *mBio* **2020**, *11*, e01192-20. [CrossRef]
157. Dean, C.R.; Poole, K. Expression of the ferric enterobactin receptor (PfeA) of Pseudomonas aeruginosa: Involvement of a two-component regulatory system. *Mol. Microbiol.* **1993**, *8*, 1095–1103. [CrossRef]
158. Boudes, M.; Lazar, N.; Graille, M.; Durand, D.; Gaidenko, T.A.; Stewart, V.; van Tilbeurgh, H. The structure of the NasR transcription antiterminator reveals a one-component system with a NIT nitrate receptor coupled to an ANTAR RNA-binding effector. *Mol. Microbiol.* **2012**, *85*, 431–444. [CrossRef]
159. Bay, D.C.; Chan, C.S.; Turner, R.J. NarJ subfamily system specific chaperone diversity and evolution is directed by respiratory enzyme associations. *BMC Evol. Biol.* **2015**, *15*, 110. [CrossRef] [PubMed]
160. Bhargava, P.; Collins, J.J. Boosting bacterial metabolism to combat antibiotic resistance. *Cell. Metab.* **2015**, *21*, 154–155. [CrossRef]
161. Shen, C.; Shen, Y.; Zhang, H.; Xu, M.; He, L.; Qie, J. Comparative Proteomics Demonstrates Altered Metabolism Pathways in Cotrimoxazole- Resistant and Amikacin-Resistant Klebsiella pneumoniae Isolates. *Front. Microbiol.* **2021**, *12*, 773829. [CrossRef]
162. Zhu, Y.; Zhao, J.; Maifiah, M.H.M.; Velkov, T.; Schreiber, F.; Li, J. Metabolic Responses to Polymyxin Treatment in *Acinetobacter baumannii* ATCC 19606: Integrating Transcriptomics and Metabolomics with Genome-Scale Metabolic Modeling. *Msystems* **2019**, *4*, e00157-18. [CrossRef] [PubMed]
163. Yee, R.; Cui, P.; Shi, W.; Feng, J.; Wang, J.; Zhang, Y. Identification of a Novel Gene *argJ* involved in Arginine Biosynthesis Critical for Persister Formation in *Staphylococcus aureus*. *Discov. Med.* **2020**, *29*, 65–77. [PubMed]
164. Sun, L.; Rasmussen, P.K.; Bai, Y.; Chen, X.; Cai, T.; Wang, J.; Guo, X.; Xie, Z.; Ding, X.; Niu, L.; et al. Proteomic Changes of Klebsiella pneumoniae in Response to Colistin Treatment and *crrB* Mutation-Mediated Colistin Resistance. *Antimicrob. Agents Chemother.* **2020**, *64*, e02200-19. [CrossRef]
165. Guo, Y.; Liu, N.; Lin, Z.; Ba, X.; Zhuo, C.; Li, F.; Wang, J.; Li, Y.; Yao, L.; Liu, B.; et al. Mutations in porin LamB contribute to ceftazidime-avibactam resistance in KPC-producing Klebsiella pneumoniae. *Emerg. Microbes Infect.* **2021**, *10*, 2042–2051. [CrossRef]
166. Nakar, A.; Pistiki, A.; Ryabchykov, O.; Bocklitz, T.; Rösch, P.; Popp, J. Label-free differentiation of clinical E. coli and Klebsiella isolates with Raman spectroscopy. *J. Biophotonics* **2022**, *15*, e202200005. [CrossRef]

167. Levy-Blitchtein, S.; Roca, I.; Plasencia-Rebata, S.; Vicente-Taboada, W.; Velásquez-Pomar, J.; Muñoz, L.; Moreno-Morales, J.; Pons, M.J.; del Valle-Mendoza, J.; Vila, J. Emergence and spread of carbapenem-resistant *Acinetobacter baumannii* international clones II and III in Lima, Peru. *Emerg. Microbes Infect.* **2018**, *7*, 1–9. [CrossRef]
168. Tacconelli, E.; Carrara, E.; Savoldi, A.; Harbarth, S.; Mendelson, M.; Monnet, D.L.; Pulcini, C.; Kahlmeter, G.; Kluytmans, J.; Carmeli, Y.; et al. Discovery, research, and development of new antibiotics: The WHO priority list of antibiotic-resistant bacteria and tuberculosis. *Lancet Infect. Dis.* **2018**, *18*, 318–327. [CrossRef]
169. Nordmann, P.; Poirel, L. Epidemiology and Diagnostics of Carbapenem Resistance in Gram-negative Bacteria. *Clin. Infect. Dis.* **2019**, *69*, S521–S528. [CrossRef] [PubMed]
170. Piperaki, E.T.; Tzouvelekis, L.S.; Miriagou, V.; Daikos, G.L. Carbapenem-resistant *Acinetobacter baumannii*: In pursuit of an effective treatment. *Clin. Microbiol. Infect.* **2019**, *25*, 951–957. [CrossRef] [PubMed]
171. Garnacho-Montero, J.; Timsit, J.-F. Managing Acinetobacter baumannii infections. *Curr. Opin. Infect. Dis.* **2019**, *32*, 69–76. [CrossRef] [PubMed]
172. Karakonstantis, S.; Kritsotakis, I.E.; Gikas, A. Treatment options for K. pneumoniae, P. aeruginosa and A. baumannii co-resistant to carbapenems, aminoglycosides, polymyxins and tigecycline: An approach based on the mechanisms of resistance to carbapenems. *Infection* **2020**, *48*, 835–851. [CrossRef]
173. Mulani, M.S.; Kamble, E.E.; Kumkar, S.N.; Tawre, M.S.; Pardesi, K.R. Emerging Strategies to Combat ESKAPE Pathogens in the Era of Antimicrobial Resistance: A Review. *Front. Microbiol.* **2019**, *10*, 539. [CrossRef]
174. Cabral, M.P.; Soares, N.C.; Aranda, J.; Parreira, J.R.; Rumbo, C.; Poza, M.; Valle, J.; Calamia, V.; Lasa, Í.; Bou, G. Proteomic and Functional Analyses Reveal a Unique Lifestyle for *Acinetobacter baumannii* Biofilms and a Key Role for Histidine Metabolism. *J. Proteome Res.* **2011**, *10*, 3399–3417. [CrossRef]
175. Tiwari, V.; Rajeswari, M.R.; Tiwari, M. Proteomic analysis of iron-regulated membrane proteins identify FhuE receptor as a target to inhibit siderophore-mediated iron acquisition in *Acinetobacter baumannii*. *Int. J. Biol. Macromol.* **2019**, *125*, 1156–1167. [CrossRef]
176. Soares, N.C.; Spät, P.; Méndez, J.A.; Nakedi, K.; Aranda, J.; Bou, G. Ser/Thr/Tyr phosphoproteome characterization of *Acinetobacter baumannii*: Comparison between a reference strain and a highly invasive multidrug-resistant clinical isolate. *J. Proteom.* **2014**, *102*, 113–124. [CrossRef]
177. Ghebremedhin, M.; Heitkamp, R.; Yesupriya, S.; Clay, B.; Crane, N.J. Accurate and Rapid Differentiation of *Acinetobacter baumannii* Strains by Raman Spectroscopy: A Comparative Study. *J. Clin. Microbiol.* **2017**, *55*, 2480–2490. [CrossRef]
178. Farrell, P.M.; Collins, J.; Broderick, L.S.; Rock, M.J.; Li, Z.; Kosorok, M.R.; Laxova, A.; Gershan, W.M.; Brody, A.S. Association between Mucoid Pseudomonas Infection and Bronchiectasis in Children with Cystic Fibrosis. *Radiology* **2009**, *252*, 534–543. [CrossRef]
179. Silby, M.W.; Winstanley, C.; Godfrey, S.A.C.; Levy, S.B.; Jackson, R.W. Pseudomonas genomes: Diverse and adaptable. *FEMS Microbiol. Rev.* **2011**, *35*, 652–680. [CrossRef] [PubMed]
180. Høiby, N.; Bjarnsholt, T.; Givskov, M.; Molin, S.; Ciofu, O. Antibiotic resistance of bacterial biofilms. *Int. J. Antimicrob. Agents* **2010**, *35*, 322–332. [CrossRef]
181. Murphy, T.F. Pseudomonas aeruginosa in adults with chronic obstructive pulmonary disease. *Curr. Opin. Pulm. Med.* **2009**, *15*, 138–142. [CrossRef]
182. Breidenstein, E.B.; de la Fuente-Núñez, C.; Hancock, R.E. Pseudomonas aeruginosa: All roads lead to resistance. *Trends Microbiol.* **2011**, *19*, 419–426. [CrossRef]
183. Drenkard, E. Antimicrobial resistance of Pseudomonas aeruginosa biofilms. *Microbes Infect.* **2003**, *5*, 1213–1219. [CrossRef] [PubMed]
184. Mulcahy, L.R.; Burns, J.L.; Lory, S.; Lewis, K. Emergence of Pseudomonas aeruginosa strains producing high levels of persister cells in patients with cystic fibrosis. *J. Bacteriol.* **2010**, *192*, 6191–6199. [CrossRef] [PubMed]
185. Pesci, E.C.; Pearson, J.P.; Seed, P.C.; Iglewski, B.H. Regulation of las and rhl quorum sensing in Pseudomonas aeruginosa. *J. Bacteriol.* **1997**, *179*, 3127–3132. [CrossRef]
186. de Kievit, T.R.; Iglewski, B. Bacterial quorum sensing in pathogenic relationships. *Infect. Immun.* **2000**, *68*, 4839–4849. [CrossRef]
187. Cámara, M.; Williams, P.; Hardman, A. Controlling infection by tuning in and turning down the volume of bacterial small-talk. *Lancet Infect. Dis.* **2002**, *2*, 667–676. [CrossRef]
188. Tang, H.B.; DiMango, E.; Bryan, R.; Gambello, M.; Iglewski, B.H.; Goldberg, J.B.; Prince, A. Contribution of specific Pseudomonas aeruginosa virulence factors to pathogenesis of pneumonia in a neonatal mouse model of infection. *Infect. Immun.* **1996**, *64*, 37–43. [CrossRef]
189. Tan, M.W.; Mahajan-Miklos, S.; Ausubel, F.M. Killing of Caenorhabditis elegans by Pseudomonas aeruginosa used to model mammalian bacterial pathogenesis. *Proc. Natl. Acad. Sci. USA* **1999**, *96*, 715–720. [CrossRef] [PubMed]
190. Wu, H.; Song, Z.; Givskov, M.; Doring, G.; Worlitzsch, D.; Mathee, K.; Rygaard, J.; Høiby, N. Pseudomonas aeruginosa mutations in lasI and rhlI quorum sensing systems result in milder chronic lung infection. *Microbiology* **2001**, *147*, 1105–1113. [CrossRef] [PubMed]
191. Nouwens, A.S.; Beatson, S.A.; Whitchurch, C.B.; Walsh, B.J.; Schweizer, H.P.; Mattick, J.S.; Cordwell, S.J. Proteome analysis of extracellular proteins regulated by the las and rhl quorum sensing systems in Pseudomonas aeruginosa PAO1. *Microbiology* **2003**, *149*, 1311–1322. [CrossRef]

192. Passador, L.; Cook, J.M.; Gambello, M.J.; Rust, L.; Iglewski, B.H. Expression of Pseudomonas aeruginosa virulence genes requires cell-to-cell communication. *Science* **1993**, *260*, 1127–1130. [CrossRef] [PubMed]
193. Pearson, J.P.; Pesci, E.; Iglewski, B.H. Roles of Pseudomonas aeruginosa las and rhl quorum-sensing systems in control of elastase and rhamnolipid biosynthesis genes. *J. Bacteriol.* **1997**, *179*, 5756–5767. [CrossRef]
194. Chapon-Hervé, V.; Akrim, M.; Latifi, A.; Williams, P.; Lazdunski, A.; Bally, M. Regulation of the xcp secretion pathway by multiple quorum-sensing modulons in Pseudomonas aeruginosa. *Mol. Microbiol.* **1997**, *24*, 1169–1178. [CrossRef]
195. Ding, J.; Gao, X.; Gui, H.; Ding, X.; Lu, Y.; An, S.; Liu, Q. Proteomic Analysis of Proteins Associated with Inhibition of Pseudomonas aeruginosa Resistance to Imipenem Mediated by the Chinese Herbal Medicine Qi Gui Yin. *Microb. Drug Resist.* **2021**, *27*, 462–470. [CrossRef]
196. Kempf, M.; Bakour, S.; Flaudrops, C.; Berrazeg, M.; Brunel, J.M.; Drissi, M.; Mesli, E.; Touati, A.; Rolain, J.M. Rapid detection of carbapenem resistance in *Acinetobacter baumannii* using matrix-assisted laser desorption ionization-time of flight mass spectrometry. *PLoS ONE* **2012**, *7*, e31676. [CrossRef]
197. Burckhardt, I.; Zimmermann, S. Using Matrix-Assisted Laser Desorption Ionization-Time of Flight Mass Spectrometry to Detect Carbapenem Resistance within 1 to 2.5 Hours. *J. Clin. Microbiol.* **2011**, *49*, 3321–3324. [CrossRef]
198. Hrabák, J.; Studentová, V.; Walková, R.; Zemlicková, H.; Jakubu, V.; Chudácková, E.; Gniadkowski, M.; Pfeifer, Y.; Perry, J.D.; Wilkinson, K.; et al. Detection of NDM-1, VIM-1, KPC, OXA-48, and OXA-162 carbapenemases by matrix-assisted laser desorption ionization-time of flight mass spectrometry. *J. Clin. Microbiol.* **2012**, *50*, 2441–2443. [CrossRef]
199. Ledeboer, N.A.; Hodinka, R.L. Molecular Detection of Resistance Determinants. *J. Clin. Microbiol.* **2011**, *49*, S20–S24. [CrossRef]
200. Sparbier, K.; Schubert, S.; Weller, U.; Boogen, C.; Kostrzewa, M. Matrix-assisted laser desorption ionization-time of flight mass spectrometry-based functional assay for rapid detection of resistance against β-lactam antibiotics. *J. Clin. Microbiol.* **2012**, *50*, 927–937. [CrossRef] [PubMed]
201. Kamath, K.S.; Krisp, C.; Chick, J.; Pascovici, D.; Gygi, S.P.; Molloy, M.P. Pseudomonas aeruginosa Proteome under Hypoxic Stress Conditions Mimicking the Cystic Fibrosis Lung. *J. Proteome Res.* **2017**, *16*, 3917–3928. [CrossRef]
202. Mezzatesta, M.L.; Gona, F.; Stefani, S. Enterobacter cloacae complex: Clinical impact and emerging antibiotic resistance. *Future Microbiol.* **2012**, *7*, 887–902. [CrossRef] [PubMed]
203. Osei Sekyere, J.; Govinden, U.; Bester, L.A.; Essack, S.Y. Colistin and tigecycline resistance in carbapenemase-producing Gram-negative bacteria: Emerging resistance mechanisms and detection methods. *J. Appl. Microbiol.* **2016**, *121*, 601–617. [CrossRef] [PubMed]
204. Aghapour, Z.; Gholizadeh, P.; Ganbarov, K.; Bialvaei, A.Z.; Mahmood, S.S.; Tanomand, A.; Yousefi, M.; Asgharzadeh, M.; Yousefi, B.; Kafil, H.S. Molecular mechanisms related to colistin resistance in Enterobacteriaceae. *Infect. Drug Resist.* **2019**, *12*, 965–975. [CrossRef] [PubMed]
205. Hindler, J.A.; Humphries, R. Colistin MIC Variability by Method for Contemporary Clinical Isolates of Multidrug-Resistant Gram-Negative Bacilli. *J. Clin. Microbiol.* **2013**, *51*, 1678–1684. [CrossRef] [PubMed]
206. Poirel, L.; Jayol, A.; Nordmann, P. Polymyxins: Antibacterial Activity, Susceptibility Testing, and Resistance Mechanisms Encoded by Plasmids or Chromosomes. *Clin. Microbiol. Rev.* **2017**, *30*, 557–596. [CrossRef] [PubMed]
207. Landman, D.; Salamera, J.; Quale, J. Irreproducible and Uninterpretable Polymyxin B MICs for Enterobacter cloacae and Enterobacter aerogenes. *J. Clin. Microbiol.* **2013**, *51*, 4106–4111. [CrossRef] [PubMed]
208. Bauer, K.A.; Perez, K.K.; Forrest, G.N.; Goff, D.A. Review of Rapid Diagnostic Tests Used by Antimicrobial Stewardship Programs. *Clin. Infect. Dis.* **2014**, *59*, S134–S145. [CrossRef]
209. Sorensen, M.; Chandler, C.E.; Gardner, F.M.; Ramadan, S.; Khot, P.D.; Leung, L.M.; Farrance, C.E.; Goodlett, D.R.; Ernst, R.K.; Nilsson, E. Rapid microbial identification and colistin resistance detection via MALDI-TOF MS using a novel on-target extraction of membrane lipids. *Sci. Rep.* **2020**, *10*, 21536. [CrossRef] [PubMed]
210. Leung, L.M.; Fondrie, W.E.; Doi, Y.; Johnson, J.K.; Strickland, D.K.; Ernst, R.K.; Goodlett, D.R. Identification of the ESKAPE pathogens by mass spectrometric analysis of microbial membrane glycolipids. *Sci. Rep.* **2017**, *7*, 6403. [CrossRef]
211. Band, V.I.; Satola, S.W.; Smith, R.D.; Hufnagel, D.A.; Bower, C.; Conley, A.B.; Rishishwar, L.; Dale, S.E.; Hardy, D.J.; Vargas, R.L.; et al. Colistin Heteroresistance Is Largely Undetected among Carbapenem-Resistant Enterobacterales in the United States. *mBio* **2021**, *12*, e02881-20. [CrossRef]
212. Furniss, R.C.D.; Dortet, L.; Bolland, W.; Drews, O.; Sparbier, K.; Bonnin, R.A.; Filloux, A.; Kostrzewa, M.; Mavridou, D.A.I.; Larrouy-Maumus, G. Detection of Colistin Resistance in Escherichia coli by Use of the MALDI Biotyper Sirius Mass Spectrometry System. *J. Clin. Microbiol.* **2019**, *57*, e01427-19. [CrossRef]
213. Joyce, S.A.; Shanahan, F.; Hill, C.; Gahan, C.G. Bacterial bile salt hydrolase in host metabolism: Potential for influencing gastrointestinal microbe-host crosstalk. *Gut Microbes* **2014**, *5*, 669–674. [CrossRef] [PubMed]
214. Rangan, K.J.; Pedicord, V.A.; Wang, Y.C.; Kim, B.; Lu, Y.; Shaham, S.; Mucida, D.; Hang, H.C. A secreted bacterial peptidoglycan hydrolase enhances tolerance to enteric pathogens. *Science* **2016**, *353*, 1434–1437. [CrossRef] [PubMed]
215. Van Spaendonk, H.; Ceuleers, H.; Witters, L.; Patteet, E.; Joossens, J.; Augustyns, K.; Lambeir, A.M.; De Meester, I.; De Man, J.G.; De Winter, B.Y. Regulation of intestinal permeability: The role of proteases. *World J. Gastroenterol.* **2017**, *23*, 2106–2123. [CrossRef]

216. Singh, S.; Kumbhar, D.; Reghu, D.; Venugopal, S.J.; Rekha, P.T.; Mohandas, S.; Rao, S.; Rangaiah, A.; Chunchanur, S.K.; Saini, D.K.; et al. Culture-Independent Raman Spectroscopic Identification of Bacterial Pathogens from Clinical Samples Using Deep Transfer Learning. *Anal. Chem.* **2022**, *94*, 14745–14754. [CrossRef]
217. Zhang, W.; Sun, H.; He, S.; Chen, X.; Yao, L.; Zhou, L.; Wang, Y.; Wang, P.; Hong, W. Compound Raman microscopy for rapid diagnosis and antimicrobial susceptibility testing of pathogenic bacteria in urine. *Front. Microbiol.* **2022**, *13*, 874966. [CrossRef]
218. Putty, S.; Vemula, H.; Bobba, S.; Gutheil, W.G. A liquid chromatography-tandem mass spectrometry assay for d-Ala-d-Lac: A key intermediate for vancomycin resistance in vancomycin-resistant enterococci. *Anal. Biochem.* **2013**, *442*, 166–171. [CrossRef]
219. Quintela-Baluja, M.; Jobling, K.; Graham, D.W.; Tabraiz, S.; Shamurad, B.; Alnakip, M.; Böhme, K.; Barros-Velázquez, J.; Carrera, M.; Calo-Mata, P. Rapid Proteomic Characterization of Bacteriocin-Producing *Enterococcus faecium* Strains from Foodstuffs. *Int. J. Mol. Sci.* **2022**, *23*, 13830. [CrossRef]
220. Yan, J.; Xia, Y.; Yang, M.; Zou, J.; Chen, Y.; Zhang, D.; Ma, L. Quantitative Proteomics Analysis of Membrane Proteins in Enterococcus faecalis With Low-Level Linezolid-Resistance. *Front. Microbiol.* **2018**, *9*, 1698. [CrossRef] [PubMed]
221. Griffin, P.M.; Price, G.R.; Schooneveldt, J.M.; Schlebusch, S.; Tilse, M.H.; Urbanski, T.; Hamilton, B.; Venter, D. Use of Matrix-Assisted Laser Desorption Ionization–Time of Flight Mass Spectrometry to Identify Vancomycin-Resistant Enterococci and Investigate the Epidemiology of an Outbreak. *J. Clin. Microbiol.* **2012**, *50*, 2918–2931. [CrossRef]
222. Bøhle, L.A.; Riaz, T.; Egge-Jacobsen, W.; Skaugen, M.; Busk, Ø.L.; Eijsink, V.G.H.; Mathiesen, G. Identification of surface proteins in Enterococcus faecalis V583. *BMC Genom.* **2011**, *12*, 135. [CrossRef]
223. Suriyanarayanan, T.; Qingsong, L.; Kwang, L.T.; Mun, L.Y.; Truong, T.; Seneviratne, C.J. Quantitative Proteomics of Strong and Weak Biofilm Formers of Enterococcus faecalis Reveals Novel Regulators of Biofilm Formation. *Mol. Cell. Proteom.* **2018**, *17*, 643–654, Correction in *Mol. Cell. Proteom.* **2018**, *17*, 2081. [CrossRef] [PubMed]
224. Josten, M.; Dischinger, J.; Szekat, C.; Reif, M.; Al-Sabti, N.; Sahl, H.G.; Parcina, M.; Bekeredjian-Ding, I.; Bierbaum, G. Identification of agr-positive methicillin-resistant Staphylococcus aureus harbouring the class A mec complex by MALDI-TOF mass spectrometry. *Int. J. Med. Microbiol.* **2014**, *304*, 1018–1023. [CrossRef]
225. Enany, S.; Yoshida, Y.; Yamamoto, T. Exploring extra-cellular proteins in methicillin susceptible and methicillin resistant Staphylococcus aureus by liquid chromatography–tandem mass spectrometry. *World J. Microbiol. Biotechnol.* **2014**, *30*, 1269–1283. [CrossRef]
226. Neil, J.R.; Verma, A.; Kronewitter, S.R.; McGee, W.M.; Mullen, C.; Viirtola, M.; Kotovuori, A.; Friedrich, H.; Finell, J.; Rannisto, J.; et al. Rapid MRSA detection via tandem mass spectrometry of the intact 80 kDa PBP2a resistance protein. *Sci. Rep.* **2021**, *11*, 18309. [CrossRef]
227. Rebrošová, K.; Šiler, M.; Samek, O.; Růžička, F.; Bernatová, S.; Holá, V.; Ježek, J.; Zemánek, P.; Sokolová, J.; Petráš, P. Rapid identification of staphylococci by Raman spectroscopy. *Sci. Rep.* **2017**, *7*, 14846. [CrossRef] [PubMed]
228. Pistiki, A.; Monecke, S.; Shen, H.; Ryabchykov, O.; Bocklitz, T.W.; Rösch, P.; Ehricht, R.; Popp, J. Comparison of Different Label-Free Raman Spectroscopy Approaches for the Discrimination of Clinical MRSA and MSSA Isolates. *Microbiol. Spectr.* **2022**, *10*, e0076322. [CrossRef]
229. Wang, H.Y.; Lien, F.; Liu, T.P.; Chen, C.H.; Chen, C.J.; Lu, J.J. Application of a MALDI-TOF analysis platform (ClinProTools) for rapid and preliminary report of MRSA sequence types in Taiwan. *PeerJ* **2018**, *6*, e5784. [CrossRef] [PubMed]
230. Majcherczyk, P.A.; McKenna, T.; Moreillon, P.; Vaudaux, P. The discriminatory power of MALDI-TOF mass spectrometry to differentiate between isogenic teicoplanin-susceptible and teicoplanin-resistant strains of methicillin-resistant Staphylococcus aureus. *FEMS Microbiol. Lett.* **2006**, *255*, 233–239. [CrossRef]
231. Tu, H.; Xu, F.; Cheng, Y.; Pan, Q.; Cai, X.; Wang, S.; Ge, S.; Cao, M.; Su, D.; Li, Y. Proteomic profiling of the endogenous peptides of MRSA and MSSA. *PeerJ* **2021**, *9*, e12508. [CrossRef]
232. Cordwell, S.J.; Larsen, M.R.; Cole, R.T.; Walsh, B.J. Comparative proteomics of Staphylococcus aureus and the response of methicillin-resistant and methicillin-sensitive strains to Triton X-100aaThe identifications for the spots shown in Fig. 1F1 can be found as supplementary data in Microbiology Online (http://mic.sgmjournals.org). *Microbiology* **2002**, *148*, 2765–2781.
233. Ji, X.; Liu, X.; Peng, Y.; Zhan, R.; Xu, H.; Ge, X. Comparative analysis of methicillin-sensitive and resistant Staphylococcus aureus exposed to emodin based on proteomic profiling. *Biochem. Biophys. Res. Commun.* **2017**, *494*, 318–324. [CrossRef] [PubMed]
234. Solis, N.; Parker, B.L.; Kwong, S.M.; Robinson, G.; Firth, N.; Cordwell, S.J. Staphylococcus aureus surface proteins involved in adaptation to oxacillin identified using a novel cell shaving approach. *J. Proteome Res.* **2014**, *13*, 2954–2972. [CrossRef]
235. Suh, M.-J.; Keasey, S.L.; Brueggemann, E.E.; Ulrich, R.G. Antibiotic-dependent perturbations of extended spectrum beta-lactamase producing Klebsiella pneumoniae proteome. *Proteomics* **2017**, *17*, 1700003. [CrossRef] [PubMed]
236. Wang, Y.; Cong, S.; Zhang, Q.; Li, R.; Wang, K. iTRAQ-Based Proteomics Reveals Potential Anti-Virulence Targets for ESBL-Producing Klebsiella pneumoniae. *Infect. Drug Resist.* **2020**, *13*, 2891–2899. [CrossRef]
237. Lovison, O.A.; Rau, R.B.; Lima-Morales, D.; Almeida, E.K.; Crispim, M.N.; Barreto, F.; Barth, A.L.; Martins, A.F. High-performance method to detection of Klebsiella pneumoniae Carbapenemase in Enterobacterales by LC-MS/MS. *Braz. J. Microbiol.* **2020**, *51*, 1029–1035. [CrossRef]
238. Hoyos-Mallecot, Y.; Cabrera-Alvargonzalez, J.J.; Miranda-Casas, C.; Rojo-Martín, M.D.; Liebana-Martos, C.; Navarro-Marí, J.M. MALDI-TOF MS, a useful instrument for differentiating metallo-β-lactamases in Enterobacteriaceae and *Pseudomonas* spp. *Lett. Appl. Microbiol.* **2014**, *58*, 325–329. [CrossRef]

239. Huang, Y.; Li, J.; Wang, Q.; Tang, K.; Li, C. Rapid detection of KPC-producing Klebsiella pneumoniae in China based on MALDI-TOF MS. *J. Microbiol. Methods* **2022**, *192*, 106385. [CrossRef] [PubMed]
240. Lee, W.; Chung, H.S.; Lee, Y.; Yong, D.; Jeong, S.H.; Lee, K.; Chong, Y. Comparison of matrix-assisted laser desorption ionization-time-of-flight mass spectrometry assay with conventional methods for detection of IMP-6, VIM-2, NDM-1, SIM-1, KPC-1, OXA-23, and OXA-51 carbapenemase-producing Acinetobacter spp., Pseudomonas aeruginosa, and Klebsiella pneumoniae. *Diagn. Microbiol. Infect Dis.* **2013**, *77*, 227–230.
241. Jung, H.J.; Sorbara, M.; Pamer, E.G. TAM mediates adaptation of carbapenem-resistant Klebsiella pneumoniae to antimicrobial stress during host colonization and infection. *PLoS Pathog.* **2021**, *17*, e1009309. [CrossRef] [PubMed]
242. Yun, S.H.; Choi, C.W.; Park, S.H.; Lee, J.C.; Leem, S.H.; Choi, J.S.; Kim, S.; Kim, S.I. Proteomic analysis of outer membrane proteins from *Acinetobacter baumannii* DU202 in tetracycline stress condition. *J. Microbiol.* **2008**, *46*, 720–727. [CrossRef]
243. Lee, H.-Y.; Chen, C.-L.; Wang, S.-B.; Su, L.-H.; Chen, S.-H.; Liu, S.-Y.; Wu, T.-L.; Lin, T.-Y.; Chiu, C.-H. Imipenem heteroresistance induced by imipenem in multidrug-resistant *Acinetobacter baumannii*: Mechanism and clinical implications. *Int. J. Antimicrob. Agents* **2011**, *37*, 302–308. [CrossRef]
244. Vashist, J.; Tiwari, V.; Kapil, A.; Rajeswari, M.R. Quantitative Profiling and Identification of Outer Membrane Proteins of β-Lactam Resistant Strain of *Acinetobacter baumannii*. *J. Proteome Res.* **2010**, *9*, 1121–1128. [CrossRef]
245. Tiwari, V.; Vashistt, J.; Kapil, A.; Moganty, R.R. Comparative Proteomics of Inner Membrane Fraction from Carbapenem-Resistant *Acinetobacter baumannii* with a Reference Strain. *PLoS ONE* **2012**, *7*, e39451. [CrossRef] [PubMed]
246. Wang, P.; Li, R.-Q.; Wang, L.; Yang, W.-T.; Zou, Q.-H.; Xiao, D. Proteomic Analyses of *Acinetobacter baumannii* Clinical Isolates to Identify Drug Resistant Mechanism. *Front. Cell. Infect. Microbiol.* **2021**, *11*, 625430. [CrossRef]
247. Mencacci, A.; Monari, C.; Leli, C.; Merlini, L.; Carolis, E.D.; Vella, A.; Cacioni, M.; Buzi, S.; Nardelli, E.; Bistoni, F.; et al. Typing of Nosocomial Outbreaks of *Acinetobacter baumannii* by Use of Matrix-Assisted Laser Desorption Ionization–Time of Flight Mass Spectrometry. *J. Clin. Microbiol.* **2013**, *51*, 603–606. [CrossRef]
248. Sharma, M.; Singhal, L.; Gautam, V.; Ray, P. Distribution of *carbapenemase* genes in clinical isolates of *Acinetobacter baumannii* & a comparison of MALDI-TOF mass spectrometry-based detection of *carbapenemase* production with other phenotypic methods. *Indian J. Med. Res.* **2020**, *151*, 585–591.
249. Tiwari, V.; Tiwari, M. Quantitative proteomics to study carbapenem resistance in *Acinetobacter baumannii*. *Front. Microbiol.* **2014**, *5*, 512. [CrossRef] [PubMed]
250. Maquelin, K.; Dijkshoorn, L.; van der Reijden, T.J.; Puppels, G.J. Rapid epidemiological analysis of Acinetobacter strains by Raman spectroscopy. *J. Microbiol. Methods* **2006**, *64*, 126–131. [CrossRef] [PubMed]
251. Kumar, S.; Anwer, R.; Yadav, M.; Sehrawat, N.; Singh, M.; Kumar, V.; Anil, S. MALDI-TOF MS and Molecular methods for identifying Multidrug resistant clinical isolates of *Acinetobacter baumannii*. *Res. J. Biotechnol.* **2021**, *16*, 47–52.
252. Chopra, S.; Ramkissoon, K.; Anderson, D. A systematic quantitative proteomic examination of multidrug resistance in *Acinetobacter baumannii*. *J. Proteom.* **2013**, *84*, 17–39. [CrossRef] [PubMed]
253. Yun, S.-H.; Choi, C.-W.; Kwon, S.-O.; Park, G.W.; Cho, K.; Kwon, K.-H.; Kim, J.Y.; Yoo, J.S.; Lee, J.C.; Choi, J.-S.; et al. Quantitative Proteomic Analysis of Cell Wall and Plasma Membrane Fractions from Multidrug-Resistant *Acinetobacter baumannii*. *J. Proteome Res.* **2011**, *10*, 459–469. [CrossRef]
254. Chan, K.-G.; Cheng, H.J.; Chen, J.W.; Yin, W.-F.; Ngeow, Y.F. Tandem Mass Spectrometry Detection of Quorum Sensing Activity in Multidrug Resistant Clinical Isolate *Acinetobacter baumannii*. *Sci. World J.* **2014**, *2014*, 891041. [CrossRef]
255. Xu, Y.; Duan, K.; Shen, L. Quorum Sensing in Pseudomonas aeruginosa. *J. Pure Appl. Microbiol.* **2013**, *7*, 2003–2015.
256. Peng, X.; Xu, C.; Ren, H.; Lin, X.; Wu, L.; Wang, S. Proteomic Analysis of the Sarcosine-Insoluble Outer Membrane Fraction of Pseudomonas aeruginosa Responding to Ampicilin, Kanamycin, and Tetracycline Resistance. *J. Proteome Res.* **2005**, *4*, 2257–2265. [CrossRef]
257. Schaumann, R.; Knoop, N.; Genzel, G.H.; Losensky, K.; Rosenkranz, C.; Stîngu, C.S.; Schellenberger, W.; Rodloff, A.C.; Eschrich, K. A step towards the discrimination of beta-lactamase-producing clinical isolates of Enterobacteriaceae and Pseudomonas aeruginosa by MALDI-TOF mass spectrometry. *Med. Sci. Monit.* **2012**, *18*, Mt71-7. [CrossRef]
258. Hemamalini, R.; Khare, S. A proteomic approach to understand the role of the outer membrane porins in the organic solvent-tolerance of Pseudomonas aeruginosa PseA. *PLoS ONE* **2014**, *9*, e103788. [CrossRef]
259. Arévalo-Ferro, C.; Hentzer, M.; Reil, G.; Görg, A.; Kjelleberg, S.; Givskov, M.; Riedel, K.; Eberl, L. Identification of quorum-sensing regulated proteins in the opportunistic pathogen Pseudomonas aeruginosa by proteomics. *Environ. Microbiol.* **2003**, *12*, 1350–1369. [CrossRef]
260. Machado, I.; Coquet, L.; Jouenne, T.; Pereira, M.O. Proteomic approach to Pseudomonas aeruginosa adaptive resistance to benzalkonium chloride. *J. Proteom.* **2013**, *89*, 273–279. [CrossRef]
261. Bodelón, G.; Montes-García, V.; Pérez-Juste, J.; Pastoriza-Santos, I. Surface-Enhanced Raman Scattering Spectroscopy for Label-Free Analysis of *P. aeruginosa* Quorum Sensing. *Front. Cell. Infect. Microbiol.* **2018**, *8*, 143. [CrossRef] [PubMed]
262. Maravić, A.; Cvjetan, S.; Konta, M.; Ladouce, R.; Martín, F.A. Proteomic response of β-lactamases-producing Enterobacter cloacae complex strain to cefotaxime-induced stress. *Pathog. Dis.* **2016**, *74*, ftw045. [CrossRef] [PubMed]

263. Bhar, S.; Edelmann, M.J.; Jones, M.K. Characterization and proteomic analysis of outer membrane vesicles from a commensal microbe, Enterobacter cloacae. *J. Proteom.* **2021**, *231*, 103994. [CrossRef]
264. De Florio, L.; Riva, E.; Giona, A.; Dedej, E.; Fogolari, M.; Cella, E.; Spoto, S.; Lai, A.; Zehender, G.; Ciccozzi, M.; et al. MALDI-TOF MS Identification and Clustering Applied to Enterobacter Species in Nosocomial Setting. *Front. Microbiol.* **2018**, *9*, 1885. [CrossRef] [PubMed]

MDPI
St. Alban-Anlage 66
4052 Basel
Switzerland
www.mdpi.com

Diagnostics Editorial Office
E-mail: diagnostics@mdpi.com
www.mdpi.com/journal/diagnostics

www.ingramcontent.com/pod-product-compliance
Lightning Source LLC
LaVergne TN
LVHW070046120526
838202LV00101B/703
* 9 7 8 3 7 2 5 8 0 3 6 1 3 *